Neuroanatomy

Second Edition

Neuroanatomy

Draw It to Know It

Adam Fisch, MD

JWM Neurology and

Adjunct Professor of Neurology

Indiana University School of Medicine

Indianapolis, IN

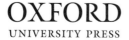

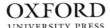
UNIVERSITY PRESS

Oxford University Press, Inc., publishes works that further
Oxford University's objective of excellence
in research, scholarship, and education.

Oxford   New York
Auckland   Cape Town   Dar es Salaam   Hong Kong   Karachi
Kuala Lumpur   Madrid   Melbourne   Mexico City   Nairobi
New Delhi   Shanghai   Taipei   Toronto

With offices in
Argentina   Austria   Brazil   Chile   Czech Republic   France   Greece
Guatemala   Hungary   Italy   Japan   Poland   Portugal   Singapore
South Korea   Switzerland   Thailand   Turkey   Ukraine   Vietnam

Published by Oxford University Press, Inc.
198 Madison Avenue, New York, New York 10016
www.oup.com

Oxford is a registered trademark of Oxford University Press

Library of Congress Cataloging-in-Publication Data

Fisch, Adam.
Neuroanatomy : draw it to know it/Adam Fisch.—2nd ed.
    p.; cm.
Includes bibliographical references and index.
ISBN 978-0-19-984571-2 (pbk.)
I. Title.
[DNLM: 1. Nervous System—anatomy & histology. 2. Anatomy, Artistic—methods.
3. Medical Illustration. WL 101]
611.'8—dc23   2011037944

This material is not intended to be, and should not be considered, a substitute for medical or other professional advice.
Treatment for the conditions described in this material is highly dependent on the individual circumstances. And, while this
material is designed to offer accurate information with respect to the subject matter covered and to be current as of the time it
was written, research and knowledge about medical and health issues is constantly evolving and dose schedules for medications
are being revised continually, with new side effects recognized and accounted for regularly. Readers must therefore always check
the product information and clinical procedures with the most up-to-date published product information and data sheets
provided by the manufacturers and the most recent codes of conduct and safety regulation. The publisher and the authors make
no representations or warranties to readers, express or implied, as to the accuracy or completeness of this material. Without
limiting the foregoing, the publisher and the authors make no representations or warranties as to the accuracy or efficacy of the
drug dosages mentioned in the material. The authors and the publisher do not accept, and expressly disclaim, any responsibility
for any liability, loss or risk that may be claimed or incurred as a consequence of the use and/or application of any of the
contents of this material.

9 8 7 6 5 4 3 2 1

Printed in the United States of America
on acid-free paper

The first edition of this book was dedicated to the memory of my younger brother, David.

This edition is dedicated to my children, Ava and Ezra, who were born during the rewrite of this book and who renew my faith that good things still happen.

Foreword from the First Edition

Neuroanatomy is a nightmare for most medical students. The complex array of nuclei, ganglia, tracts, lobes, Brodmann areas and cortical layers seem to the uninitiated as the height of useless trivia. My own memory of my neuroanatomy class in medical school is vivid. Our professor ordered each member of the class to buy a set of colored pencils—the kind you had in third grade. Each color was coded for particular structures (red for the caudate, green for the putamen, yellow for the claustrum and burnt sienna for the globus pallidus). At our senior play, which poked fun at our professors, a beleaguered medical student was asked to name the components of the basal ganglia. Without knowing what the structures even were or did, he responded "red, green, yellow, and burnt sienna." Almost forty years later, this remains a class joke. Except for the handful of us who went into neurology, neurosurgery, and psychiatry, the basal ganglia to the rest of my class is just a fading joke from the distant past.

And yet, no one can practice even rudimentary neurology without some basic understanding of the neuroanatomy. Non-neurologists in particular, many of whom see large numbers of patients with neurological complaints, have no hope of sorting out common problems such as headache, dizziness, tiredness, fatigue, sleep disorders, numbness and tingling, and pain, without a reasonable grasp of how the nervous system is organized. Despite all of the marvelous advances in neuroscience, genetics, and neuroimaging, the actual practice of neurology, whether it is done by a neurologist or a non-neurologist, involves localizing the problem. The nervous system is just too complicated to skip this step. Without an organized approach based on a reasonable understanding of functional neuroanatomy, clinical neurology becomes incomprehensible.

In his wonderful book, *Neuroanatomy: Draw It to Know It*, neurologist Adam Fisch applies my old neuroanatomy professor's colored pencil idea in a manner that actually works, and it's fun! Over the course of 39 chapters, most of the clinically important neuroanatomically important subjects are covered, ranging through the overall organization of the nervous system, the coverings of the brain, the peripheral nervous system, the spinal cord, the brainstem, the cerebellum, and the cerebral cortex. It is clear that the book was written by an experienced neurologist, as the topics are organized in a fashion that illuminates the principle of anatomical pathophysiological correlation, which is the tool with which neurologists approach clinical problems.

This book should be of great interest to all neurologists, neurosurgeons, neurology residents, and students of neurology. Others who see patients with neurological complaints, such as internists, emergency physicians and obstetrician-gynecologists should also review their neuroanatomy if they wish to provide excellent care to their patients.

As any experienced teacher knows, one only really knows a subject when one can teach it oneself. By drawing the anatomy, the reader of this book literally teaches the subject to himself. By making it clinically relevant, the information learned in this manner is likely to stick. Adam Fisch has done us all a great service by rekindling the enjoyment in learning the relevant, elegant anatomy of the nervous system.

Martin A. Samuels, MD, DSc(hon), FAAN, MACP
Chairman, Department of Neurology
Brigham and Women's Hospital
Professor of Neurology
Harvard Medical School
Boston, MA

Preface

Neuroanatomy is at once the most fascinating and most difficult subject in the field of anatomy. When we master it, we can resolve the most perplexing diagnostic riddles in medicine, and yet we struggle with the numerous neuroanatomical structures and pathways, the intertextual inconsistencies in nomenclature and opinion, and the complex spatial relationships. So here, we bring the differences in nomenclature and opinion to the forefront to mitigate them and we present the material in an active, kinesthetic way.

In this book, we approach each neuroanatomical lesson by beginning fresh with a blank page, and from there we build our diagram in an instructive, rather than a didactic format. With each lesson, we create a schema that provides a unique place for each neuroanatomical item. This, then, allows us to rehearse the schema and in the process memorize the fundamental neuroanatomical items. And because we are all students of anatomy—and not art—our purpose with each lesson is to learn a schematic that we can reproduce in the classroom, the laboratory, or at the bedside in a way that is especially designed for the "left-brained" among us.

Some of us possess pigeon-like navigational skills, whereas others of us find ourselves getting lost in our own houses. The ease with which we learn anatomy is inherently related to the strength of our spatial cognition, which makes it harder for those of us who struggle with complex spatial relationships to master the subject matter[1]. When it comes to the task of deciphering a complicated illustration, specifically in studying the details of an illustration, it has been shown that we rely heavily on the right frontoparietal network[2-4]. In *Neuroanatomy: Draw It to Know It*, we shift the process of learning neuroanatomy away from the classic model of spatial de-encoding, away from the right frontoparietal network, to the formulation of memorizable scripts or schemas, which task the prefrontal cortices more intensively, instead[5,6]. In so doing, we provide the less spatially-inclined with a different entry zone into the world of neuroanatomy.

This book reconciles the most burdensome impasses to our learning: we highlight inconsistencies, remove spatial complexities, and create an active, instructive text that adheres to the principle—when we can draw a pathway step by step, we know it.

References

1. Garg, A. X., Norman, G. & Sperotable, L. How medical students learn spatial anatomy. *Lancet* 357, 363–364 (2001).
2. Walter, E. & Dassonville, P. Activation in a frontoparietal cortical network underlies individual differences in the performance of an embedded figures task. *PLoS One* 6 (2011).
3. Walter, E. & Dassonville, P. Visuospatial contextual processing in the parietal cortex: an fMRI investigation of the induced Roelofs effect. *Neuroimage* 42, 1686–1697 (2008).
4. Aradillas, E., Libon, D. J. & Schwartzman, R. J. Acute loss of spatial navigational skills in a case of a right posterior hippocampus stroke. *J Neurol Sci* 308 (2011).
5. Knutson, K. M., Wood, J. N. & Grafman, J. Brain activation in processing temporal sequence: an fMRI study. *Neuroimage* 23, 1299–1307 (2004).
6. Rushworth, M. F., Johansen-Berg, H., Gobel, S. M. & Devlin, J. T. The left parietal and premotor cortices: motor attention and selection. *Neuroimage* 20 Suppl 1, S89–100 (2003).

Acknowledgments

I'd like to thank my wife, Kate, and the rest of my family and friends for putting up with my decision to rewrite this book, and I'd like to thank my editor, Craig Panner, and the rest of the Oxford University Press team for all of their hard work.

To rewrite this book, I started over entirely. I spent the first year creating a muscle–nerve directory and the following year creating a brain atlas, and then I went to work on rewriting the book, itself. I threw out all of the original illustrations and redrafted them as I wrote the individual tutorials. Taking advantage of the ability to keyword search the massive library of books now available online and taking advantage of several fundamental reference materials I'd used during the creation of the muscle–nerve directory and brain atlas, I was able to create detailed illustrations and scripts that maintained the simplicity of the original book but greatly improved upon its level of detail. As well, feedback from the first edition helped me understand how to provide the information a student of neuroanatomy needs without sacrificing the clinical relevance a clinician is looking for. In creating the tutorials, I came to understand that the text should serve as a play-by-play manual that tersely defines each step in the drawing—only after the steps were solidified did I flesh out the material, itself. When the tutorials were written and finalized, I then broke them down into their individual steps, which served as an invaluable editorial process.

Rewriting this book was all-consuming and I am eternally grateful to those closest to me for giving me the time and space to see it to completion. There are many, many people who have helped me along the way and I hope the end product of this book will prove your patience and efforts worthwhile. I believe this book represents the best that neuroanatomy education has to offer and I am exceedingly grateful to those around me who gave me the opportunity and freedom to have a second crack at it.

Contents

Neuroanatomy

General Organization

Overview of Neuroanatomy

Orientational Terminology

Divisions & Signs

Know-It Points

Orientational Terminology

- The top of the cerebral hemisphere is dorsal and the bottom is ventral.
- The anterior aspect of the cerebral hemisphere is rostral and the posterior aspect is caudal.
- The top of the brainstem is rostral and the bottom is caudal.
- The anterior aspect of the brainstem is ventral and the posterior aspect is dorsal.
- Towards midline is medial and towards the outside is lateral.
- Sagittal view is side-on.
- Coronal view is front-on.
- Axial view is horizontal.

Divisions & Signs

- Cerebral cortical pyramidal cells are upper motor neuron.
- Cranial nerve nuclei and spinal motor neurons are lower motor neuron.
- Upper motor neuron injury causes spastic muscle tone, hyperactive muscle stretch reflexes, and pathologic reflexes (eg, positive Babinski's sign).
- Lower motor neuron injury causes flaccid muscle tone, hypoactive muscle stretch reflexes, and absent pathologic reflexes (eg, negative Babinski's sign).

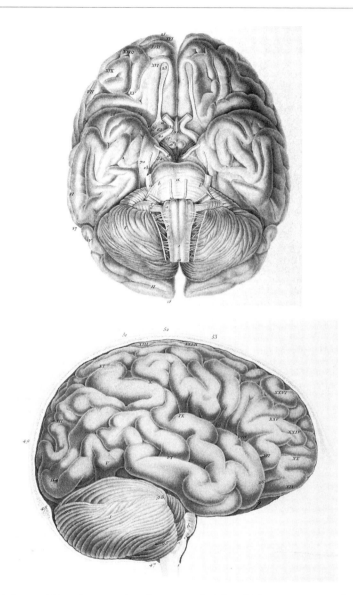

FIGURE 1-1 Plate 4 (top) and plate 8 (bottom) from the 1810 atlas of Franz Joseph Gall and Johann Kaspar Spurzheim—*Anatomie et physiologie du systeme nerveux.*

Overview of Neuroanatomy

To begin, we will draw an overview of the anatomy of the nervous system. First, we will address the brain, brainstem, and cerebellum. Begin with a coronal section through the brain. From outside to inside, label the meninges, which protect and nourish the nervous system; the cortex, which constitutes the outer, cellular gray matter portion of the brain; the subcortical white matter, which constitutes the underlying nerve axons; the basal ganglia, which are most notably involved in motor function but are also important for behavioral and cognitive functions; the thalamus, which in combination with the metathalamus relays most of the afferent information that enters the nervous system to various regions throughout the cerebral cortex; the hypothalamus, which lies along the third ventricle and is the center for autonomic nervous system function; and the cerebrospinal fluid system, which assists the meninges in supporting and nourishing the nervous system.

Below the brain, draw the brainstem. From superior to inferior, show the midbrain, identified by its crus cerebri, then the pons, identified by its bulbous basal outpouching, and finally the medulla. The brainstem contains cranial nerve nuclei, which command oculobulbar motility, facial sensation, and many craniofacial and thoracoabdominal autonomic functions. And the brainstem also contains many additional neuronal pools essential for survival as well as the fiber tracts that pass between the brain and spinal cord. On the posterior aspect of the brainstem, draw the leafy hemispheres of the cerebellum; the cerebellum is important for balance and orientation, postural stability, and coordination.

Next, we will address the spinal cord and peripheral nervous system. Draw the long, thin spinal cord with its cervical and lumbosacral enlargements. Label the segments of the spinal cord from top to bottom as follows: cervical, thoracic, lumbosacral, and coccygeal. The cervical segment mostly communicates with the upper extremities, upper trunk, head, and neck; the thoracic segment mostly communicates with the trunk and abdomen; and the lumbosacral segment communicates with the abdominal-pelvic region and the lower extremities.

Draw a dorsal nerve root off of the posterior spinal cord; identify it with its dorsal root ganglion, which houses the sensory cell bodies. Then, draw the ventral root from the anterior surface of the spinal cord; it contains the motor fibers that exit from the gray matter of the spinal cord. Next, show that the motor and sensory roots meet to form a mixed spinal nerve within a neural foramen. Then, show that the cervical nerves interweave to form the cervical and brachial plexuses. Now, indicate that the lower lumbosacral nerve roots descend through the lumbar cistern and exit the spinal canal to form the lumbosacral plexus. Next, indicate that the majority of the thoracic nerves remain unmixed. Then, show that after the nerves exit their plexuses, they continue as peripheral nerve fibers. Now, draw a representative neuromuscular junction and a sensory cell receptor and attach muscle fibers to them. Neurotransmissions pass across the neuromuscular junctions to stimulate muscle fibers, and peripheral nerve receptors detect sensory impulses from the musculoskeletal system and skin.

Lastly, to represent the divisions of the autonomic nervous system, draw a parasympathetic ganglion and a sympathetic paravertebral chain segment; the parasympathetic nervous system is active in states of rest whereas the sympathetic nervous system is active in states of heightened awareness—it produces the "fight-or-flight" response.

Brain, Brainstem, & Cerebellum

Spinal Cord & Peripheral Nervous System

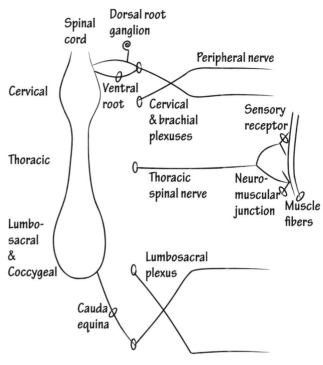

Meninges

Cortex

Subcortical
white matter

Basal
ganglia

Cerebro-
spinal
fluid

Hypo-
thalamus

Thalamus

Midbrain

Cere-
bellum

Pons

Medulla

Spinal
cord

Dorsal root
ganglion

Peripheral nerve

Cervical

Ventral
root

Cervical
& brachial
plexuses

Sensory
receptor

Thoracic

Thoracic
spinal nerve

Neuro-
muscular
junction

Muscle
fibers

Lumbo-
sacral
&
Coccygeal

Lumbosacral
plexus

Cauda
equina

Peripheral Autonomic Nervous System

Sympathetic
chain

Parasympathetic
ganglion

DRAWING 1-1 **Overview of Neuroanatomy**

Orientational Terminology

Here, we will draw the orientational planes of the nervous system. To begin, draw intersecting horizontal and vertical lines. Label the left side of the horizontal line as anterior and right side as posterior. Label the top of the vertical line as superior and the bottom as inferior. Throughout the nervous system, front is always anterior and behind is always posterior, top is always superior and bottom is always inferior. The anteroposterior and superoinferior planes and medial-lateral planes, which we will introduce later, are static: they do not change orientation—unlike the rostral-caudal and dorsal-ventral planes, which we introduce next.

Next, let's draw a side-on, sagittal view of the oblong cerebral hemisphere. Label the top of the cerebral hemisphere as dorsal and the bottom as ventral: the dorsal fin of a shark is on its back whereas a shark's underbelly is its ventral surface. Label the anterior portion of the cerebral hemisphere as rostral and the posterior portion as caudal. Rostral relates to the word "beak" and caudal relates to the word "tail."

Now, draw a sagittal view of the brainstem at a negative 80-degree angle to the cerebral hemisphere. During embryogenesis, human forebrains undergo an 80-degree flexion at the junction of the brainstem and the cerebral hemispheres. Label the posterior aspect of the brainstem as dorsal and the anterior aspect as ventral. Then, label the superior aspect of the brainstem as rostral and the inferior aspect as caudal.

Next, draw a coronal section through the brain—a coronal view of the brain bears resemblance to an ornate *crown*. Indicate that the top of the brain is dorsal (also superior) and the bottom is ventral (also inferior). For this view, we need to additionally introduce the lateral–medial and left-right planes of orientation. Label the midline as medial and the outside edges of the hemispheres as lateral. For the left–right planes of orientation we need to include both the anatomic and radiographic perspectives. Label the left-hand side of the page as radiographic right and anatomic left and the right-hand side as radiographic left and anatomic right. These planes refer to the standardized ways in which coronal radiographic images and anatomic sections are viewed: in radiographic images, the head is viewed face-forward and in anatomic sections, the head is viewed from behind.

Lastly, draw an axial (aka horizontal or transverse) section through the brain — the top of the page is the front of the brain and the bottom is the back. Label the front of the section as rostral (also anterior) and the back as caudal (also posterior). Label the left-hand side of the section as radiographic right and anatomic left and the right-hand side as radiographic left and anatomic right. Radiographic axial images are viewed from below (as if the patient's feet are coming out at you) whereas anatomic axial sections are viewed from above (as if the patient's head is coming up at you). Label the center of the cerebral hemispheres as medial and their periphery as lateral.[1-8]

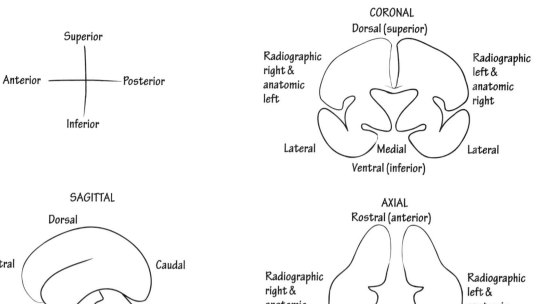

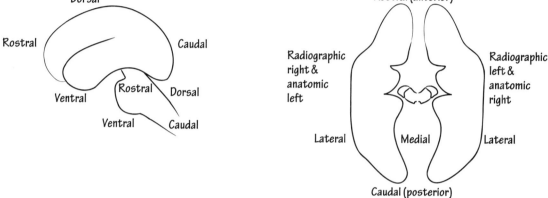

DRAWING 1-2 **Orientational Terminology**

Divisions & Signs

Here, we will learn the central and peripheral divisions of the nervous system and the meaning of upper and lower motor neuron signs; note that we exclude the autonomic division of the nervous system, here, for simplicity. First, let's draw the central nervous system. Draw a brain, brainstem and cerebellum, and spinal cord. Next, in order to label the upper motor neuron and nerve components of the central nervous system, draw a cerebral cortical neuron and label it as an upper motor neuron, and then show a white matter tract descend from it, and label the tract as an upper motor neuron fiber.

Now, let's draw the peripheral nervous system. From the brainstem, draw a cranial nerve and from the spinal cord, draw a spinal nerve. Next, in order to label the lower motor neuron and nerve components of the peripheral nervous system, draw a spinal motor neuron and label it as a lower motor neuron and label the spinal nerve as a lower motor neuron fiber. Note that a common point of confusion is when the lower motor neuron lies within the central nervous system, as it does here. For this reason, it's easier to determine whether a neuron is upper motor or lower motor, if we think about the fiber type the neuron projects rather than the location of the neuron, itself. Generally, cerebral cortical pyramidal cells are upper motor neuron whereas cranial nerve nuclei and spinal motor neurons are lower motor neuron.

Next, we will use three different locations of nervous system injury to learn the exam findings in upper and lower motor neuron lesions. Let's start by creating a small table. Across the top, write the words: injury type, muscle tone, muscle stretch reflexes, and pathologic reflexes (eg, the Babinski sign). Now, for the first injury type, show that injury to the cerebral cortex, such as from a stroke, disrupts the brain and the related white matter tracts. Indicate that it causes an upper motor neuron pattern of injury: there is spastic muscle tone, hyperactive muscle stretch reflexes, and the presence of pathologic reflexes. Second, show that injury to the spinal nerve fiber, such as from neuropathy, causes a lower motor neuron pattern of injury: there is flaccid muscle tone, hypoactive muscle stretch reflexes, and the absence of pathologic reflexes.

The third pattern of injury, spinal cord injury, is mixed. Transect the cervical spinal cord. Then, indicate that above the level of lesion, the patient is normal. Below the level of lesion, there is damage to the upper motor neuron fibers, so show that below the level of lesion, there is an upper motor neuron pattern of injury. Then, at the level of lesion, the spinal motor neuron and its emanating fibers are affected, so show that at the level of lesion, there is a lower motor neuron pattern of injury.

Note that upper motor neuron findings often evolve over hours to weeks. Initially, in a spinal cord injury, for instance, the observed pattern of deficit below the level of injury may be more characteristic of lower motor neuron injury than upper motor neuron injury—there may be loss of muscle tone and areflexia; however, over hours to weeks, the patient's tone and reflexes will become pathologically increased and take on a more typical upper motor neuron injury pattern. This initial phase is called spinal shock in acute spinal cord injury and cerebral shock in acute brain injury.[1-4,6,7,9]

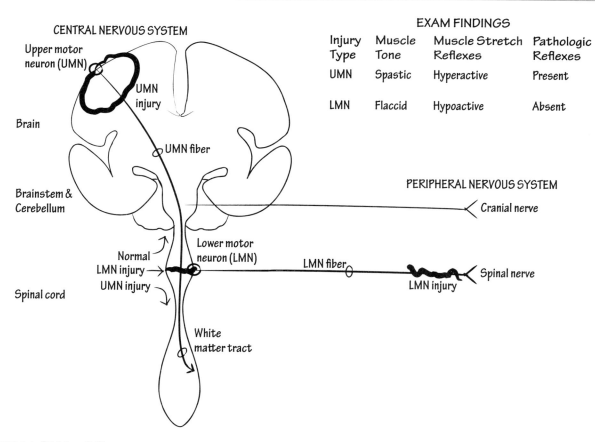

CENTRAL NERVOUS SYSTEM

Upper motor neuron (UMN)

UMN injury

Brain

UMN fiber

Brainstem & Cerebellum

EXAM FINDINGS

Injury Type	Muscle Tone	Muscle Stretch Reflexes	Pathologic Reflexes
UMN	Spastic	Hyperactive	Present
LMN	Flaccid	Hypoactive	Absent

PERIPHERAL NERVOUS SYSTEM

Cranial nerve

Lower motor neuron (LMN)

Normal

LMN injury

UMN injury

LMN fiber

Spinal nerve

LMN injury

Spinal cord

White matter tract

DRAWING 1-3 **Divisions & Signs**

References

1. Bruni, J. E. & Montemurro, D. G. *Human neuroanatomy: a text, brain atlas, and laboratory dissection guide* (Oxford University Press, 2009).

2. Campbell, W. W., DeJong, R. N. & Haerer, A. F. *DeJong's the neurologic examination: incorporating the fundamentals of neuroanatomy and neurophysiology*, 6th ed. (Lippincott Williams & Wilkins, 2005).

3. DeMyer, W. *Neuroanatomy,* 2nd ed. (Williams & Wilkins, 1998).

4. Haines, D. E. & Ard, M. D. *Fundamental neuroscience: for basic and clinical applications,* 3rd ed. (Churchill Livingstone Elsevier, 2006).

5. Leestma, J. E. *Forensic neuropathology,* 2nd ed. (CRC Press/Taylor & Francis, 2009).

6. Netter, F. H. & Dalley, A. F. *Atlas of human anatomy*, 2nd ed., Plates 4–7 (Novartis, 1997).

7. Standring, S. & Gray, H. *Gray's anatomy: the anatomical basis of clinical practice,* 40th ed. (Churchill Livingstone/Elsevier, 2008).

8. Troncoso, J. C., Rubio, A. & Fowler, D. R. *Essential forensic neuropathology* (Wolters Kluwer Lippincott Williams & Wilkins, 2010).

9. Nielsen, J. B., Crone, C. & Hultborn, H. The spinal pathophysiology of spasticity—from a basic science point of view. *Acta Physiol (Oxf)* 189, 171–180 (2007).

2

Meninges and Ventricular System

Meninges

Cerebrospinal Fluid Flow

Cerebral Ventricles

Cisterns, Sinuses, & Veins (Advanced)

Hemorrhages & Innervation (Advanced)

Know-It Points

Meninges

- From outside to inside, the meningeal layers are the dura mater, arachnoid mater, and pia mater.
- From outside to inside, the meningeal spaces are the epidural space, subdural space, and subarachnoid space.
- The falx cerebri separates the cerebral hemispheres.
- The tentorium cerebelli separates the cerebellum from the overlying occipital lobes.
- The falx cerebelli separates the cerebellar hemispheres.
- The superior sagittal dural venous sinus forms within the falx cerebri.
- The transverse sinuses form within the tentorium cerebelli.
- The tentorium cerebelli divides the cranial vault into supratentorial and infratentorial compartments.

Cerebrospinal Fluid Flow

- Cerebrospinal fluid flow pattern:
  - The lateral ventricles empty through the paired foramina of Monro into the third ventricle.
  - The third ventricle empties into the fourth ventricle.
  - The fourth ventricle empties down the central canal of the spinal cord and also through the foramen of Magendie, in midline, and the foramina of Luschka, laterally, into the subarachnoid space.
- Cerebrospinal fluid is produced and reabsorbed at a rate of roughly 0.35 milliliters per minute.
- There is roughly 150 milliliters of cerebrospinal fluid in the nervous system at any given time.

Cerebral Ventricles

- Each lateral ventricle has a frontal horn, occipital horn, and temporal horn.
- The bend of the lateral ventricle is the body.
- The atrium of the lateral ventricle is the confluence where the body and the occipital and temporal horns meet.
- The borders of the fourth ventricle include the floor of the fourth ventricle, the superior medullary velum, the inferior medullary velum, cerebellar peduncles, and cerebellum.
- Choroid plexus lies centrally within the cerebral ventricles: in the body, atrium, and temporal horn of the lateral ventricle, third ventricle, and fourth ventricle.

Cisterns, Sinuses, & Veins *(Advanced)*

- Collectively, the subarachnoid cisterns at the base of the brain are referred to as the basal cisterns.
- The notable cisterns are the suprasellar, interpeduncular, ambient, quadrigeminal, prepontine, pontocerebellar, premedullary, lateral cerebellomedullary, and posterior cerebellomedullary cisterns, and the cistern of the velum interpositum.
- The notable dural venous sinuses are the superior sagittal sinus, confluence of sinuses, bilateral transverse sinuses, inferior sagittal sinus, straight sinus, and also the sigmoid sinuses, which drain into the internal jugular veins.
- The notable deep cerebral veins are the vein of Galen, the basal veins of Rosenthal, and the internal cerebral veins.
- The superficial cerebral veins drain the superficial cerebrum.

Hemorrhages & Innervation *(Advanced)*

- In epidural hematoma, blood collects between the periosteal dura and skull.
- Epidural hematoma assumes a biconvex lens shape.
- In subdural hematoma, blood collects within the dural border cell layer, external to the underlying arachnoid layer.
- Subdural hematoma assumes a crescent shape.
- Epidural hematomas are unaffected by the dural folds whereas subdural hematomas pool at the site of dural reflections.

- The trigeminal nerve innervates the supratentorial meninges, which includes the meninges of the anterior and middle cranial fossae.
- Posterior cranial fossa meningeal innervation is derived, most notably, from the second and third cervical spinal nerves and a minor branch of the vagus nerve.

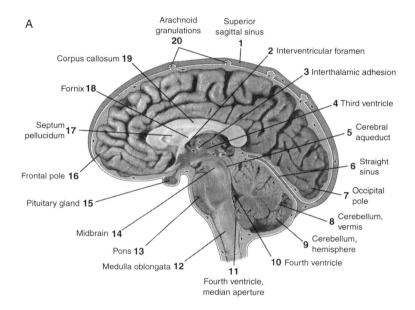

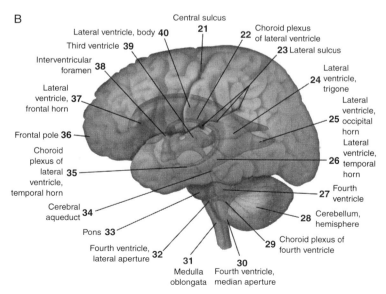

FIGURE 2-1 **A. Flow pattern of cerebrospinal fluid. B. Anatomy of the ventricular system.** Used with permission from Woolsey, Thomas A., Joseph Hanaway, and Mokhtar H. Gado. *The Brain Atlas: A Visual Guide to the Human Central Nervous System.* 3rd ed. Hoboken, NJ: Wiley, 2008.

Menges

Here, we will draw the meninges, which comprises the dura mater, arachnoid mater, and pia mater. First draw an outline of the skull and upper spinal canal. Intracranially, draw the outermost meningeal layer: the dura mater, directly underlying the skull. Then, within the spinal canal, show that space exists between the dura mater and the vertebral column, which creates a true epidural space. Epidural hematoma more commonly occurs in the spinal canal, because of its true epidural space, than in the cranial vault, where the dura mater directly adheres to the skull. The classic example of intracranial epidural hematoma is that which occurs from trauma to the temporal bone—the fractured bone severs the underlying middle meningeal artery and the high pressure of this arterial vessel rips the dura away from the skull so that blood collects between the dura and the cranium.

Clinically, we commonly discuss the dura mater as a single layer, but within the cranium, it actually comprises two separate anatomic sublayers. Label the layer we just drew as the periosteal dural sublayer, which tightly adheres to the skull. Next, label the underlying meningeal sublayer. The periosteal layer ends within the cranium; within the spinal canal, only the meningeal dural sublayer exists. Indicate that for much of the cranial dura mater, the periosteal and meningeal sublayers closely adhere; however, show that meningeal dural sublayer reflections also exist. These reflections form the falx cerebri, which separates the cerebral hemispheres; the tentorium cerebelli, which separates the cerebellum from the overlying occipital lobes; and the falx cerebelli (not shown here), which separates the cerebellar hemispheres. Then, show that the superior sagittal dural venous sinus forms within the falx cerebri and that the transverse sinuses form within the tentorium cerebelli. These dural venous sinuses function in cerebrospinal fluid absorption and blood-flow return; we discuss them in detail elsewhere.[1] Next, indicate that the tentorium cerebelli divides the cranial vault into a supratentorial compartment, which contains the cerebral hemispheres (note that we grossly distort the cerebral hemispheric proportions for diagrammatic purposes, here), and an infratentorial compartment, which contains the cerebellum and brainstem. Intracranial herniation syndromes involve pathologic displacement of central nervous system structures. Three forms of supratentorial herniation exist. Indicate that in subfalcine herniation, one hemisphere herniates underneath the falx cerebri (this shift is also called cingulate herniation because it is the cingulate gyrus that first herniates under the falx); next, show that in uncal herniation, the medial temporal lobe (the uncus) herniates over the tentorium cerebelli; and then, show that in central herniation (aka transtentorial herniation), the diencephalon herniates directly down through the tentorium cerebelli. Next, let's show the two forms of infratentorial herniation that exist. Indicate that in upward cerebellar herniation, the cerebellum herniates upward into the supratentorial cavity, and then, show that in tonsillar herniation, the cerebellar tonsils undergo downward herniation through the foramen magnum.[2,3]

Now, label the next innermost meningeal layer as the arachnoid mater and then show that a potential space exists between the dura and arachnoid mater layers: the subdural space. Show that this space is actually filled with the loosely arranged dural border cell layer. The classic cause of subdural hematoma is from rupture of low-pressure bridging veins as they run within this space.

Next, show that the pia mater directly contacts the central nervous system parenchyma; it is the delicate, innermost layer of the meninges. Then, label the space between the pia and arachnoid mater layers as the subarachnoid space. Unlike the subdural space, this is a true (actual) space, which bathes the nervous system. The subarachnoid space contains cisternal fluid collections, which we draw in Drawing 2-4.[4-8]

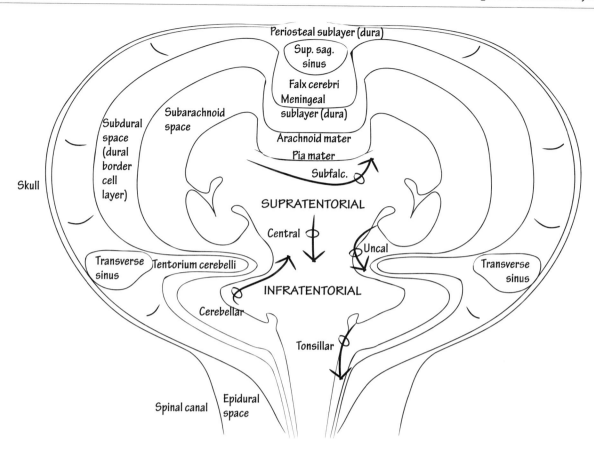

DRAWING 2-1 **Meninges**

Cerebrospinal Fluid Flow

Here, we will draw the flow of cerebrospinal fluid through the nervous system in coronal view. First, establish the relevant meningeal layers: draw the outermost dural sublayer—the periosteal sublayer, and then the innermost layer—the meningeal sublayer. Show that together they form the dura mater, which contains dural venous sinuses within the dural reflections. Next, move inward and draw the arachnoid mater. Between the arachnoid mater and the overlying meningeal sublayer, label the subdural space, which is constituted by the dural border cell layer. Now, draw the pia mater as the layer directly adhering to the nervous system parenchyma. Between the pia mater and the arachnoid mater, label the subarachnoid space.

Next, let's draw the cerebral ventricles. Show a T-shaped coronal view of the paired lateral ventricles, third ventricle, and fourth ventricle, and then, show the central canal of the spinal cord. Also, show some representative choroid plexus, the secretory epithelial tissue that produces cerebrospinal fluid, in the lateral ventricles; we show the ventricular locations of the choroid plexus in Drawing 2-3. The choroid plexus is formed where invaginations of vascularized meninges, called tela choroidea, merge with ventricular ependyma. The tela choroidea are variably defined histologically as either combinations of pia and ependyma or double pial layers. The tight junctions within the choroid plexus cuboidal epithelium form an important blood–cerebrospinal fluid barrier.[9–12]

Now, show that cerebrospinal fluid empties through the paired foramina of Monro into the third ventricle, then into the fourth ventricle, and then down the central canal, which is mostly obliterated by middle adulthood. Next, show that cerebrospinal fluid empties from the fourth ventricle through the foramen of Magendie, in midline, and the foramina of Luschka, laterally, to enter the subarachnoid space. Then, show that fluid descends into the spinal canal to bathe the spinal cord, and show that it also ascends into the cranial vault to bathe the rest of the brain.

Next, show a representative arachnoid villus extend from the subarachnoid space through the subdural space into a dural venous sinus. Finally, indicate that cerebrospinal fluid passes into the arachnoid villus to be reabsorbed within the dural venous sinus. Neoplastic arachnoid villi cells form meningiomas, a common brain tumor type; the greatest concentration of meningiomas is found where there is the greatest concentration of arachnoid villi: at the cerebral convexity, falx cerebri, and base of the skull.

Note that although we have highlighted the cerebrospinal fluid resorption into the dural venous sinuses, here, the majority of fluid within these dural venous channels is blood. This is because the rate of cerebrospinal fluid production and resorption is far slower than the rate of blood entrance and reabsorption into and out of the cranial vault. Cerebrospinal fluid is produced and reabsorbed at a rate of roughly 0.35 milliliters per minute, which equals about 20 milliliters per hour. In a typical lumbar puncture, anywhere from 10 to 20 milliliters of fluid are withdrawn; thus, this fluid is replaced within a half-hour to one hour after the procedure. There is roughly 150 milliliters of cerebrospinal fluid in the nervous system at any given time.[4–8]

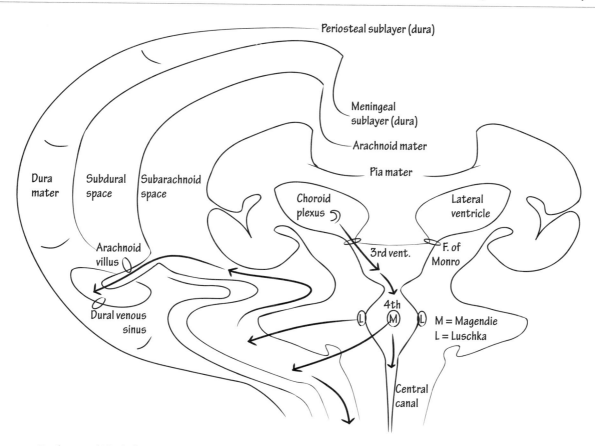

DRAWING 2-2 **Cerebrospinal Fluid Flow**

Cerebral Ventricles

Here, we will draw the cerebral ventricles in sagittal view. First, draw the C-shaped appearance of one of the bilateral lateral ventricles and include its posterior tail. Next, label the individual horns of the representative lateral ventricle. Label the supero-anterior-lying horn as the frontal horn, the posterior-lying horn as the occipital horn, and the infero-anterior-lying horn as the temporal horn. The head of the caudate constitutes the majority of the lateral wall of the frontal horn, the occipital horn extends deep into the occipital lobe, and the hippocampus constitutes the anterior medial wall of the temporal horn (the amygdala sits just in front of it and forms the anterior border of the temporal horn). Next, label the long superior bend of the lateral ventricle as its body and label the region where the temporal and occipital horns and body come together as the atrium (aka trigone). Now, show that through the bilateral foramina of Monro, the lateral ventricles empty into the third ventricle, which lies in the midline of the nervous system and which is flanked by the hypothalamus, inferiorly, and the bilateral thalami, superiorly. Next, show that the third ventricle empties into the narrow cerebral aqueduct (of Sylvius), which empties into the diamond-shaped fourth ventricle. Then, show that at the inferior angle of the fourth ventricle, at the level of the gracile tubercle (the swelling formed by the gracile nucleus in the posterior wall of the medulla), the fourth ventricle becomes the obex, and descends as the central canal of the spinal cord.[13]

Next, let's label the midline borders of the fourth ventricle. First, label the anterior border as the floor of the fourth ventricle. The floor of the fourth ventricle is an important anatomic site because it forms the posterior border of the tegmentum of the pons and medulla and many important anatomic structures lie within or near to it, including certain lower cranial nerve nuclei and certain neurobehavioral cell groups (eg, the locus coeruleus and the area postrema). Next, label the superior–posterior border of the fourth ventricle as the superior medullary velum (aka anterior medullary velum) and then the inferior–posterior border as the inferior medullary velum (aka posterior medullary velum). The cerebellar peduncles form the lateral borders of the fourth ventricle and the cerebellum helps form the rest of the posterior border (the roof). Medulloblastoma tumors often lie along the superior medullary velum.

Now, let's include the choroid plexus. Show that it lies within the central regions of the cerebral ventricles: in the body and atrium of the lateral ventricle, temporal horn of the lateral ventricle, third ventricle, and fourth ventricle. The lack of choroid plexus in the frontal and occipital horns allows neurosurgeons to place intraventricular drains in these horns without injuring the highly vascularized choroid plexus.

The shape of the lateral ventricles bears resemblance to many major cerebral structures—the cerebral hemispheres, the caudate–putamen, and the fornix–hippocampus. During embryogenesis, all of these structures undergo a backward, downward, and forward migration, which we will demonstrate with our arms, now. First, create a coronal view of the developing brain as follows. Hold your arms together with your elbows bent and extend your wrists so you could set a plate on your palms. Your hyper-extended palms represent the flat surface of the brain when it first forms. Next, curl your fingertips to demonstrate that during early development, there is inrolling of the walls of the hemispheres. Then, continue to curl your fingers in so that they touch your palms to form the bilateral lateral ventricles and the small midline third ventricle. Next, initiate the backward, downward, and forward evagination of the ventricles. Bring your forearms back toward your chest, then fan your elbows apart as you bring your hands downward, and then extend your arms forward. This completes our demonstration. We can imagine how each of the horns takes shape during the different steps of lateral ventricular development: the frontal horns take shape during the origination of the ventricular system, the occipital horns are created during the backward migration, and the temporal horns form during the downward and forward migration.[4–8]

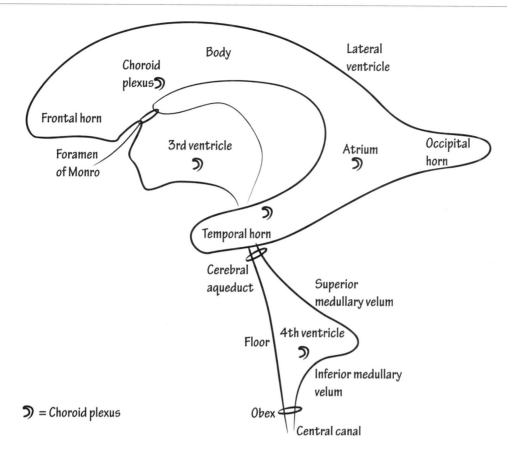

Body

Choroid
plexus⟩

Lateral
ventricle

Frontal horn

3rd ventricle
⟩

Foramen
of Monro

Atrium
⟩

Occipital
horn

⟩

Temporal horn

Cerebral
aqueduct

Superior
medullary velum

Floor

4th ventricle
⟩

Inferior medullary
velum

⟩ = Choroid plexus

Obex

Central canal

DRAWING 2-3 **Cerebral Ventricles**

Cisterns, Sinuses, & Veins (*Advanced*)

Here, we will draw the subarachnoid cisterns, dural venous sinuses, and cerebral veins. Begin with the cisterns. Draw a few key anatomic landmarks; first, the brainstem: label the midbrain, pons, and medulla; then, the thalamus; next, the splenium of the corpus callosum; and lastly, the sella turcica. First, above the sella turcica, label the suprasellar cistern. The optic chiasm lies within this cistern and, thus, it is also referred to as the chiasmatic cistern. Next, in front of the midbrain, in between the cerebral peduncles, label the interpeduncular cistern; then, along the lateral midbrain, label the ambient cistern; and finally, behind the midbrain, label the quadrigeminal cistern, which is also called the cistern of the great vein because it contains the great cerebral vein (aka vein of Galen).

Next, label the cistern of the velum interpositum in between the thalamus and the splenium of the corpus callosum. Note that this small cistern actually lies between the tela choroidea that lines the inferior surface of the fornix and splenium of the corpus callosum and the superior surface of the third ventricle and thalamus. Within the velum interpositum lie the internal cerebral veins (drawn later). Now, in front of the pons, label the prepontine cistern and lateral to it, label the pontocerebellar cistern. Next, in front of the medulla, label the premedullary cistern and, lateral to it, label the lateral cerebellomedullary cistern. Then, underneath the cerebellum, label the posterior cerebellomedullary cistern (aka cisterna magna); this is the cerebrospinal extraction site during cisternal puncture.[14–16]

Collectively, the subarachnoid cisterns at the base of the brain are referred to as the basal cisterns. Obliteration of the basal cisterns on radiographic imaging suggests brainstem swelling or compression, which is life-threatening—see Figures 2-3 and 2-4.

Next, let's draw the dural venous sinuses. First show that the superior sagittal sinus runs along the superficial midline surface of the cerebrum. Then, indicate that at the occiput, lies the confluence of sinuses (torcular Herophili). Next, show that the confluence of sinuses merges with the bilateral transverse sinuses, which wrap horizontally along the tentorium cerebelli. Note that often the right transverse sinus is larger than the left. Now, show that the confluence of sinuses also receives the straight sinus, which as we will later indicate, drains the deep cerebral veins. Note that an occipital sinus also exists, which drains inferiorly from the confluence of sinuses; we leave it out of our diagram for simplicity.

Next, draw the inferior sagittal sinus; it runs inferior to the superior sagittal sinus along the same midline course, just above the corpus callosum, and it empties into the straight sinus. Now, indicate that each transverse sinus empties into a sigmoid sinus, which forms an S-shaped curve along the intracranial surface of the mastoid portion of the temporal bone. Then, show that at the jugular bulb, each sigmoid sinus empties into its respective internal jugular vein.

Now, let's introduce a few key deep cerebral veins. First, show that the vein of Galen (aka the great cerebral vein) lies posterior to the splenium of the corpus callosum and drains directly into the straight sinus. Then, indicate that each of the bilateral basal veins of Rosenthal passes around the midbrain to drain into the vein of Galen, and that each of the bilateral internal cerebral veins passes through the cistern of the velum interpositum to drain into the vein of Galen, as well.

Finally, show a representative superficial cerebral vein—the superior cerebral vein, which drains into the superior sagittal sinus. The superficial cerebral veins divide into superior, middle, and inferior groups of veins, which drain the superficial cerebrum.[4–8,17]

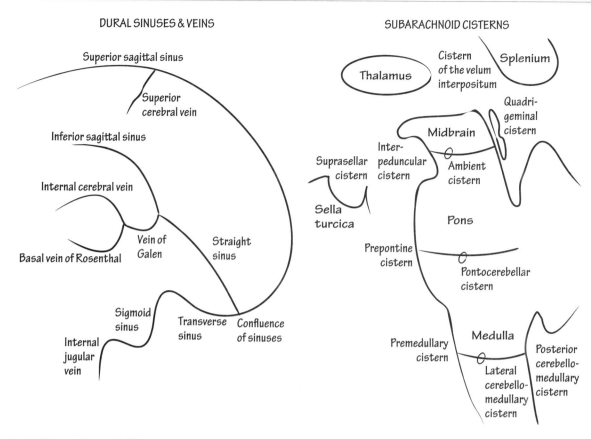

DURAL SINUSES & VEINS

Superior sagittal sinus

Superior cerebral vein

Inferior sagittal sinus

Internal cerebral vein

Basal vein of Rosenthal

Vein of Galen

Straight sinus

Sigmoid sinus

Internal jugular vein

Transverse sinus

Confluence of sinuses

SUBARACHNOID CISTERNS

Thalamus

Cistern of the velum interpositum

Splenium

Quadri-geminal cistern

Midbrain

Inter-peduncular cistern

Ambient cistern

Suprasellar cistern

Sella turcica

Pons

Prepontine cistern

Pontocerebellar cistern

Premedullary cistern

Medulla

Lateral cerebello-medullary cistern

Posterior cerebello-medullary cistern

DRAWING 2-4 **Cisterns, Sinuses, & Veins**

Hemorrhages & Innervation *(Advanced)*

Here, let's learn a few important clinical correlates to the meninges. First, let's learn how to distinguish epidural and subdural hematomas (Fig. 2-2). In epidural hematoma, blood collects between the periosteal dura and skull. As it collects, it pushes aside the spongy brain parenchyma and forms a biconvex lens-shaped fluid collection with one side of the convexity displacing brain matter and the other side layering against the cranium. In subdural hematoma, blood collects within the dural border cell layer, external to the underlying arachnoid layer. The dural border cell layer is less resistant than the brain tissue, so blood spreads along the border cell layer in a crescent shape.

Next, let's distinguish these two hematoma types based on whether or not they respect the dural folds. Epidural hematomas form external to the periosteal sublayer, and therefore, they are unaffected by the dural folds (the falx cerebri, tentorium cerebelli, and falx cerebelli), which lie deep to them. On the contrary, subdural hematomas form underneath the meningeal sublayer and pool at the site of the dural reflections: they do not cross the dural folds.

Lastly, consider the effect of the cranial sutures (the junctions between the skull bones) on both types of hematoma. Because epidural hematomas lie between the dura and skull, they are stopped at the cranial sutures; in contrast, subdural hematomas lie underneath the dura mater and are unaffected by the cranial sutures.[18,19]

Figures 2-3 and 2-4, each contain subarachnoid hemorrhage; the subarachnoid space was described in the previous lesson — *CISTERNS, SINUSES, & VEINS.*

Next, let's consider the innervation pattern of the meninges. Most meningeal innervation comes from the trigeminal nerve, which innervates the supratentorial meninges, including the meninges of the anterior and middle cranial fossae. Posterior cranial fossa meningeal innervation is derived, most notably, from the second and third cervical spinal nerves and a minor branch of the vagus nerve. Note that the facial and glossopharyngeal nerves potentially play a role in meningeal innervation, as well.[8,11]

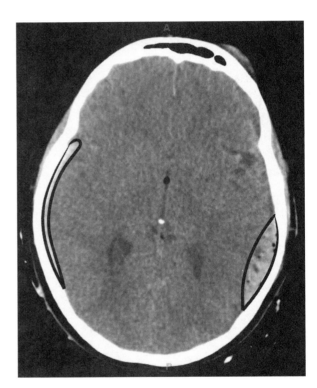

FIGURE 2-2 **Subdural hematoma on left side of page (right side of brain) and epidural hematoma on right side of page (left side of brain).**

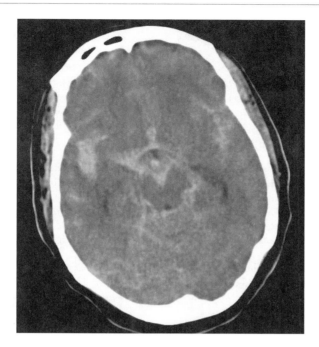

FIGURE 2-3 **Subarachnoid hemorrhage. Hemorrhage fills the subarachnoid space but spares the cerebral aqueduct and temporal horns of the lateral ventricles.**

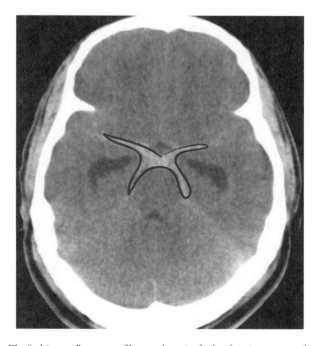

FIGURE 2-4 **Subarachnoid hemorrhage.** The "white star" pattern of hemorrhage in the basilar cisterns is outlined.

References

1. Watson, C., Paxinos, G., Kayalioglu, G. & Christopher & Dana Reeve Foundation. *The spinal cord: a Christopher and Dana Reeve Foundation text and atlas,* 1st ed. (Elsevier/Academic Press, 2009).

2. Gilroy, J. *Basic neurology,* 3rd ed., Chapter 2 (McGraw-Hill, Health Professions Division, 2000).

3. Schünke, M., Schulte, E. & Schumacher, U. *Thieme atlas of anatomy. Head and neuroanatomy* (Thieme, 2007).

4. Afifi, A. K. & Bergman, R. A. *Functional neuroanatomy: text and atlas,* 2nd ed. (Lange Medical Books/McGraw-Hill, 2005).

5. DeMyer, W. *Neuroanatomy,* 2nd ed. (Williams & Wilkins, 1998).

6. Haines, D. E. & Ard, M. D. *Fundamental neuroscience: for basic and clinical applications,* 3rd ed. (Churchill Livingstone Elsevier, 2006).

7. Netter, F. H. & Dalley, A. F. *Atlas of human anatomy,* 2nd ed., Plates 4–7 (Novartis, 1997).

8. Standring, S. & Gray, H. *Gray's anatomy: the anatomical basis of clinical practice,* 40th ed. (Churchill Livingstone/Elsevier, 2008).

9. Bruni, J. E. & Montemurro, D. G. *Human neuroanatomy: a text, brain atlas, and laboratory dissection guide* (Oxford University Press, 2009).

10. Cottrell, J. E. & Young, W. L. *Cottrell and Young's neuroanesthesia,* 5th ed. (Mosby/Elsevier, 2010).

11. Jinkins, R. *Atlas of neuroradiologic embryology, anatomy, and variants* (Lippincott Williams & Wilkins, 2000).

12. Kiernan, J. A. & Barr, M. L. *Barr's the human nervous system: an anatomical viewpoint,* 9th ed. (Wolters Kluwer/Lippincott, Williams & Wilkins, 2009).

13. Sekhar, L. N. a. F., Richard G. *Atlas of neurosurgical techniques: Brain* (Thieme, 2006).

14. Duvernoy, H. M. & Cattin, F. *The human hippocampus: functional anatomy, vascularization and serial sections with MRI,* 3rd ed. (Springer, 2005).

15. Ryan, S., McNicholas, M. & Eustace, S. J. *Anatomy for diagnostic imaging,* 2nd ed. (Saunders, 2004).

16. Thapar, K. *Diagnosis and management of pituitary tumors* (Humana Press, 2001).

17. Swartz, J. D. & Loevner, L. A. *Imaging of the temporal bone,* 4th ed., Chapter 4 (Thieme, 2009).

18. Evans, R. W. *Neurology and trauma,* 2nd ed., Chapter 3 (Oxford University Press, 2006).

19. Zasler, N. D., Katz, D. I. & Zafonte, R. D. *Brain injury medicine: principles and practice* (Demos, 2007).

3

Peripheral Nervous System

Upper Extremity

Brachial Plexus

Median Nerve

Ulnar Nerve

Radial Nerve

Cervical Plexus (Advanced)

Know-It Points

Brachial Plexus

- Rami. The brachial plexus is most commonly formed from the C5–T1 ventral rami.
- Trunks. C7 makes up the middle trunk; C5 and C6 form the upper trunk; and C8 and T1 form the lower trunk.
- Divisions & Cords. The posterior divisions form the posterior cord; the anterior division (lower trunk) forms the medial cord; the anterior division (upper trunk) and the anterior division (middle trunk) form the lateral cord.
- Major terminal nerves. The lateral and medial cords form the median nerve; the medial cord becomes the ulnar nerve; the posterior cord becomes the radial nerve.

Median Nerve

- The median nerve is formed from the lateral cord (C6, C7) and the medial cord (C8, T1).
- The superficial forearm group comprises pronator teres and flexor carpi radialis (C6, C7) and flexor digitorum superficialis and palmaris longus (C7, C8).
- The anterior interosseous group (C7–T1) comprises pronator quadratus, flexor pollicis longus, and flexor digitorum profundus 2 and 3.
- The thenar group (C8, T1) comprises abductor pollicis brevis, opponens pollicis, and flexor pollicis brevis.
- The terminal motor group (C8, T1) comprises the first and second lumbricals.

Ulnar Nerve

- The ulnar nerve is formed from the medial cord (C8, T1).
- The forearm muscle group comprises flexor carpi ulnaris and flexor digitorum profundus 4 and 5.
- The superficial sensory division is purely sensory except that it provides motor innervation to palmaris brevis.
- The deep branch is purely motor and innervates muscle groups across the hand:
  - The hypothenar group: abductor digiti minimi, opponens digiti minimi, and flexor digiti minimi
  - The intrinsic hand group: lumbricals 3 and 4, palmar interossei, and dorsal interossei
  - The thenar group: flexor pollicis brevis and adductor pollicis

Radial Nerve

- The radial nerve is formed from the posterior cord (C5–C8).
- The radial nerve innervates the triceps muscle (primarily, C6, C7).
- The elbow group comprises brachioradialis (C5, C6), extensor carpi radialis longus and brevis (C6, C7), and anconeus (C6–C8).
- The posterior interosseous nerve branch supplies the supinator muscle (C6, C7), extensor carpi ulnaris (C7, C8) abductor pollicis longus (C7, C8), and the finger and thumb extensors (C7, C8).

Cervical Plexus *(Advanced)*

- The cervical plexus (C1–C4) innervates the anterior and posterior cervical triangles and the floor of the mouth.
- The four major sensory nerves of the cervical plexus are the lesser occipital, greater auricular, and transverse cervical nerves (C2, C3), and the supraclavicular nerve (C3, C4).

- The phrenic nerve innervates the diaphragm; it is supplied by C3 and C4 from the cervical plexus and C5 from the brachial plexus.
- The cervical spinal ventral rami form the cervical plexus; the dorsal ramus of C2 supplies the greater occipital nerve.

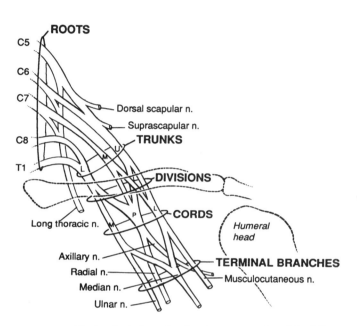

FIGURE 3-1 The brachial plexus. Used with permission from Mendell, Jerry R., John T. Kissel, and David R. Cornblath. *Diagnosis and Management of Peripheral Nerve Disorders*, Contemporary Neurology Series. Oxford: Oxford University Press, 2001.

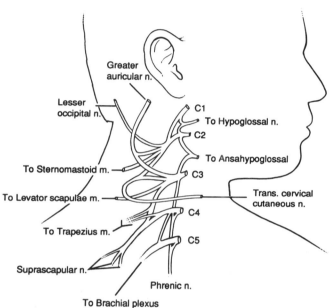

FIGURE 3-2 Cervical plexus. Used with permission from Mendell, Jerry R., John T. Kissel, and David R. Cornblath. *Diagnosis and Management of Peripheral Nerve Disorders*, Contemporary Neurology Series. Oxford: Oxford University Press, 2001.

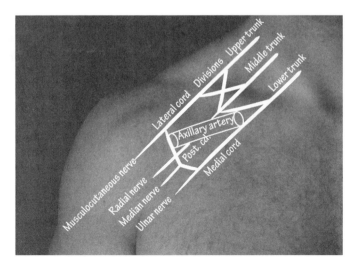

FIGURE 3-3 The brachial plexus and the axillary artery.

Brachial Plexus

Here, we will draw the brachial plexus. First, draw three horizontal lines. Label them from top to bottom as the upper, middle, and lower trunks. Next, indicate that C7 makes up the middle trunk, and then that C5 and C6 form the upper trunk (C5 and C6 join at Erb's point and a shoulder injury here is called an Erb's palsy). Then, show that C8 and T1 form the lower trunk. The brachial plexus is typically formed from the C5–T1 ventral rami.

The trunks divide into anterior and posterior divisions as follows. Show that the posterior divisions all join to form the posterior cord. At the bottom, label the anterior division (lower trunk) and then the medial cord. Next, label the anterior division (upper trunk) and show that the anterior division (middle trunk) joins it to form the lateral cord. The cords are named by their relationship to the second portion of the axillary artery: the lateral cord lies lateral to the axillary artery, the medial cord lies medial to it, and the posterior cord lies posterior to it.

Now, connect the distal lateral and medial cords and label their union as the median nerve. Then, show that the medial cord becomes the ulnar nerve and that the posterior cord becomes the radial nerve.

Next, just distal to the lateral cord, label the musculocutaneous nerve, which most notably innervates the biceps brachii (C5, C6). Biceps brachii is an important elbow flexor and also an important supinator. The role of the biceps brachii in supination explains why supination is at least partially preserved in radial nerve injury (when the radial-innervated supinator muscle, itself, becomes weakened). We'll include the lesser muscles innervated by the musculocutaneous nerve later.

Now, show that C5, C6, and C7 derive the long thoracic nerve, which innervates the serratus anterior muscle: it pulls the scapula forward (protracts it). Then, show that the dorsal scapular nerve originates from C5 and C4 (not shown) and that it innervates the rhomboid muscles, which pull the scapula in the opposite direction of the serratus anterior muscle: toward midline and downward. Injury to either serratus anterior, the rhomboids, or the trapezius, which cranial nerve 11 innervates, results in scapular winging. Note that the nerves to the serratus anterior and rhomboids are derived directly from the nerve roots, themselves—not from the brachial plexus, which means that in a pure brachial plexopathy, the serratus anterior and rhomboids are spared.

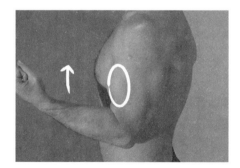

FIGURE 3-4 **Biceps brachii.**

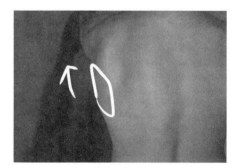

FIGURE 3-5 **Serratus anterior.**

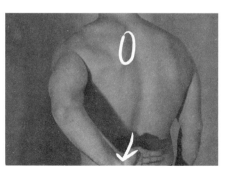

FIGURE 3-6 **Rhomboids.**

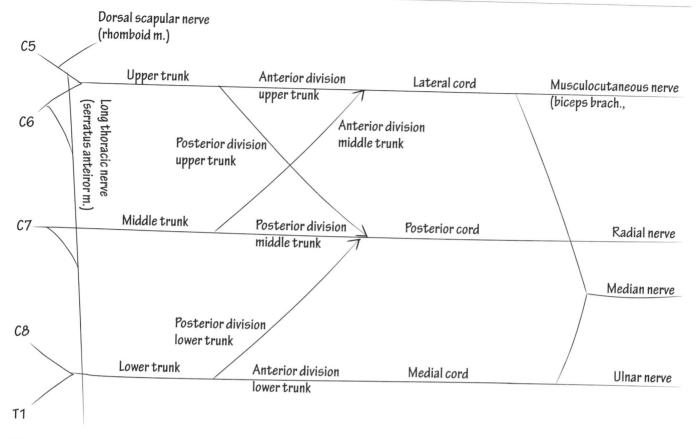

Dorsal scapular nerve
(rhomboid m.)

C5

Upper trunk

Long thoracic nerve
(serratus anteiror m.)

Anterior division
upper trunk

Lateral cord

Musculocutaneous nerve
(biceps brach.,

C6

Posterior division
upper trunk

Anterior division
middle trunk

C7   Middle trunk

Posterior division
middle trunk

Posterior cord

Radial nerve

Median nerve

C8

Posterior division
lower trunk

Lower trunk

Anterior division
lower trunk

Medial cord

Ulnar nerve

T1

DRAWING 3-1 **Brachial Plexus—Partial**

Brachial Plexus (Cont.)

Next, show that the suprascapular nerve originates from the upper trunk and indicate that it innervates the supraspinatus muscle (C5, C6), which is responsible for the first 20 to 30 degrees of arm abduction, and also show that the suprascapular nerve innervates the infraspinatus muscle (C5, C6), which is the primary external rotator of the arm (the other is teres minor).

Draw the axillary nerve off the posterior cord and show that it innervates the deltoid muscle. Whereas supraspinatus is responsible for the first 20 to 30 degrees of arm abduction, the deltoid muscle (C5, C6) is responsible for the latter 70 to 80 degrees of arm abduction. We will complete the musculature innervated by the axillary nerve at the end.

Next, more proximally off the posterior cord, draw the thoracodorsal nerve; it innervates latissimus dorsi (C6, C7, C8), which provides shoulder adduction, most notably.

Now, we will draw the pectoral nerves. Off the lateral cord, draw the lateral pectoral nerve, and off the medial cord, draw the medial pectoral nerve; they innervate the pectoralis major muscle, which as a whole, provides shoulder adduction and shoulder internal rotation. The lateral pectoral nerve innervates the clavicular head of pectoralis major (C5 (most notably) and C6), which additionally provides shoulder flexion and the medial pectoral nerve innervates the sternal head of the pectoralis major muscle (C6, C7 (most notably), C8, and T1), which additionally provides shoulder extension. For completeness, show that the pectoral nerves (mostly the medial pectoral nerve) also innervate pectoralis minor, which provides scapula depression.

Now, draw the medial brachial cutaneous and medial antebrachial cutaneous nerves; they are sensory nerves that cover the medial aspect of the upper arm and forearm, respectively. In ulnar nerve injuries, medial arm and forearm sensation is spared due to sparing of these cutaneous nerves; in contrast, in medial cordopathies, these nerves are often injured and medial upper arm and forearm sensation is impaired.

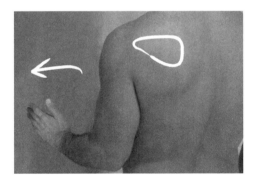

FIGURE 3-7 **Infraspinatus.**

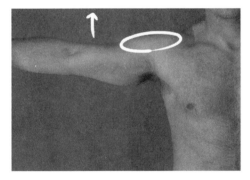

FIGURE 3-8 **Deltoid.**

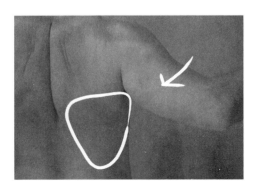

FIGURE 3-9 **Latissimus dorsi.**

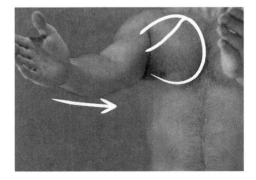

FIGURE 3-10 **Pectoralis major.**

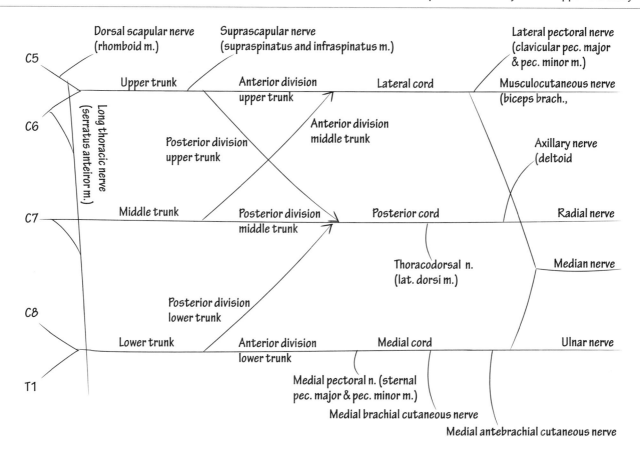

DRAWING 3-2 **Brachial Plexus—Partial**

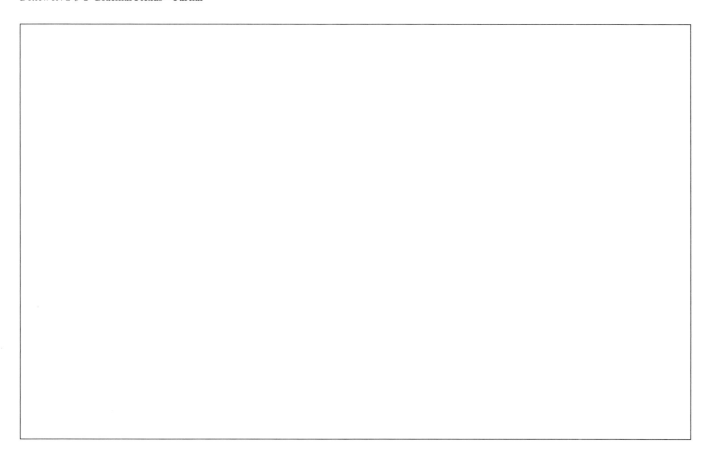

Brachial Plexus (Cont.)

Now, let's include some of the less often clinically tested brachial plexus structures. First, where the fifth and sixth cervical roots join together, indicate the nerve to the subclavius muscle. The subclavius provides clavicle depression.

Next, show that in addition to the biceps brachii, the musculocutaneous nerve also innervates the brachialis muscle, which lies deep within the anterior upper arm, and flexes the elbow with the forearm in any position; also show that the musculocutaneous nerve innervates the coracobrachialis muscle, which assists the clavicular head of the pectoralis major muscle in shoulder flexion.

Proximal and distal to the thoracodorsal nerve, respectively, draw the upper subscapular and lower subscapular nerves. Show that they both innervate the subscapularis muscle, which assists in shoulder internal rotation. Then, show that the lower subscapular nerve also innervates teres major, which assists in shoulder internal rotation, as well.

Next, return to the axillary nerve and show that the more "minor" muscle it innervates is teres minor, which assists in shoulder external rotation. The action of teres minor is best remembered by its relationship to the action of the axillary-innervated deltoid muscle, which provides shoulder abduction.

Lastly, show that if the brachial plexus is shifted up one level and receives substantial innervation from C4, it is called a prefixed plexus, and if it is shifted down one level and receives substantial innervation from T2, it is called a postfixed plexus.

Note that we have only listed the major actions of each muscle—refer to a kinesiology textbook for a listing of additional muscle actions.[1-6]

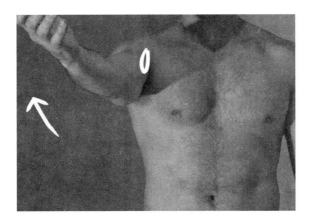

FIGURE 3-11 **Coracobrachialis.**

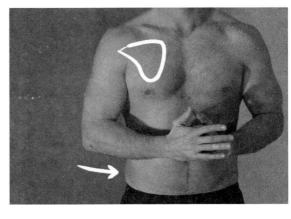

FIGURE 3-12 **Subscapularis.**

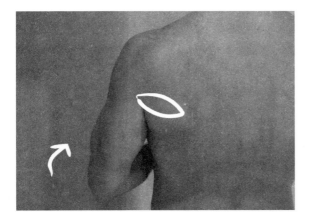

FIGURE 3-13 **Teres major.**

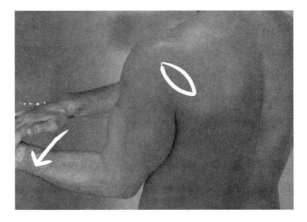

FIGURE 3-14 **Teres minor.**

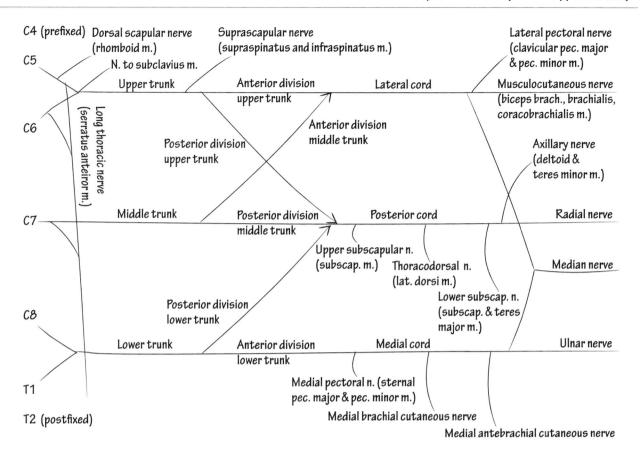

C4 (prefixed)

C5

C6

C7

C8

T1

T2 (postfixed)

Dorsal scapular nerve
(rhomboid m.)

N. to subclavius m.

Upper trunk

Long thoracic nerve
(serratus anterior m.)

Posterior division
upper trunk

Middle trunk

Posterior division
lower trunk

Lower trunk

Suprascapular nerve
(supraspinatus and infraspinatus m.)

Anterior division
upper trunk

Anterior division
middle trunk

Posterior division
middle trunk

Upper subscapular n.
(subscap. m.)

Anterior division
lower trunk

Medial pectoral n. (sternal
pec. major & pec. minor m.)

Medial brachial cutaneous nerve

Medial antebrachial cutaneous nerve

Lateral cord

Posterior cord

Thoracodorsal n.
(lat. dorsi m.)

Lower subscap. n.
(subscap. & teres
major m.)

Medial cord

Lateral pectoral nerve
(clavicular pec. major
& pec. minor m.)

Musculocutaneous nerve
(biceps brach., brachialis,
coracobrachialis m.)

Axillary nerve
(deltoid &
teres minor m.)

Radial nerve

Median nerve

Ulnar nerve

DRAWING 3-3 **Brachial Plexus—Complete**

Median Nerve

Here, we will draw the median nerve. To localize each form of median nerve injury, learn at least one muscle from each muscle group. First, divide the page into the ventral rami and brachial plexus, upper arm, forearm, and hand. Next, draw a line across the page to represent the course of the median nerve down the upper extremity. At the left-hand side of the page, underneath the brachial plexus segment, show that the lateral and medial cords form the median nerve. Indicate that the lateral cord rami that supply the median nerve are C6 and C7, which are mostly sensory, and that the medial cord rami that supply the median nerve are C8 and T1, which are mostly motor.

Next, show that the median nerve does not innervate any of the muscles of the upper arm or provide any of its sensory coverage.

Now, in the proximal forearm, draw the branch to the superficial forearm group. At the bottom of the page, we will keep track of the muscle groups, their nerve roots, and the muscles they comprise. Show that the superficial forearm group is derived from roots C6 and C7 and also from roots C7 and C8. The C6, C7 innervated muscles are pronator teres and flexor carpi radialis. Pronator teres provides forearm pronation when the elbow is extended and flexor carpi radialis provides wrist flexion with lateral deviation (towards the radius bone).

Next, show that the C7, C8 innervated muscles are flexor digitorum superficialis and palmaris longus. Flexor digitorum superficialis flexes digits 2 through 5 at their proximal interphalangeal joints. It receives additional supply from T1. Palmaris longus corrugates the skin over the wrist; you can see the palmaris longus tendon pop out in midline when you flex your wrist.

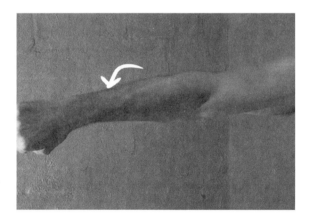

FIGURE 3-15 **Pronator teres.**

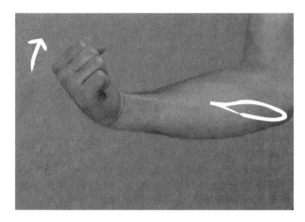

FIGURE 3-16 **Flexor carpi radialis.**

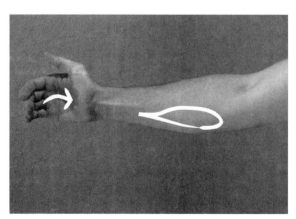

FIGURE 3-17 **Flexor digitorum superficialis.**

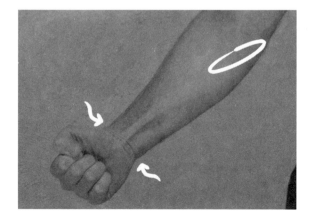

FIGURE 3-18 **Palmaris longus.**

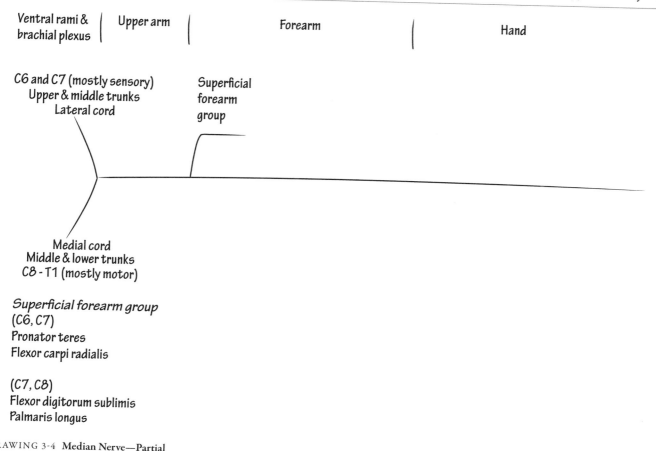

| Ventral rami & brachial plexus | Upper arm | Forearm | Hand |

C6 and C7 (mostly sensory)
Upper & middle trunks
Lateral cord

Superficial
forearm
group

Medial cord
Middle & lower trunks
C8 - T1 (mostly motor)

Superficial forearm group
(C6, C7)
Pronator teres
Flexor carpi radialis

(C7, C8)
Flexor digitorum sublimis
Palmaris longus

DRAWING 3-4 **Median Nerve—Partial**

Median Nerve (Cont.)

There are two important proximal entrapment sites for the median nerve, which we will indicate now. First, show that proximal to the superficial forearm group, lies the ligament of Struthers. All of the components of the median nerve lie downstream of this ligament; therefore, when the median nerve is entrapped in the ligament of Struthers, all of the median nerve components are affected. Next, indicate the heads of the pronator teres muscles. When the median nerve becomes entrapped in these muscle heads, everything downstream of them is affected. Note, however, that the components of the superficial forearm group, including the pronator teres muscle, itself, are unaffected when the nerve is entrapped in the heads of the pronator teres muscles, because innervation to the superficial forearm group lies proximal to the entrapment site.

Now, draw the anterior interosseous nerve branch. Show that it innervates the anterior interosseous group.

Indicate that the anterior interosseous group is derived from roots C7–T1, which comprises pronator quadratus, flexor pollicis longus, and flexor digitorum profundus 2 and 3. Pronator quadratus pronates the forearm with the elbow in flexion. Flexor pollicis longus flexes the interphalangeal joint of the thumb; it is the "long" flexor of the thumb in that it passes the metacarpal–phalangeal joint to flex the interphalangeal joint. Flexor digitorum profundus 2 and 3 flexes the distal interphalangeal joints of the second and third digits.

Now, draw the carpal tunnel at the wrist; this is the most common entrapment site of the median nerve. Show that the median sensory branch to the proximal palm, the palmar cutaneous nerve, takes off proximal to the carpal tunnel, and therefore it and everything else we have drawn so far is unaffected in carpal tunnel syndrome.

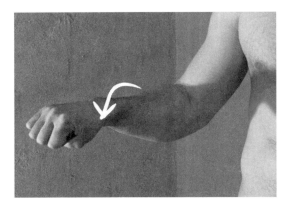

FIGURE 3-19 **Pronator quadratus.**

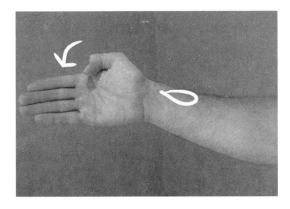

FIGURE 3-20 **Flexor pollicis longus.**

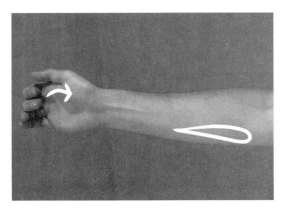

FIGURE 3-21 **Flexor digitorum profundus 2 and 3.**

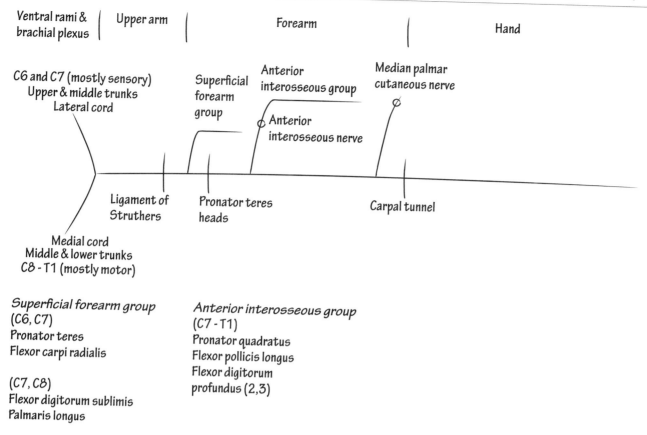

| Ventral rami & brachial plexus | Upper arm | Forearm | Hand |

C6 and C7 (mostly sensory)
Upper & middle trunks
Lateral cord

Superficial forearm group

Anterior interosseous group

Median palmar cutaneous nerve

Anterior interosseous nerve

Ligament of Struthers

Pronator teres heads

Carpal tunnel

Medial cord
Middle & lower trunks
C8 - T1 (mostly motor)

Superficial forearm group
(C6, C7)
Pronator teres
Flexor carpi radialis

(C7, C8)
Flexor digitorum sublimis
Palmaris longus

Anterior interosseous group
(C7 - T1)
Pronator quadratus
Flexor pollicis longus
Flexor digitorum
profundus (2,3)

DRAWING 3-5 **Median Nerve—Partial**

Median Nerve (Cont.)

Next, show that the recurrent motor branch of the thumb innervates the thenar group, supplied by C8 and T1. Show that this group comprises abductor pollicis brevis, opponens pollicis, and flexor pollicis brevis. Abductor pollicis brevis provides thumb abduction perpendicular to the plane of the palm (in other words, when the palm is up, it raises the thumb toward the ceiling). Abductor pollicis brevis provides the Up component of the Up, In, Out triad, which is as follows. The median-innervated abductor pollicis brevis moves the thumb perpendicular to the plane of the palm: with the palm up, it raises the thumb up toward the ceiling. The ulnar-innervated adductor pollicis and the radial-innervated abductor pollicis longus move the thumb in the plane of the palm: adductor pollicis draws the thumb in toward the side of the palm and abductor pollicis longus moves the thumb out away from the side of the palm.

Both the median and ulnar nerves produce the action of thumb to little finger opposition; the median nerve supplies the opponens pollicis muscle, which directs the thumb to the little finger, and the ulnar nerve supplies the opponens digiti minimi muscle, which directs the little finger to the thumb. Flexor pollicis brevis attaches to the proximal phalanx of the thumb and flexes the thumb against the palm. Its tendon length is shorter (more "brief") than that of flexor pollicis longus, which acts at the more distal-lying interphalangeal joint. Both the median and ulnar nerves supply flexor pollicis brevis.

Now, show the most distal median nerve motor group: the terminal motor group. Indicate that it is derived from C8–T1 and that it comprises the first and second lumbricals, which have dual actions on the second and third digits; they extend their proximal interphalangeal joints and flex their metacarpal–phalangeal joints.

Finally, show that the median nerve provides distal sensory innervation via digital sensory branches, which we map along with the rest of the median nerve's sensory coverage of the hand in Drawing 5-1.[1–4,7–11]

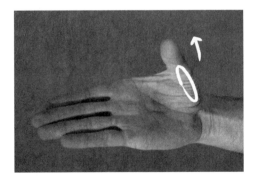

FIGURE 3-22 **Abductor pollicis brevis.**

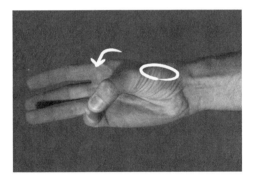

FIGURE 3-23 **Opponens pollicis.**

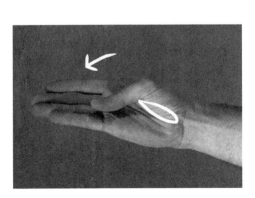

FIGURE 3-24 **Flexor pollicis brevis.**

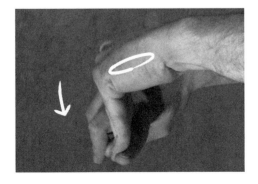

FIGURE 3-25 **Lumbricals.**

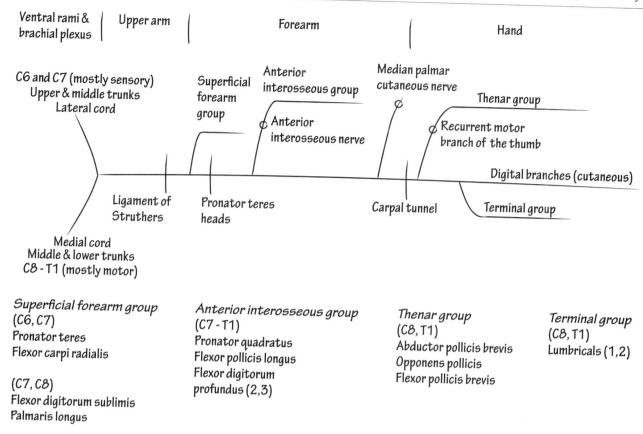

Ventral rami & brachial plexus	Upper arm	Forearm	Hand

C6 and C7 (mostly sensory)
Upper & middle trunks
Lateral cord

Superficial forearm group

Anterior interosseous group

Median palmar cutaneous nerve

Thenar group

Anterior interosseous nerve

Recurrent motor branch of the thumb

Digital branches (cutaneous)

Ligament of Struthers

Pronator teres heads

Carpal tunnel

Terminal group

Medial cord
Middle & lower trunks
C8 - T1 (mostly motor)

Superficial forearm group
(C6, C7)
Pronator teres
Flexor carpi radialis

(C7, C8)
Flexor digitorum sublimis
Palmaris longus

Anterior interosseous group
(C7 - T1)
Pronator quadratus
Flexor pollicis longus
Flexor digitorum profundus (2,3)

Thenar group
(C8, T1)
Abductor pollicis brevis
Opponens pollicis
Flexor pollicis brevis

Terminal group
(C8, T1)
Lumbricals (1,2)

DRAWING 3-6 **Median Nerve—Complete**

Ulnar Nerve

Here, we will draw the ulnar nerve. To localize each form of ulnar nerve injury, learn at least one muscle from each muscle group. First, divide the page into the ventral rami and brachial plexus, upper arm, forearm, and hand. Draw a line across the page to represent the course of the ulnar nerve. Indicate that the ulnar nerve is formed from the medial cord of the brachial plexus, which the C8–T1 nerve roots of the lower trunk supply. The C8–T1 nerve roots supply all of the ulnar nerve-innervated muscles.

First, show that the medial cutaneous nerves to the arm and forearm (aka medial brachial and medial antebrachial cutaneous nerves) are direct branches from the medial cord (and are not part of the ulnar nerve); they provide sensory coverage to the medial arm and forearm. The ulnar nerve sensory coverage, itself, is confined to the medial hand.

Now, show that the most proximal muscle group the ulnar nerve innervates is the forearm muscle group, which comprises flexor carpi ulnaris and flexor digitorum profundus 4 and 5. Flexor carpi ulnaris flexes the wrist with medial deviation (in the direction of the ulna bone). Flexor digitorum profundus 4 and 5 flexes the distal interphalangeal joints of the fourth and fifth digits.

Next, at the elbow, draw the cubital tunnel—the most common ulnar nerve entrapment site. All of the motor and sensory components of the ulnar nerve lie distal to the cubital tunnel; therefore, in a cubital tunnel syndrome, all of the components of the ulnar nerve are affected.

Now, at the wrist, show that the ulnar nerve passes through Guyon's canal (aka Guyon's tunnel). This is the other major ulnar nerve entrapment site. Variations of Guyon's canal entrapments exist affecting a variety of different distal ulnar components.

Next, show that proximal to Guyon's canal, the ulnar nerve derives the palmar and dorsal ulnar cutaneous nerves; these branches are unaffected in Guyon's canal entrapments because they lie upstream from it. We map their sensory coverage, along with the sensory coverage of the rest of the hand, in Drawing 5-1.

As the ulnar nerve enters the hand, it splits into the superficial sensory division, which is purely sensory except that it provides motor innervation to palmaris brevis, which corrugates the hypothenar eminence, and the deep branch, which is purely motor and innervates muscle groups across the hand.

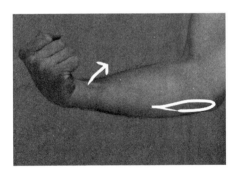

FIGURE 3-26 **Flexor carpi ulnaris.**

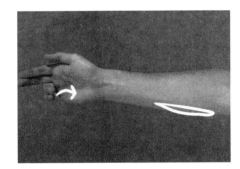

FIGURE 3-27 **Flexor digitorum profundus 4 and 5.**

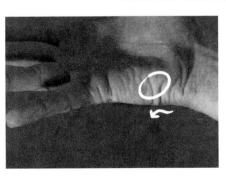

FIGURE 3-28 **Palmaris brevis.**

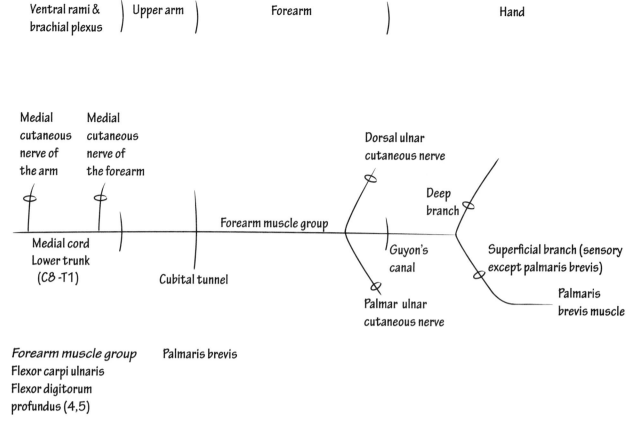

Ventral rami & brachial plexus) Upper arm) Forearm) Hand

Medial cutaneous nerve of the arm

Medial cutaneous nerve of the forearm

Dorsal ulnar cutaneous nerve

Deep branch

Forearm muscle group

Medial cord
Lower trunk
(C8 -T1)

Cubital tunnel

Guyon's canal

Superficial branch (sensory except palmaris brevis)

Palmaris brevis muscle

Palmar ulnar cutaneous nerve

Forearm muscle group
Flexor carpi ulnaris
Flexor digitorum
profundus (4,5)

Palmaris brevis

DRAWING 3-7 **Ulnar Nerve—Partial**

Ulnar Nerve (Cont.)

First, indicate that the deep branch innervates the hypothenar group, which comprises abductor digiti minimi, opponens digiti minimi, and flexor digiti minimi. Abductor digiti minimi abducts the fifth digit in the plane of the palm. In regards to opponens digiti minimi, both the median and ulnar nerves produce the action of thumb to little finger opposition: the median nerve supplies the opponens pollicis muscle, which directs the thumb to the little finger, and the ulnar nerve innervates the opponens digiti minimi muscle, which directs the little finger to the thumb. Flexor digiti minimi flexes the fifth digit toward the palm.

Now, show that the deep branch innervates the intrinsic hand group, which comprises lumbricals 3 and 4, the palmar interossei, and dorsal interossei muscles. The third and fourth lumbricals have dual actions on digits 4 and 5: they extend their proximal interphalangeal joints and flex their metacarpal–phalangeal joints. The palmar interossei bring the fingers together (they provide finger closure) whereas the dorsal interossei spread them apart. We focus on the first dorsal interosseous muscle because it is commonly clinically tested; it provides finger abduction of the second digit.

Lastly, show that the deep branch innervates the thenar group, which comprises flexor pollicis brevis and adductor pollicis. Flexor pollicis brevis flexes the thumb against the palm; the median nerve also innervates it. Adductor pollicis adducts the thumb against the side of the palm. It is the In component of the Up, In, Out triad, which is as follows. The median-innervated abductor pollicis brevis moves the thumb perpendicular to the plane of the palm: with the palm up, it raises the thumb up toward the ceiling. The ulnar-innervated adductor pollicis and the radial-innervated abductor pollicis longus move the thumb in the plane of the palm: adductor pollicis draws the thumb in toward the side of the palm and abductor pollicis longus moves the thumb out away from the side of the palm.[1–4,9,11,12]

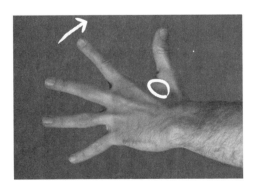

FIGURE 3-29 **Abductor digiti minimi.**

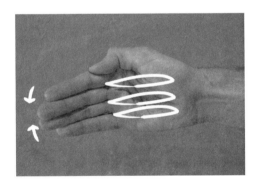

FIGURE 3-30 **Palmar interossei.**

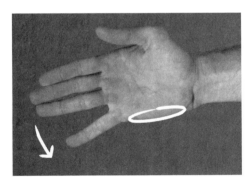

FIGURE 3-31 **First dorsal interosseous.**

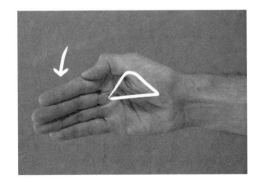

FIGURE 3-32 **Adductor pollicis.**

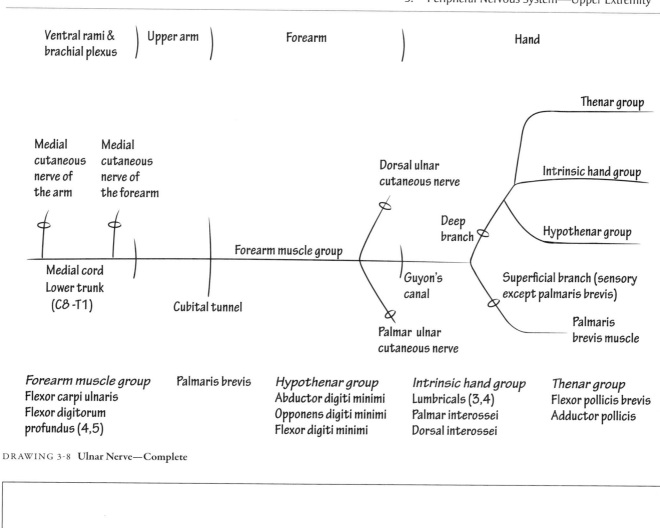

Ventral rami & brachial plexus) Upper arm) Forearm) Hand

Thenar group

Medial cutaneous nerve of the arm

Medial cutaneous nerve of the forearm

Dorsal ulnar cutaneous nerve

Intrinsic hand group

Deep branch

Hypothenar group

Forearm muscle group

Medial cord Lower trunk (C8 -T1)

Guyon's canal

Superficial branch (sensory except palmaris brevis)

Cubital tunnel

Palmaris brevis muscle

Palmar ulnar cutaneous nerve

Forearm muscle group
Flexor carpi ulnaris
Flexor digitorum profundus (4,5)

Palmaris brevis

Hypothenar group
Abductor digiti minimi
Opponens digiti minimi
Flexor digiti minimi

Intrinsic hand group
Lumbricals (3,4)
Palmar interossei
Dorsal interossei

Thenar group
Flexor pollicis brevis
Adductor pollicis

DRAWING 3-8 **Ulnar Nerve—Complete**

Radial Nerve

Here, we will draw the radial nerve. To localize each form of radial nerve injury, learn at least one muscle from each muscle group. To draw the radial nerve, divide the page into the ventral rami and brachial plexus, upper arm, forearm, and hand. First, show the proximal segment of the radial nerve. Next, indicate that the radial nerve is derived from the C5–C8 nerve roots via the posterior cord. Indicate that the axillary nerve originates from the posterior cord just proximal to the derivation of the radial nerve; the axillary nerve innervates the deltoid and teres minor muscles. Because the axillary nerve lies upstream from the radial nerve, it is unaffected in radial nerve palsy; we show it here because its anatomic proximity to the radial nerve makes it useful to test for clinical localization.

Unlike the median and ulnar nerves, the radial nerve does provide important motor and sensory branches to the upper arm. First, show that the radial nerve innervates the triceps muscle, which is supplied primarily by C6 and C7 but also by C8; it provides elbow extension.

Now, show two key anatomic sites so we can understand how to use the triceps as a localizing tool in radial nerve palsy. First, show that the axilla lies proximal to the triceps. When the radial nerve is compressed within the axilla, such as from using crutches, the triceps is affected because it lies downstream from the axilla. Next, show that the spiral groove lies distal to the triceps. Along the spiral groove, the radial nerve opposes the humerus and is susceptible to compression; injury here is called "Saturday night palsy." The triceps is unaffected in Saturday night palsy because the take-off for the triceps is proximal to the spiral groove.

Where the upper arm and forearm meet, label the elbow and show the elbow group, which the C5–C8 nerve roots supply. It comprises brachioradialis, which C5 and C6 supply, extensor carpi radialis longus and brevis, which C6 and C7 supply, and anconeus, which C6–C8 supply. In regards to brachialis, the musculocutaneous nerve innervates the C5 and C6 portion and the radial nerve innervates the small C7 portion. Brachioradialis flexes the elbow with the forearm in mid-pronation/supination position whereas brachialis flexes the elbow with the arm in any position. The extensor carpi radialis longus and brevis muscles extend the wrist with lateral deviation (toward the radius bone). Anconeus assists in elbow extension.

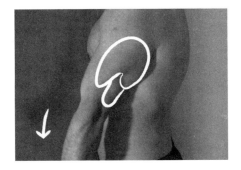

FIGURE 3-33 **Triceps.**

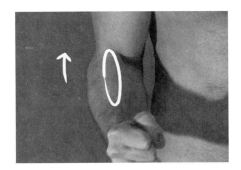

FIGURE 3-34 **Brachioradialis.**

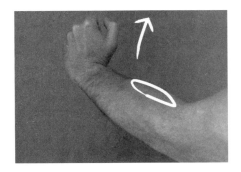

FIGURE 3-35 **Extensor carpi radialis.**

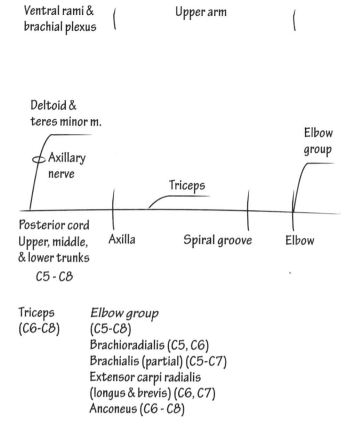

| Ventral rami & brachial plexus | (| Upper arm | (| Forearm | (| Hand |

Deltoid & teres minor m.

Axillary nerve

Triceps

Elbow group

Posterior cord
Upper, middle, & lower trunks
C5 - C8

Axilla   Spiral groove   Elbow

Triceps
(C6-C8)

Elbow group
(C5-C8)
Brachioradialis (C5, C6)
Brachialis (partial) (C5-C7)
Extensor carpi radialis
(longus & brevis) (C6, C7)
Anconeus (C6 - C8)

DRAWING 3-9 **Radial Nerve—Partial**

Radial Nerve (Cont.)

Next, show that the radial nerve branches into the posterior interosseous nerve. In the proximal segment of the posterior interosseous nerve, indicate the supinator muscle. The C6, C7 nerve roots supply the supinator; it provides outward rotation (supination) of the forearm. Note that the biceps brachii is also a major supinator of the elbow, and therefore, forearm supination is often preserved in radial neuropathy because of the unaffected musculocutaneous-innervated biceps brachii.

Now, show that the posterior interosseous nerve innervates extensor carpi ulnaris and abductor pollicis longus, which are both supplied by C7, C8. Extensor carpi ulnaris extends the wrist with medial deviation (towards the ulna bone) and abductor pollicis longus abducts the thumb in the plane of the palm. It is the Out component of the Up, In, Out triad, which is as follows. The median-innervated abductor pollicis brevis moves the thumb perpendicular to the plane of the palm: with the palm up, it raises the thumb up toward the ceiling. The ulnar-innervated adductor pollicis and the radial-innervated abductor pollicis longus move the thumb in the plane of the palm: adductor pollicis draws the thumb in toward the side of the palm and abductor pollicis longus moves the thumb out away from the side of the palm.

Finally, indicate the posterior interosseous nerve innervation of finger and thumb extensors, supplied by C7, C8; they are extensor indicis proprius, extensor digitorum communis, and extensor digiti minimi (for the fingers), and extensor pollicis longus and extensor pollicis brevis (for the thumb). Extensor indicis proprius extends the second digit; extensor digitorum communis extends the third and fourth digits; and extensor digiti minimi extends the fifth digit. The extensor pollicis muscles extend the thumb (with the palm down, they raise it up). Extensor pollicis brevis extends the thumb at the metacarpal–phalangeal joint whereas extensor pollicis longus extends the thumb at the interphalangeal joint.

This completes the motor innervation of the radial nerve; now, let's address the sensory innervation. First, just distal to the axilla, show the take-off for the proximal radial nerve branches. The proximal radial sensory nerves are the posterior cutaneous nerves to the arm and forearm and the lower lateral cutaneous nerve of the arm. These nerves cover the lower upper arm and the midline posterior arm and forearm, shown in Drawing 5-4. Next, at the take-off of the posterior interosseous nerve, draw the superficial sensory radial nerve; it provides distal radial sensory coverage, shown in Drawing 5-1.[1–4,9]

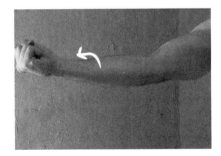

FIGURE 3-36 **Supinator.**

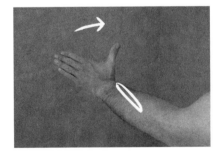

FIGURE 3-37 **Abductor pollicis longus.**

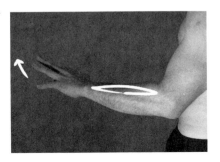

FIGURE 3-38 **Extensor digitorum communis.**

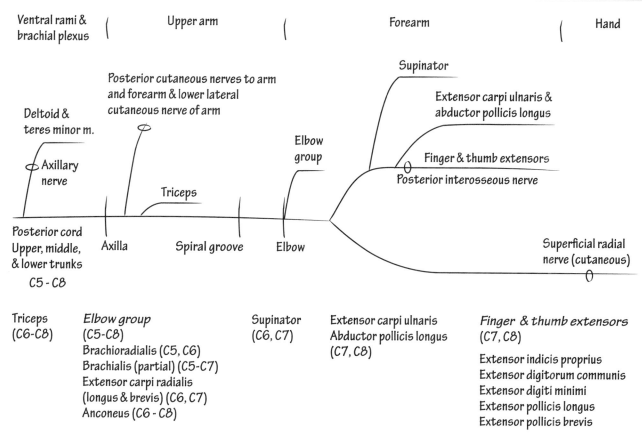

Ventral rami &
brachial plexus

Upper arm

Forearm

Hand

Deltoid &
teres minor m.

Posterior cutaneous nerves to arm
and forearm & lower lateral
cutaneous nerve of arm

Supinator

Extensor carpi ulnaris &
abductor pollicis longus

Axillary
nerve

Elbow
group

Finger & thumb extensors
Posterior interosseous nerve

Triceps

Posterior cord
Upper, middle,
& lower trunks
C5 - C8

Axilla

Spiral groove

Elbow

Superficial radial
nerve (cutaneous)

Triceps
(C6-C8)

Elbow group
(C5-C8)
Brachioradialis (C5, C6)
Brachialis (partial) (C5-C7)
Extensor carpi radialis
(longus & brevis) (C6, C7)
Anconeus (C6 - C8)

Supinator
(C6, C7)

Extensor carpi ulnaris
Abductor pollicis longus
(C7, C8)

Finger & thumb extensors
(C7, C8)

Extensor indicis proprius
Extensor digitorum communis
Extensor digiti minimi
Extensor pollicis longus
Extensor pollicis brevis

DRAWING 3-10 **Radial Nerve—Complete**

Cervical Plexus *(Advanced)*

Here, we will draw the cervical plexus; it is constituted by ventral rami from C1–C4, which emerge from underneath the sternocleidomastoid muscle and innervate structures of the anterior and posterior cervical triangles and the floor of the mouth. Begin our diagram with a few key anatomic structures: first, draw the clavicle; then, the trapezius muscle; and then, the inferior attachment of the sternocleidomastoid muscle to the anterior clavicle; and finally, the superior attachment of the sternocleidomastoid muscle to the mastoid bone. We cut out the sternocleidomastoid muscle belly because it would obstruct the view of our diagram.

Next, in midline of the page, draw seven small foramina: the jugular foramen, the hypoglossal canal, and the foramina of C1 through C5. As mentioned, the cervical plexus is formed from the C1–C4 spinal nerves, but we include the jugular foramen, hypoglossal canal, and C5 foramen, here, because they are the exit sites of related anatomic structures.

First, let's draw the four major sensory nerves of the cervical plexus, three of which we show by first drawing an anastomosis between C2 and C3. This connection forms the lesser occipital, greater auricular, and transverse cervical nerves. Show that the lesser occipital nerve provides sensory coverage to the superior pole of the pinna and posterolateral head; the greater auricular nerve provides sensory coverage to the inferior pole of the pinna and the angle of the mandible; and the transverse cervical nerve (aka the anterior cutaneous nerve of the neck) provides sensory coverage to the anterolateral neck. Next, for the fourth sensory nerve, draw an anastomosis between C3 and C4 and show that it derives the supraclavicular nerve, which provides sensory coverage to the posterolateral neck, upper chest, and shoulder. Note that minor C3 and C4 sensory branches to the trapezius muscle also exist, which we leave out of our diagram for simplicity.

Next, let's draw the motor nerves of the cervical plexus. For this, we begin with the phrenic nerve. Show that it originates from C3 and C4 from the cervical plexus and C5 from the brachial plexus. It descends through the thoracic cavity to innervate the diaphragm.

Although not part of the cervical plexus, for regional purposes also include the hypoglossal nerve, which traverses the hypoglossal canal. It innervates all of the intrinsic tongue muscles and the majority of the extrinsic tongue muscles, shown in Drawing 12-6.

Next, show that for a portion of its course, C1 joins cranial nerve 12 as part of the hypoglossal nerve. Then, show that C1 innervates both the geniohyoid and thyrohyoid muscles and that it forms the superior (aka descending) root of the ansa cervicalis, which innervates the superior belly of the omohyoid muscle.

Now, show that C2 and C3 together form the inferior root of the ansa cervicalis, and show that where the superior and inferior roots meet, the ansa cervicalis innervates sternohyoid, sternothyroid, and the inferior belly of omohyoid.

We can group the aforementioned muscles based on their anatomic compartments. Sternohyoid, sternothyroid, omohyoid, and thyrohyoid are all infrahyoid muscles (meaning they lie below the hyoid bone) and they are collectively referred to as strap muscles. On the contrary, geniohyoid is a suprahyoid muscle (meaning it lies above the hyoid bone); the other suprahyoid muscles are mylohyoid, stylohyoid, and the digastric. The digastric and stylohyoid muscles lie within the anterior triangle of the neck whereas geniohyoid and mylohyoid lie within the floor of the mouth.

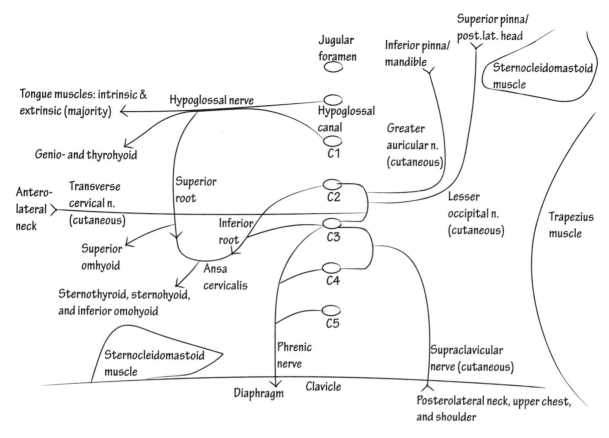

Jugular foramen

Hypoglossal nerve

Tongue muscles: intrinsic & extrinsic (majority)

Genio- and thyrohyoid

Hypoglossal canal

C1

Superior pinna/ post.lat. head

Inferior pinna/ mandible

Sternocleidomastoid muscle

Greater auricular n. (cutaneous)

Antero- lateral neck

Transverse cervical n. (cutaneous)

Superior root

C2

Lesser occipital n. (cutaneous)

Trapezius muscle

Superior omhyoid

Inferior root

C3

Ansa cervicalis

Sternothyroid, sternohyoid, and inferior omohyoid

C4

Sternocleidomastoid muscle

C5

Phrenic nerve

Diaphragm

Clavicle

Supraclavicular nerve (cutaneous)

Posterolateral neck, upper chest, and shoulder

DRAWING 3-11 **Cervical Plexus—Partial**

Cervical Plexus *(Advanced)* (Cont.)

We have completed the cervical plexus innervation of the muscles of the anterior cervical triangle and the floor of the mouth, so now let's show how the cervical plexus derives the majority of cranial nerve 11, the spinal accessory nerve, which innervates the sternocleidomastoid and trapezius muscles. Motor cells from the medulla to the sixth cervical segment are responsible for the complete supply of the spinal accessory nerve, but we will only show the cervical plexus contribution, here. Show that branches from C2–C4 ascend the spinal canal, pass through the foramen magnum, and exit the cranium through the jugular foramen as the spinal accessory nerve. The spinal accessory nerve innervates the trapezius, supplied by C3 and C4, and the sternocleidomastoid, supplied by C2–C4. Trapezius elevates the shoulders (most notably) and sternocleidomastoid turns the head.

Note that the trapezius receives additional innervation from cervical sources other than the spinal accessory nerve; and therefore, in spinal accessory nerve palsy, the trapezius muscle is partially spared.

Now, in the corner of the diagram, make a notation that the cervical plexus also provides innervation to the deep anterior vertebral muscles, which comprise the anterior and lateral rectus capitis muscles (C1, C2), longus capitis (C1, C2, C3), and longus colli (C2–C6) muscles, and that the cervical plexus also helps innervate the scalene and levator scapulae muscles.

As a final note, keep in mind that it is the cervical spinal *ventral* rami that form the cervical plexus; on the contrary, the cervical *dorsal* rami supply the posterior scalp and suboccipital region. The primary motor innervator of this region is the suboccipital nerve and the primary sensory innervator of this region is the greater occipital nerve. The dorsal ramus of C1 supplies the suboccipital nerve whereas the dorsal ramus of C2 supplies the greater occipital nerve—see Drawing 5-6.[1-4]

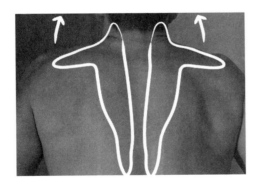

FIGURE 3-39 **Trapezius.**

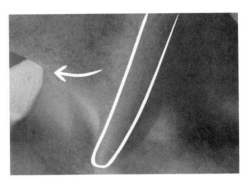

FIGURE 3-40 **Sternocleidomastoid.**

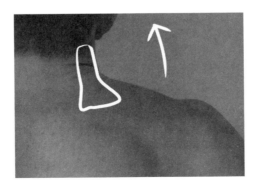

FIGURE 3-41 **Levator scapulae.**

Cervical plexus also provides innervation to the anterior vertebral muscles, scalene muscles, and the levator scapulae.

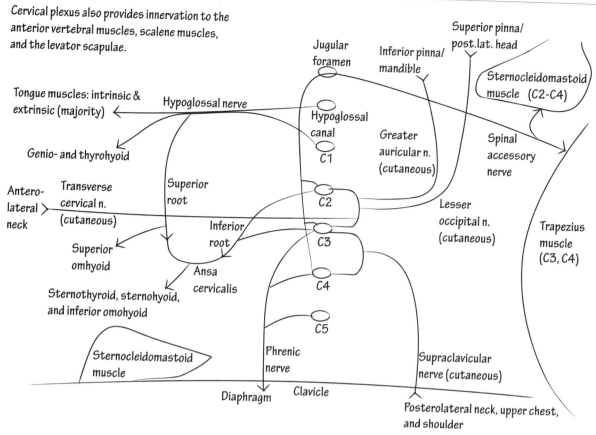

Tongue muscles: intrinsic & extrinsic (majority)

Hypoglossal nerve

Genio- and thyrohyoid

Jugular foramen

Inferior pinna/ mandible

Superior pinna/ post.lat. head

Sternocleidomastoid muscle (C2-C4)

Hypoglossal canal

C1

Greater auricular n. (cutaneous)

Spinal accessory nerve

Antero-lateral neck

Transverse cervical n. (cutaneous)

Superior root

Inferior root

C2

C3

Lesser occipital n. (cutaneous)

Trapezius muscle (C3, C4)

Superior omhyoid

Ansa cervicalis

C4

Sternothyroid, sternohyoid, and inferior omohyoid

C5

Sternocleidomastoid muscle

Phrenic nerve

Diaphragm   Clavicle

Supraclavicular nerve (cutaneous)

Posterolateral neck, upper chest, and shoulder

DRAWING 3-12 **Cervical Plexus—Complete**

References

1. Standring, S. & Gray, H. *Gray's anatomy: the anatomical basis of clinical practice*, 40th ed. (Churchill Livingstone/Elsevier, 2008).

2. Preston, D. C. & Shapiro, B. E. *Electromyography and neuromuscular disorders: clinical-electrophysiologic correlations,* 2nd ed. (Elsevier Butterworth-Heinemann, 2005).

3. Perotto, A. & Delagi, E. F. *Anatomical guide for the electromyographer: the limbs and trunk,* 4th ed. (Charles C Thomas, 2005).

4. Netter, F. H. & Dalley, A. F. *Atlas of human anatomy,* 2nd ed., Plates 4–7 (Novartis, 1997).

5. Martin, R. M. & Fish, D. E. Scapular winging: anatomical review, diagnosis, and treatments. *Curr Rev Musculoskelet Med* 1, 1–11 (2008).

6. Wilbourn, A. J. & Aminoff, M. J. AAEM minimonograph #32: the electrodiagnostic examination in patients with radiculopathies. American Association of Electrodiagnostic Medicine. *Muscle Nerve* 21, 1612–1631 (1998).

7. Stevens, J. C. AAEM minimonograph #26: the electrodiagnosis of carpal tunnel syndrome. American Association of Electrodiagnostic Medicine. *Muscle Nerve* 20, 1477–1486 (1997).

8. Rathakrishnan, R., Therimadasamy, A. K., Chan, Y. H. & Wilder-Smith, E. P. The median palmar cutaneous nerve in normal subjects and CTS. *Clin Neurophysiol* 118, 776–780 (2007).

9. Martinoli, C., et al. US of nerve entrapments in osteofibrous tunnels of the upper and lower limbs. *Radiographics* 20 Spec No. S199–213; discussion S213–197 (2000).

10. Jablecki, C. K., et al. Practice parameter: Electrodiagnostic studies in carpal tunnel syndrome. Report of the American Association of Electrodiagnostic Medicine, American Academy of Neurology, and the American Academy of Physical Medicine and Rehabilitation. *Neurology* 58, 1589–1592 (2002).

11. Furuya, H. Usefulness of manual muscle testing of pronator teres and supinator muscles in assessing cervical radiculopathy. *Fukuoka Acta Med.* 96, 319–325 (2005).

12. Palmer, B. A. & Hughes, T. B. Cubital tunnel syndrome. *J Hand Surg Am* 35, 153–163 (2010).

Peripheral Nervous System

Lower Extremity

Lumbosacral Plexus

The Leg & Foot

The Thigh

Know-It Points

Lumbosacral Plexus

- The lumbosacral plexus is formed from L1–S4.
- The sciatic nerve (L4–S3) innervates the posterior thigh.
- The femoral and obturator nerves (L2–L4) innervate the anterior thigh.
- The peroneal nerve (L4–S2) innervates the anterior and lateral leg and dorsal foot.

- The tibial nerve (L4–S3) innervates the posterior leg and plantar foot.
- The lateral cutaneous nerve of the thigh (L2, L3) provides sensory coverage to the lateral thigh.

The Leg & Foot

- The common peroneal nerve divides into the deep peroneal nerve and superficial peroneal nerve.
- The deep peroneal nerve innervates tibialis anterior (L4, L5), extensor digitorum longus, extensor hallucis longus, peroneus tertius, extensor digitorum brevis, and extensor hallucis brevis (L5, S1).
- The superficial peroneal nerve innervates peroneus longus and peroneus brevis (L5, S1).

- The major tibial-innervated muscles are the gastrocnemius and soleus (S1, S2), tibialis posterior, flexor digitorum longus, and flexor hallucis longus (L5, S1).
- The sural nerve is formed from branches of the common peroneal nerve and the tibial nerve.

The Thigh

- The femoral nerve innervates the anterior compartment (L2–L4).
- The obturator nerve innervates the medial compartment (L2–L4).
- The sciatic nerve innervates the posterior compartment (L4–S2).
- The femoral nerve innervates the quadriceps femoris muscles and we also consider it to innervate the iliopsoas (see text for details).

- The obturator nerve innervates the adductor muscles.
- The sciatic nerve innervates the hamstrings muscles.
- Within the femoral triangle, the nerve lies most laterally; medial to it is the artery; and medial to it is the vein: use the mnemonic NAVY.

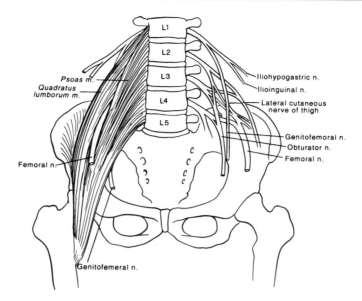

FIGURE 4-1 **The lumbar plexus.** Used with permission from Mendell, Jerry R., John T. Kissel, and David R. Cornblath. *Diagnosis and Management of Peripheral Nerve Disorders*, Contemporary Neurology Series. Oxford: Oxford University Press, 2001.

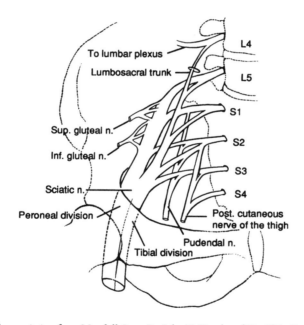

FIGURE 4-2 **The sacral plexus.** Used with permission from Mendell, Jerry R., John T. Kissel, and David R. Cornblath. *Diagnosis and Management of Peripheral Nerve Disorders*, Contemporary Neurology Series. Oxford: Oxford University Press, 2001.

Lumbosacral Plexus

Here, we will draw the lumbosacral plexus. First, label the top of the page from left to right as follows: ventral rami; pelvis, gluteal region, and hip; thigh; leg; and foot. Nine spinal nerves (L1–S4) form the lumbosacral plexus. Although more spinal nerves are involved in the lumbosacral plexus than in the brachial plexus, their courses are, generally, much simpler, which makes learning the lumbosacral plexus comparatively easier.

First, draw the innervator of the posterior thigh: the sciatic nerve, which is derived from L4–S3. Show that it passes through the pelvis and posterior thigh and then branches into the peroneal and tibial nerves, which are the innervators of the leg and foot. The peroneal nerve wraps around the fibular neck and innervates the anterior and lateral leg and dorsal foot whereas the tibial nerve innervates the posterior leg and plantar foot. Indicate that the L4–S2 roots supply the peroneal nerve and that the L4–S3 roots supply the tibial nerve. We draw the details of the sciatic, peroneal, and tibial nerves in Drawings 4-3 and 4-4.

Now, draw the innervators of the anterior thigh: the femoral and obturator nerves, derived from L2–L4. We draw their innervation pattern in Drawings 4-5 and 4-6. Note that an accessory obturator nerve branch occasionally exists.

Next, draw the innervators of the hip: the gluteal nerves. Show that the inferior gluteal nerve, derived from L5–S2, innervates gluteus maximus; and that one level above it, the superior gluteal nerve, derived from L4–S1, innervates gluteus medius, gluteus minimus, and tensor fasciae latae. Gluteus medius inserts into the ilium slightly higher than gluteus maximus, which helps us remember that the superior gluteal nerve innervates gluteus medius whereas the inferior gluteal nerve innervates gluteus maximus. Gluteus maximus provides hip extension and gluteus medius provides hip abduction. Regarding the other superior gluteal nerve-innervated muscles, gluteus minimus provides hip abduction and tensor fasciae latae provides hip abduction when the hip is in flexion.

Above the femoral and obturator nerves, draw the lateral cutaneous nerve of the thigh (aka lateral femoral cutaneous nerve), derived from L2 and L3, which provides sensory coverage to the lateral thigh.

At the bottom, draw the pudendal nerve, which is primarily supplied by S4 but which also receives contributions from S2 and S3. The pudendal nerve branches into the inferior rectal nerve, perineal nerve, and dorsal nerve to the penis or clitoris. The pudendal nerve provides motor innervation to the external urethral and anal sphincters and external genitalia and it provides sensory coverage to the anus and external genitalia, as shown in Drawing 5-6.

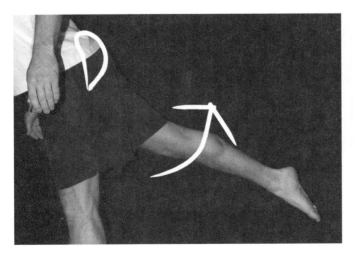

FIGURE 4-3 **Gluteus maximus.**

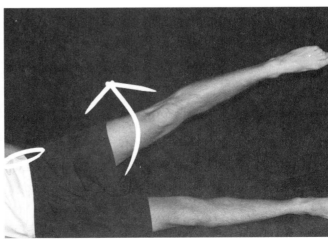

FIGURE 4-4 **Gluteus medius.**

Ventral rami	) Pelvis, gluteal region, & hip	)	Thigh		Leg	)	Foot

L2 - L3   Lateral cutaneous nerve of the thigh

L2 - L4   _____ Obturator nerve _____

                 Femoral nerve

L4 - S1   Superior gluteal nerve (gluteus med. & min., and tensor fasc. lat. m.)

L5 - S2   Inferior gluteal nerve (gluteus maximus muscle)

                                                              L4 - S2   Peroneal nerve

L4 - S3   Sciatic nerve

                                                              L4 - S3   Tibial nerve

S4 & S2/S3   Pudendal nerve (perineum and external genitalia)

DRAWING 4-1 **Lumbosacral Plexus—Partial**

Lumbosacral Plexus (Cont.)

Next, go back beneath the sciatic nerve and draw the posterior cutaneous nerve of the thigh (aka the posterior femoral cutaneous nerve), derived from S1–S3. It provides sensory coverage to the midline back of the thigh.

Now, we will draw the less commonly considered neuroanatomic components of the lumbosacral plexus. Above the lateral cutaneous nerve of the thigh, draw the genitofemoral nerve, derived from L1–L2. Show that the genital branch innervates the cremaster muscle and provides sensory coverage to the scrotum or labia and that the femoral branch is purely sensory; it provides sensory coverage to the femoral triangle.

Next, at the top of the diagram, draw the iliohypogastric and ilioinguinal nerves, derived from L1. Both nerves provide motor innervation to the internal oblique and transversus abdominis muscles. The iliohypogastric nerve provides sensory coverage to the suprapubic and upper-lateral gluteal areas, and the ilioinguinal nerve provides sensory coverage to the superior-medial portion of the thigh and proximal external genitalia.

Next, show that L5–S2 supplies the short rotators of the hip. The short rotators provide external rotation of the hip when it is in extension and hip abduction when it is in flexion. Their innervation is as follows: the nerve to quadratus femoris innervates quadratus femoris and gemellus inferior; the nerve to obturator internus innervates obturator internus and gemellus superior; the nerve to piriformis innervates piriformis; and the obturator nerve innervates obturator externus (note that obturator externus is supplied by L3, L4).

Now, from S2 and S3 show the pelvic splanchnic nerves and the perforating cutaneous nerve. And from S4 show the nerves to levator ani and coccygeus, which form the pelvic diaphragm, and also show the sphincter ani externus.[1–5]

Ventral rami	) Pelvis, gluteal region, & hip)	Thigh		Leg	)	Foot

L1 Iliohypogastric nerve
_____ (Internal oblique and transversus abdominus muscles)
Ilioinguinal nerve

L1 - L2 Genitofemoral nerve   (genital branch - cremaster muscle)
(femoral branch - sensory only)

L2 - L3 Lateral cutaneous nerve of the thigh

L2 - L4 Obturator nerve
Femoral nerve

L4 - S1 Superior gluteal nerve (gluteus med. & min., and tensor fasc. lat. m.)

L5 - S2 Inferior gluteal nerve (gluteus maximus muscle)
Short rotators of the hip

L4 - S3 Sciatic nerve

L4 - S2   Peroneal nerve

L4 - S3   Tibial nerve

S1 - S3 Posterior cutaneous nerve of the thigh

S2 - S3 Pelvic splanchnic nerves
Perforating cutaneous nerve

S4 & S2/S3 Pudendal nerve (perineum and external genitalia)

S4 Nerves to levator ani, coccygeus, and sphincter ani externus

DRAWING 4-2 **Lumbosacral Plexus—Complete**

The Leg & Foot

Here, we will draw the innervation of the leg and foot. To localize each form of peroneal or tibial nerve injury, learn at least one muscle from each muscle group. Label the top of the page from left to right as thigh, leg, and foot. First, show that the innervation of the leg and foot is derived from the sciatic nerve, supplied by L4–S3. Then, define two key anatomic structures. Indicate that the popliteal fossa is the depression behind the knee and that the fibular neck is the continuation of the head of the fibula (the top of the lateral leg bone).

Now, proximal to the popliteal fossa, let's show how the sciatic nerve unbundles to innervate the anterior, lateral, and posterior leg compartments. Show that the common peroneal nerve leaves the path of the sciatic nerve; passes inferolaterally through the popliteal fossa; wraps around the fibular neck; and then splits into the deep peroneal nerve, which innervates the muscles of the anterior leg and dorsum of the foot, and the superficial peroneal nerve, which innervates the muscles of the lateral leg. Next, show that the tibial nerve continues straight down the posterior leg to innervate the muscles of the posterior leg and plantar foot.

Now, show that the deep peroneal nerve innervates tibialis anterior, supplied by L4, L5. Tibialis anterior provides foot dorsiflexion and to a lesser extent foot inversion. Next, show that the deep peroneal nerve also innervates extensor digitorum longus, extensor hallucis longus, and peroneus tertius, supplied by L5, S1. Extensor digitorum longus extends the toes (except the great toe); extensor hallucis longus extends the great toe, only; and peroneus tertius assists in foot eversion. To a lesser extent, all three of these muscles also provide foot dorsiflexion.

Next, show that the superficial peroneal nerve innervates peroneus longus and peroneus brevis, supplied by L5, S1. They provide foot eversion and to a lesser extent foot plantar flexion.

Then, show that in addition to the aforementioned muscles, the deep peroneal nerve also innervates the short extensor muscles of the foot: extensor digitorum brevis and extensor hallucis brevis, supplied by L5, S1. Extensor digitorum brevis extends the middle three toes and extensor hallucis brevis extends only the great toe and only at the proximal phalanx.

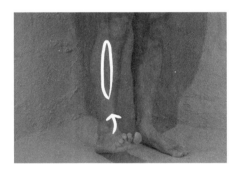

FIGURE 4-5 **Tibialis anterior.**

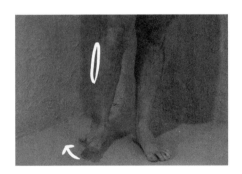

FIGURE 4-6 **Peroneus longus.**

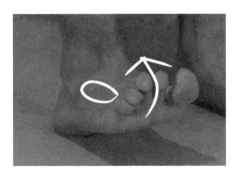

FIGURE 4-7 **Extensor digitorum brevis.**

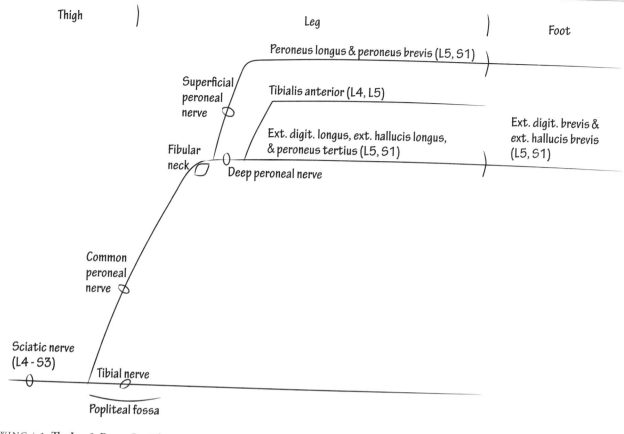

Thigh)   Leg) Foot

Peroneus longus & peroneus brevis (L5, S1)

Superficial peroneal nerve

Tibialis anterior (L4, L5)

Fibular neck

Ext. digit. longus, ext. hallucis longus, & peroneus tertius (L5, S1)

Deep peroneal nerve

Ext. digit. brevis & ext. hallucis brevis (L5, S1)

Common peroneal nerve

Sciatic nerve (L4 - S3)

Tibial nerve

Popliteal fossa

DRAWING 4-3 The Leg & Foot—Partial

The Leg & Foot (Cont.)

Now, let's show the tibial nerve-innervated muscles. First, indicate the superficial posterior compartment muscles: gastrocnemius and soleus, supplied by S1, S2. Both muscles provide foot plantar flexion: we test gastrocnemius with the knee extended and soleus with the knee flexed.

Next, show the deep posterior compartment muscles: tibialis posterior and flexor digitorum longus and flexor hallucis longus, supplied by L5, S1, primarily. Note that some texts indicate that L4 also innervates tibialis posterior and some texts indicate that S2 also innervates the flexor digitorum and hallucis muscles. Tibialis posterior provides foot inversion; flexor digitorum longus flexes the toes (except the great toe); and flexor hallucis longus flexes the great toe.

Now, add the lesser muscles that the tibial nerve innervates: popliteus and plantaris. Popliteus unlocks the knee at the beginning of knee flexion and plantaris acts in concert with gastrocnemius.

Finally, let's begin to address the sensory innervation of the leg and foot. First, show that the common peroneal nerve derives a common sensory trunk that produces

both the lateral sural cutaneous nerve and also the sural communicating branch. Show that the tibial nerve produces the medial sural cutaneous nerve, which joins the sural communicating branch to form the sural nerve. Then, show that when the sural nerve passes through the ankle, it produces both the lateral calcaneal nerve branch and also the lateral dorsal cutaneous nerve. The lateral calcaneal branch is the lateral corollary of the medial calcaneal branch, which we will draw in a moment. But first, show another important anatomic region, the tarsal tunnel, which is the medial entry zone of the tibial nerve through the ankle into the foot.

The medial malleolus and medial calcaneus form the superior and inferior boundaries of the tarsal tunnel, respectively, and the flexor retinaculum forms its roof. Show that within the tarsal tunnel, the tibial nerve divides into the plantar nerves (medial and lateral) and also the medial calcaneal sensory nerve. The plantar nerves innervate the plantar intrinsic foot muscles, supplied by S1–S3, and the plantar nerves and medial calcaneal nerve provide sensory coverage to the sole of the foot.[1–4,6–8]

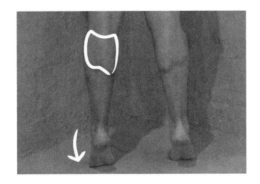

FIGURE 4-8 **Gastrocnemius.**

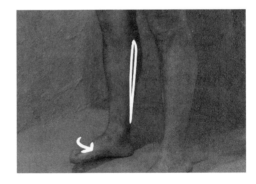

FIGURE 4-9 **Tibialis posterior.**

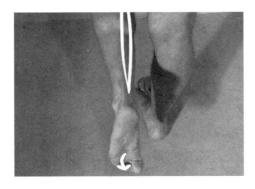

FIGURE 4-10 **Flexor digitorum longus.**

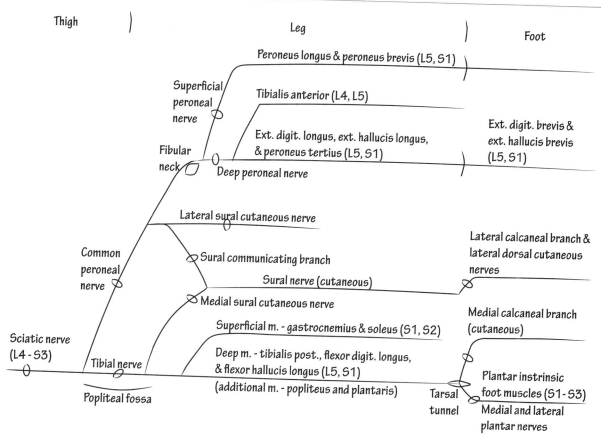

Thigh)   Leg   ) Foot

Peroneus longus & peroneus brevis (L5, S1)

Superficial peroneal nerve

Tibialis anterior (L4, L5)

Fibular neck

Ext. digit. longus, ext. hallucis longus, & peroneus tertius (L5, S1)

Deep peroneal nerve

Ext. digit. brevis & ext. hallucis brevis (L5, S1)

Lateral sural cutaneous nerve

Common peroneal nerve

Sural communicating branch

Sural nerve (cutaneous)

Lateral calcaneal branch & lateral dorsal cutaneous nerves

Medial sural cutaneous nerve

Sciatic nerve (L4 - S3)

Tibial nerve

Superficial m. - gastrocnemius & soleus (S1, S2)

Medial calcaneal branch (cutaneous)

Popliteal fossa

Deep m. - tibialis post., flexor digit. longus, & flexor hallucis longus (L5, S1)
(additional m. - popliteus and plantaris)

Tarsal tunnel

Plantar intrinsic foot muscles (S1- S3)

Medial and lateral plantar nerves

DRAWING 4-4 **The Leg & Foot—Complete**

The Thigh

Here, we will draw the innervation of the thigh. To localize each form of femoral, sciatic, or obturator nerve injury, learn at least one muscle from each muscle group. First, label across the top of the page from left to right: abdomen and pelvis, thigh, and leg. The thigh divides into three compartments: anterior, medial, and posterior, which supply the extensor, adductor, and flexor muscles, respectively. In accordance with the "one compartment—one nerve" principle, indicate that the femoral nerve innervates the anterior compartment, which the L2–L4 nerve roots supply; the obturator nerve innervates the medial compartment, which is also supplied by L2–L4; and the sciatic nerve innervates the posterior compartment, which, again, is supplied by L4–S2. Note, though, that the tibial division of the sciatic nerve receives additional supply from S3 for its innervation of the foot.

Now, let's show the innervation of each compartment's primary muscle groups. First, indicate that proximally, the femoral nerve innervates the iliopsoas muscle, which comprises iliacus and the psoas major and minor muscles. Iliopsoas is the primary hip flexor and attaches within the "iliac region;" when it is weak, patients have difficulty climbing upstairs or rising from a low chair. Next, indicate that distally, the femoral nerve innervates the quadriceps femoris muscles, which are rectus femoris and the vastus muscles: vastus medialis, vastus intermedius, and vastus lateralis. The quadriceps femoris muscles provide knee extension, and when they are weak, patients have difficulty walking downstairs.

Next, show that the obturator nerve innervates the adductor muscles, which are adductor longus, adductor brevis, and adductor magnus; note that adductor magnus is also supplied by the sciatic nerve, as we will later show. We test the adductor muscles through hip adduction but these muscles provide a variety of actions intrinsic to gait and stability.

Now, show that the sciatic nerve innervates the hamstrings muscles, which are semimembranosus, semitendinosus, and the short and long heads of the biceps femoris muscle. The hamstrings muscles provide knee flexion and hip extension.

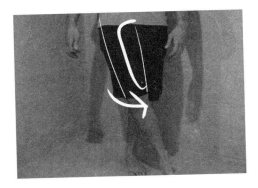

FIGURE 4-11 **Iliopsoas.**

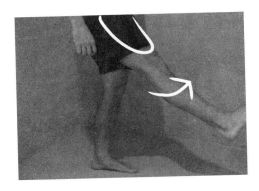

FIGURE 4-12 **Quadriceps femoris.**

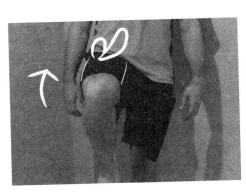

FIGURE 4-13 **Adductor muscles.**

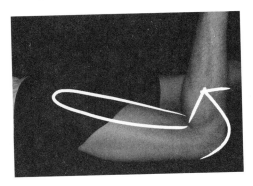

FIGURE 4-14 **Hamstrings.**

Abdomen & pelvis   )   Thigh   )   Leg

Iliopsoas

Femoral nerve   Quadriceps femoris: rectus femoris, vastus medialis,
(L2 - L4)   vastus intermedius, & vastus lateralis
Anterior compartment

Obturator nerve
(L2 - L4)   Adductor muscles: longus, brevis, (magnus)
Medial compartment

Sciatic nerve   Hamstrings: semimembranosus, semitendinosus,
(L4 - S2)   biceps femoris (short and long heads)
Posterior compartment

DRAWING 4-5 **The Thigh—Partial**

The Thigh (Cont.)

Next, let's consider some of the finer details regarding the primary muscles of the thigh. First, note that in regards to the iliopsoas muscle, the psoas muscles (psoas major and minor) are actually innervated by direct branches from ventral lumbar rami from L1 to L3 (and not the femoral nerve). However, because the psoas muscles cannot be isolated and tested clinically, they are lumped in with the iliacus muscle, and all three are considered collectively as the femoral nerve-innervated iliopsoas muscle.

Now, show the sciatic nerve's innervation to the adductor magnus muscle, and indicate that the adductor magnus has both an adductor portion, supplied by L2–L4, and a hamstrings portion, supplied by L4, L5.

Finally, note that the peroneal division of the sciatic nerve innervates the short head of the biceps femoris and that the tibial division innervates the other hamstrings muscles: the long head of biceps femoris, semitendinosus, and semimembranosus. The peroneal innervation of the short head of the biceps femoris is especially important in localization because a peroneal neuropathy at the fibular head (the most common peroneal nerve entrapment site) will spare the short head of the biceps femoris, but a peroneal neuropathy proximal to the fibular head will affect the short head of the biceps femoris.

Now, let's include the lesser clinical muscles of the thigh. First, show that the femoral nerve innervates the sartorius muscle, which is the longest muscle in the body. It is a superficial muscle that crosses the thigh: it spans from the anterior superior iliac spine to the medial knee. Think of someone checking the bottom of his or her shoe to imagine the sartorius' action; it provides knee flexion in combination with hip abduction and lateral rotation. Functionally, it serves to decelerate the lower extremity during climbing movements.

Next, show that the obturator nerve innervates the gracilis muscle, supplied by L2, L3. It also lies superficially and spans the medial line of the thigh, and it provides hip adduction and also knee flexion and medial rotation.

Then, show that the femoral nerve innervates the pectineus muscle, which lies in the femoral triangle; occasionally, the obturator nerve helps innervate the pectineus muscle, as well. The pectineus assists in both hip flexion and adduction. It cannot be isolated and tested clinically.

Finally, show that the obturator nerve innervates the obturator externus muscle, which is one of the short rotators of the hip and which provides external rotation of the hip in hip extension and hip abduction in hip flexion.

Now, let's include the sensory branches of the thigh; we map their sensory coverage in Drawing 5-5. First, draw the lateral femoral cutaneous nerve (aka the lateral cutaneous nerve of the thigh), supplied by L2, L3. It provides sensory coverage to the lateral aspect of the thigh.

Then, from the femoral nerve, draw the medial and intermediate cutaneous nerves of the thigh, which cover the anterior thigh and which are collectively known as the anterior femoral cutaneous nerve. Then, draw the saphenous nerve, which extends down the medial leg to the instep of the foot and provides sensory coverage to that same area. Lastly, show that the saphenous nerve produces the small but clinically important sensory branch called the infrapatellar branch, which innervates the anterior knee and which can be injured in knee arthroscopy.

Now, draw the posterior cutaneous nerve of the thigh, which S1–S3 supply; it covers the posterior thigh, and also some of the pelvic and proximal leg regions. Finally, note that the obturator nerve, itself, covers a small cutaneous area on the medial thigh.

Before we conclude, let's consider the anatomic relationships of the neurovascular structures of the femoral triangle because they are critical to know when performing femoral venous cannulation. Within the femoral triangle, the nerve lies most laterally; medial to it is the artery; and medial to it is the vein. The mnemonic NAVY is helpful because it incorporates the position of the midline genitalia, the "Y," into the acronym.[1–4]

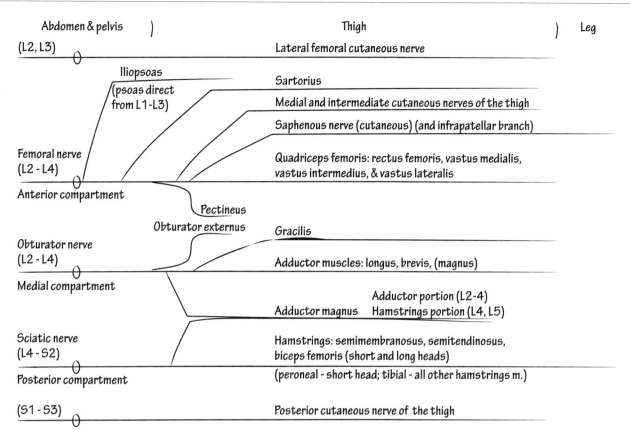

Abdomen & pelvis) Thigh) Leg

(L2, L3) Lateral femoral cutaneous nerve

Iliopsoas
(psoas direct
from L1-L3) Sartorius

Medial and intermediate cutaneous nerves of the thigh

Saphenous nerve (cutaneous) (and infrapatellar branch)

Femoral nerve
(L2 - L4) Quadriceps femoris: rectus femoris, vastus medialis,
vastus intermedius, & vastus lateralis

Anterior compartment

Pectineus

Obturator externus Gracilis

Obturator nerve
(L2 - L4) Adductor muscles: longus, brevis, (magnus)

Medial compartment

Adductor portion (L2-4)

Adductor magnus   Hamstrings portion (L4, L5)

Sciatic nerve
(L4 - S2) Hamstrings: semimembranosus, semitendinosus,
biceps femoris (short and long heads)

Posterior compartment (peroneal - short head; tibial - all other hamstrings m.)

(S1 - S3) Posterior cutaneous nerve of the thigh

DRAWING 4-6 The Thigh—Complete

References

1. Standring, S. & Gray, H. *Gray's anatomy: the anatomical basis of clinical practice,* 40th ed. (Churchill Livingstone/Elsevier, 2008).
2. Preston, D. C. & Shapiro, B. E. *Electromyography and neuromuscular disorders: clinical-electrophysiologic correlations,* 2nd ed. (Elsevier Butterworth-Heinemann, 2005).
3. Perotto, A. & Delagi, E. F. *Anatomical guide for the electromyographer: the limbs and trunk,* 4th ed. (Charles C Thomas, 2005).
4. Netter, F. H. & Dalley, A. F. *Atlas of human anatomy,* 2nd ed., Plates 4–7 (Novartis, 1997).
5. Wilbourn, A. J. & Aminoff, M. J. AAEM minimonograph #32: the electrodiagnostic examination in patients with radiculopathies. American Association of Electrodiagnostic Medicine. *Muscle Nerve* 21, 1612–1631 (1998).
6. Takakura, Y., Kitada, C., Sugimoto, K., Tanaka, Y. & Tamai, S. Tarsal tunnel syndrome. Causes and results of operative treatment. *J Bone Joint Surg Br* 73, 125–128 (1991).
7. Stewart, J. D. Foot drop: where, why and what to do? *Pract Neurol* 8, 158–169, doi:10.1136/jnnp.2008.149393 (2008).
8. Antoniadis, G. & Scheglmann, K. Posterior tarsal tunnel syndrome: diagnosis and treatment. *Dtsch Arztebl Int* 105, 776–781, doi:10.3238/arztebl.2008.0776 (2008).

5

Peripheral Nervous System

Sensory Maps

Know-It Points

Sensory Map of the Hand

- The median nerve covers the ball of the thumb, the lateral palm, and the palmar surface and dorsal tips of the lateral digits.
- The ulnar nerve covers the palmar and dorsal surfaces of the medial one third of the hand and digits.
- The radial nerve covers the dorsal lateral two thirds of the hand and proximal dorsal surface of the lateral digits.

Sensory Map of the Foot

- Tibial nerve branches cover the plantar foot.
- Peroneal nerve branches cover the dorsal foot.
- The plantar nerves cover the plantar foot and the medial calcaneal nerve covers the heel.
- The superficial peroneal nerve covers the dorsum of the foot, except that the deep peroneal nerve covers the webbing between the great toe and second digit and except for the distal sural branches.
- The distal branches of the sural nerve cover the lateral malleolus, lateral foot, and little toe.
- The saphenous nerve covers the instep of the foot.

Dermatomes

- C7 covers the middle finger, C8 the medial hand, C6 the lateral hand and lateral forearm, C5 the upper lateral arm, T1 the medial forearm, and T2 the medial upper arm.
- T4 covers the nipple line and T10 the umbilicus.
- L3 and L4 cover the knee, L5 covers the great toe, and S1 covers the ankle and little toe.
- The coccyx covers the center of the anus; S5 through S1 form rings around it.
- S2 covers the posteromedial lower limb and S1 covers the posterolateral lower limb.
- C2 covers the back of the head.

Cutaneous Nerves—Upper Limb

- The medial and lateral cutaneous nerves of the forearm and arm cover the medial and lateral forearm and arm, respectively.
- The intercostobrachial nerve covers the axilla.
- The supraclavicular nerve covers the shoulder.
- The posterior cutaneous nerves to the forearm and arm cover the midline posterior forearm and arm, respectively.

Cutaneous Nerves—Lower Limb

- The lateral femoral cutaneous nerve covers the lateral thigh, the posterior femoral cutaneous nerve covers the posterior thigh, and the anterior femoral cutaneous nerve covers the anterior and medial thigh.
- The lateral sural cutaneous nerve and the superficial peroneal nerve cover the upper lateral and lower lateral leg, respectively.
- The sural nerve covers the posterior leg.
- The saphenous nerve covers the medial leg.

Cutaneous Nerves—Trunk (Advanced)

- The posterior ramus derives the posterior cutaneous branch.
- The anterior ramus derives the intercostal nerve, which provides the lateral cutaneous branch and the anterior cutaneous branch.
- The thoracic anterior and lateral cutaneous branches cover the midline thorax and abdomen and the lateral thorax and abdomen, respectively.

- The iliohypogastric, ilioinguinal, genitofemoral, and pudendal nerves cover the abdomino-pelvic region.
- The posterior cutaneous rami cover the posterior trunk, posterior neck, and posterior head.
- The greater occipital nerve, specifically, covers the back of the head.

Referred Pain

- Innervation of the diaphragm comes from C3, C4, and C5, which cover the neck, shoulders, and upper lateral arm.
- Use the mnemonic: C3, C4, C5 keeps the diaphragm alive!

- Innervation of the heart comes from T1–T5, which cover the chest and medial upper arm and forearm.
- Innervation of the appendix comes from T10, which covers the umbilicus.

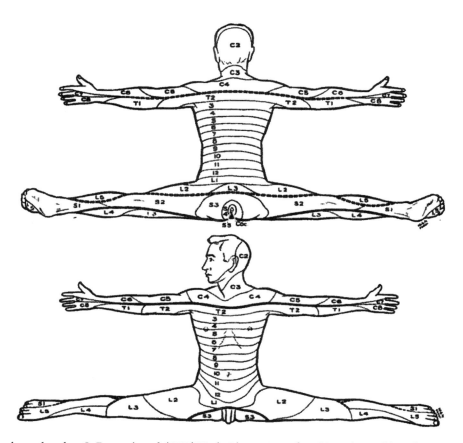

FIGURE 5-1 **Dermatomal maps based on O. Foerster's work (1933).Used with permission from Haymaker, Webb, and Barnes Woodhall.** *Peripheral Nerve Injuries, Principles of Diagnosis.* **2nd ed. Philadelphia: Saunders, 1953.**

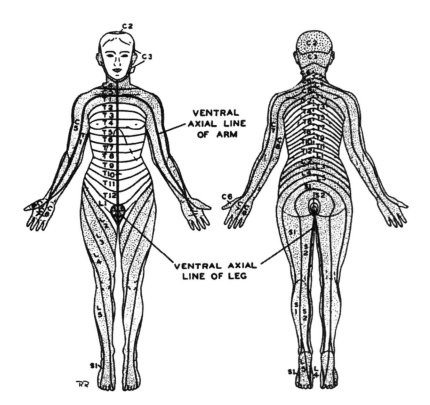

FIGURE 5-2 **Dermatomal maps based on Keegan & Garrett's work (1948). Used with permission from Haymaker, Webb, and Barnes Woodhall.** *Peripheral Nerve Injuries, Principles of Diagnosis.* 2nd ed. Philadelphia: Saunders, 1953.

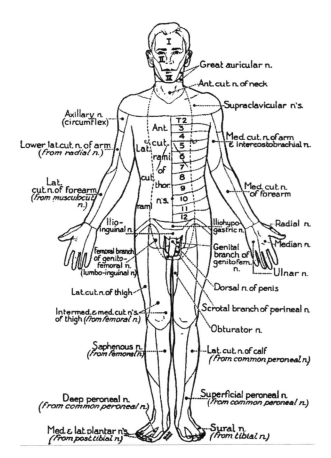

FIGURE 5-3 **Anterior peripheral nerve map. Used with permission from Haymaker, Webb, and Barnes Woodhall.** *Peripheral Nerve Injuries, Principles of Diagnosis.* 2nd ed. Philadelphia: Saunders, 1953.

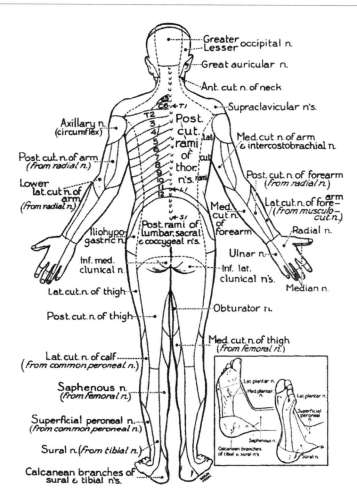

FIGURE 5-4 **Posterior peripheral nerve map.** Used with permission from Haymaker, Webb, and Barnes Woodhall. *Peripheral Nerve Injuries, Principles of Diagnosis.* 2nd ed. Philadelphia: Saunders, 1953.

Sensory Map of the Hand

Here, we will create a diagram for the sensory coverage of the hand. Begin with the median nerve's sensory coverage. Trace both sides of your hand. On the palm-up tracing, square off the ball of the thumb to indicate the sensory coverage of the palmar cutaneous nerve. Then, show that the median nerve digital sensory branches cover the lateral palm, lateral half of the ring finger, middle and index fingers, and the palmar thumb. Next, on the dorsal surface of the hand, show that the median nerve provides sensory coverage to the dorsal tips of the thumb, index and middle fingers, and lateral half of the ring finger.

Next, let's show the ulnar nerve's sensory coverage. On the dorsal surface tracing, show that the dorsal ulnar cutaneous nerve covers the medial one third of the hand and the medial half of the fourth digit and fifth digit.

Then, on the palm-up tracing, show that the palmar ulnar cutaneous nerve covers the hypothenar eminence. Remember that both of these sensory nerves branch proximal to Guyon's canal. Lastly, still on the palm-up tracing, show that the superficial sensory division covers the medial half of the fourth digit and the fifth digit. This sensory branch passes through Guyon's canal.

Now, to map the superficial sensory radial nerve coverage, first, on the dorsal surface tracing, show that the superficial sensory radial nerve covers the lateral two thirds of the dorsum of the hand, the proximal thumb, proximal second and third digits, and proximal lateral half of the fourth digit. And then on the palm-up tracing, show that the radial nerve's sensory coverage wraps around to the proximal palmar thumb.[1-8]

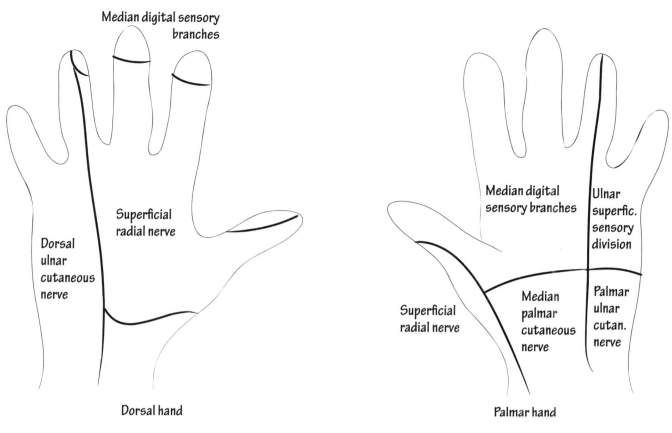

Median digital sensory branches

Superficial radial nerve

Dorsal ulnar cutaneous nerve

Dorsal hand

Median digital sensory branches

Ulnar superfic. sensory division

Superficial radial nerve

Median palmar cutaneous nerve

Palmar ulnar cutan. nerve

Palmar hand

DRAWING 5-1 Sensory Map of the Hand

Sensory Map of the Foot

Here, let's sketch the sensory coverage of the feet. Despite the following details, bear in mind that generally, quite simply, the tibial nerve covers the plantar foot and the peroneal nerve covers the dorsal foot. Now, trace your feet. Label one tracing as the dorsal foot and the other as the plantar foot. On the plantar foot, show that the medial calcaneal nerve covers the heel. Then, draw a line down the center of the fourth toe and through the sole. Indicate that the medial plantar nerve covers the medial foot and that the lateral plantar nerve covers the lateral foot.

Next, turn to the dorsal foot tracing. Indicate that the superficial peroneal nerve covers the dorsum of the foot except for the following areas: the deep peroneal nerve covers the webbing between the great toe and second digit, and the distal branches of the sural nerve (the lateral calcaneal branch and lateral dorsal cutaneous nerve) cover the lateral malleolus, lateral foot, and little toe.

Finally, on the plantar and dorsal surfaces, show that the femoral-derived saphenous nerve covers the instep (or medial surface) of the foot.[1-4,8]

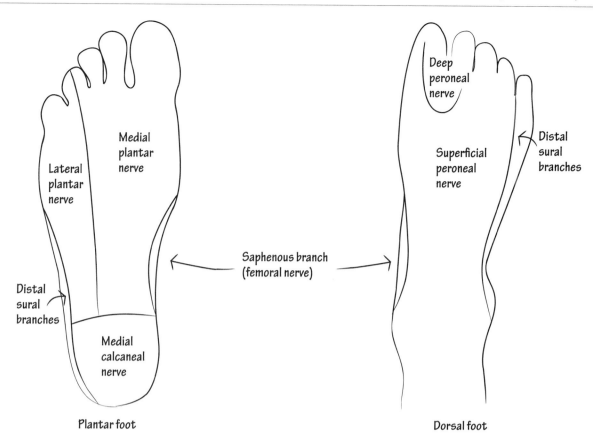

DRAWING 5-2 **Sensory Map of the Foot**

Dermatomes

Here, we will draw the dermatomal sensory innervation of the limbs and trunk. Note that the dermatomal maps have broader clinical significance and are simpler than the cutaneous nerve maps of the limbs and trunk.

Draw the anterior and posterior outlines of the body. Then begin with the hand; show that C7 covers the middle finger, C8 the medial hand, and C6 the lateral hand and lateral forearm. Next, show that C5 covers the upper lateral arm. Then, show that T1 covers the medial forearm and T2 the medial upper arm.

Next, to show the important dermatomes of the thorax, abdomen, and pelvis, indicate that T4 covers the nipple line, T10 covers the umbilicus, T12 covers the suprapubic area, L1 covers the inguinal region, S2 covers the proximal external genitalia, and S3 covers the distal external genitalia.

Now, show the sloping dermatomal coverage of the anterior lower extremity. First, indicate that L2 begins its descent from the superolateral anterior lower extremity; then, indicate that the coverage of L3 and L4 crosses the knee; then, show that L5 covers the great toe; and then, that S1 covers the ankle and little toe.

Next, let's draw the posterior lower extremity and gluteal coverage. First, show that the coccyx covers the center of the anus and then show the dermatomal rings that surround it: the innermost is S5, then going outward is S4, then S3, and then show that S2 encircles S3 but also extends down the posteromedial lower limb. And lastly, show that S1 extends down the posterolateral lower limb and covers the Achilles.

Finally, show that C2 covers the back of the head, C3 and C4 cover the posterior neck, and T2–L5 cover the upper back to the buttocks (note that L2 is sometimes listed as the lowest lumbar dermatome).

We show the trigeminal nerve sensory innervation to the face in Drawing 13-1.[1-4,8]

Anterior dermatomal map   **Posterior dermatomal map**

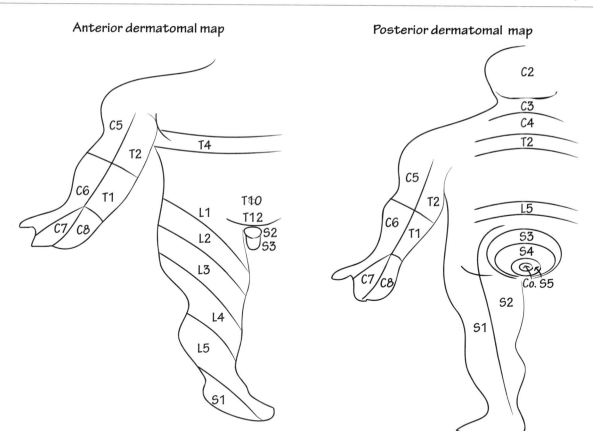

DRAWING 5-3 **Dermatomes**

Cutaneous Nerves—Upper Limb

Here, we will draw the cutaneous nerve innervation of the upper limb. First, draw an anterior upper limb. Show that the medial cord-derived medial cutaneous nerves of the forearm and arm cover the medial forearm and arm, respectively. And then show that the intercostobrachial nerve covers the axilla. In our discussion of the sensory innervation of the trunk, we discuss the T2 lateral cutaneous intercostal origins of the intercostobrachial nerve.

Next, show that the musculocutaneous nerve-derived lateral cutaneous nerve of the forearm covers the anterior lateral forearm; the radial nerve-derived lower lateral cutaneous nerve of the arm covers the lower lateral anterior upper arm; the axillary nerve-derived upper lateral cutaneous nerve of the arm covers the upper lateral anterior arm; and the supraclavicular nerve covers the shoulder.

Next, draw the posterior upper limb. The posterior upper limb sensory coverage is nearly identical to the anterior upper limb coverage, so, first, simply redraw the anterior limb. Next, indicate that the radial nerve-derived posterior cutaneous nerves to the forearm and arm cover the midline forearm and arm, respectively.[1–4,8]

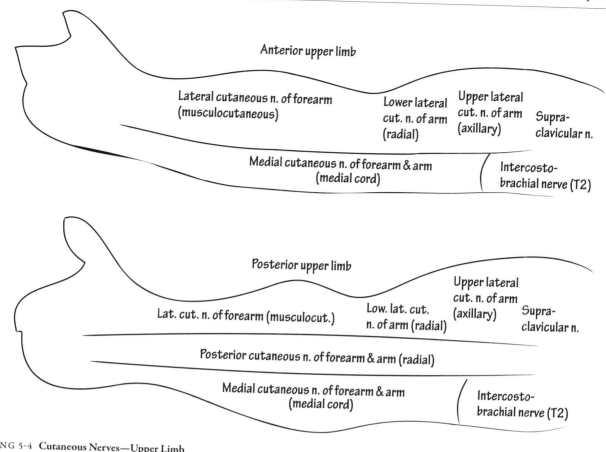

Anterior upper limb

Lateral cutaneous n. of forearm
(musculocutaneous)

Lower lateral
cut. n. of arm
(radial)

Upper lateral
cut. n. of arm
(axillary)

Supra-
clavicular n.

Medial cutaneous n. of forearm & arm
(medial cord)

Intercosto-
brachial nerve (T2)

Posterior upper limb

Lat. cut. n. of forearm (musculocut.)

Low. lat. cut.
n. of arm (radial)

Upper lateral
cut. n. of arm
(axillary)

Supra-
clavicular n.

Posterior cutaneous n. of forearm & arm (radial)

Medial cutaneous n. of forearm & arm
(medial cord)

Intercosto-
brachial nerve (T2)

DRAWING 5-4 **Cutaneous Nerves—Upper Limb**

Cutaneous Nerves—Lower Limb

Here, we will map the cutaneous innervation of the lower limb. First, let's draw the anterior and posterior aspects of the lower limb and label their medial and lateral surfaces. Begin with the thigh. Indicate that the lateral cutaneous nerve of the thigh (aka lateral femoral cutaneous nerve) covers the lateral aspect of the complete thigh. Then, show that the posterior cutaneous nerve of the thigh (aka posterior femoral cutaneous nerve) covers the back of thigh. Next, show that the anterior femoral cutaneous nerve covers the anterior and medial thigh. And finally, show that the obturator nerve covers a small sensory patch on the medial aspect of the thigh. Note that the lateral and posterior cutaneous nerves of the thigh are direct branches from the lumbosacral plexus, whereas the anterior femoral cutaneous nerve is a branch of the femoral nerve. The anterior femoral cutaneous nerve is often subdivided into the intermediate and medial femoral cutaneous nerves.

Now, move to the leg. Show that the lateral sural cutaneous nerve, which is derived from the common peroneal nerve, covers the upper lateral aspect of the leg and that the superficial peroneal nerve covers the lower lateral aspect of the leg. The superficial peroneal nerve also covers the dorsum of the foot except as follows: the deep peroneal nerve covers the webbing between the great toe and second digit, and the distal sural branches cover the extreme lateral foot. Next, indicate that the medial calcaneal nerve covers the heel.

Show that the sural nerve, which is derived from both the common peroneal and tibial nerves, covers the posterior leg. The medial sural cutaneous branch of the tibial nerve provides the upper sural coverage and the distal sural branches (the lateral calcaneal and lateral dorsal cutaneous nerves) provide the distal coverage.

To complete the leg, show that the femoral-derived saphenous nerve covers the medial aspect of the leg and instep of the foot. Include the clinically important infrapatellar branch of the saphenous nerve, which covers the anterior knee; this small branch is sometimes injured during arthroscopic knee surgery.[1–4,8–10]

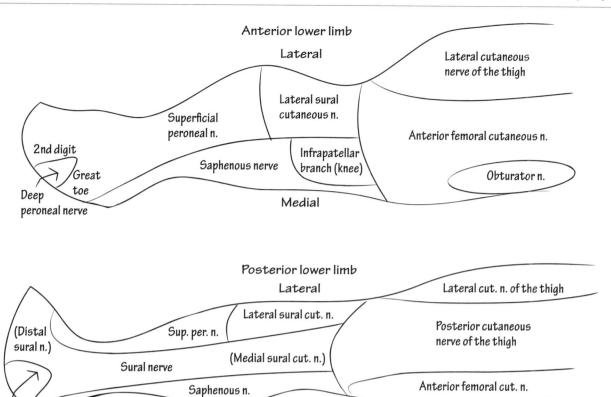

Anterior lower limb

Lateral

Lateral cutaneous nerve of the thigh

Lateral sural cutaneous n.

Superficial peroneal n.

Anterior femoral cutaneous n.

2nd digit

Infrapatellar branch (knee)

Great toe

Saphenous nerve

Obturator n.

Deep peroneal nerve

Medial

Posterior lower limb

Lateral

Lateral cut. n. of the thigh

Lateral sural cut. n.

(Distal sural n.)

Sup. per. n.

Posterior cutaneous nerve of the thigh

(Medial sural cut. n.)

Sural nerve

Saphenous n.

Anterior femoral cut. n.

Medial

Medial calcaneal nerve

DRAWING 5-5 **Cutaneous Nerves—Lower Limb**

Cutaneous Nerves—Trunk *(Advanced)*

Here, we will map the cutaneous innervation of the trunk and related anatomic regions. Before sketching their sensory coverage, let's address the origins of the sensory nerves of the thorax, abdomen, and back. Show that the anterior and posterior nerve roots form a mixed spinal nerve, which splits into posterior and anterior rami. The posterior ramus derives the posterior cutaneous sensory branch and the anterior ramus derives the intercostal nerve, which provides the lateral cutaneous branch and the anterior cutaneous branch.

Now, draw the anterior trunk (the thorax and abdomen) and posterior trunk (the back). Also include the pelvic and gluteal junctional zones in our posterior trunk diagram and also the back of the head and neck, as well, given their regional relevance. Show that the supraclavicular nerve covers the supraclavicular chest and also the posterior shoulders. Then, show that thoracic anterior cutaneous branches cover the midline thorax and abdomen, and then that the thoracic lateral cutaneous branches cover the lateral thorax and abdomen. Note that T1 is uninvolved in sensory coverage of the trunk: it supplies the medial cutaneous nerves of the arm and forearm, instead; also, note that the lateral cutaneous branch of T2 is called the intercostobrachial nerve and it covers the axilla; and, finally, note that T12 is called the subcostal nerve, which innervates the upper/lateral buttock, and has important connections with the cutaneous branches of the lower abdomen, which we draw next.

Now, show that the iliohypogastric nerve provides sensory coverage to the suprapubic area and the upper-lateral gluteal region. Next, show that the ilioinguinal nerve provides sensory coverage to the superior-medial thigh and proximal external genitalia. Then, show that the genital branch of the genitofemoral nerve provides additional sensory coverage to the proximal external genitalia and that the femoral branch of the genitofemoral nerve covers the femoral triangle. Next, show that the lateral cutaneous nerve of the thigh covers the lateral thigh. And finally, show that the pudendal nerve covers the distal external genitalia, provides even further coverage to the proximal external genitalia, and also covers the anus.

Next, show that the posterior cutaneous rami provide most of the sensory innervation to the posterior trunk. First, indicate that the thoracic rami cover from the scapulae to the iliac crests and then that the lumbosacral and coccygeal rami cover the buttocks. Note that the sensory innervators of the buttocks are often called the cluneal nerves. Now, show that the inferior aspect of each buttock receives additional coverage from the anterior rami-derived posterior cutaneous nerve of the thigh and perforating cutaneous nerve.

Finally, show that the posterior cervical rami cover the back of the neck and that the greater occipital nerve, which is supplied by the posterior ramus of C2, covers the back of the head.[1,2,4,8,11]

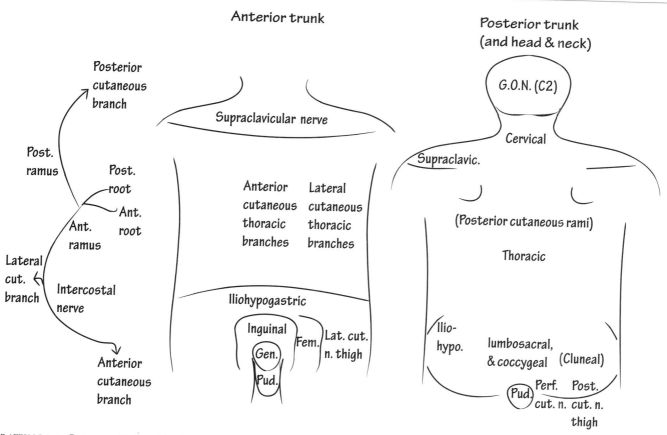

Anterior trunk

Posterior cutaneous branch

Post. ramus

Post. root

Ant. root

Ant. ramus

Lateral cut. branch

Intercostal nerve

Anterior cutaneous branch

Supraclavicular nerve

Anterior cutaneous thoracic branches

Lateral cutaneous thoracic branches

Iliohypogastric

Inguinal

Gen.

Pud.

Fem.

Lat. cut. n. thigh

Posterior trunk (and head & neck)

G.O.N. (C2)

Cervical

Supraclavic.

(Posterior cutaneous rami)

Thoracic

Ilio-hypo.

lumbosacral, & coccygeal

(Cluneal)

Pud.

Perf. cut. n.

Post. cut. n. thigh

DRAWING 5-6 **Cutaneous Nerves—Trunk**

Referred Pain

Here, we will draw a map for referred pain, which is the physiologic process whereby internal organs manifest with body surface pain. Since Sir Henry Head wrote about this subject in the late 1800s and early 1900s, many accounts of the dermatomal distribution of visceral pain have been published; however, the true pathophysiologic mechanism of visceral pain remains to be determined. It results either from direct intermingling of visceral and somatic afferent fibers or from indirect somatic fiber sensitization. Also, it either occurs peripherally (ie, in the peripheral nerves) or centrally (ie, in the spinal cord). Regardless of the exact pathophysiologic mechanism of referred pain, it is clear that visceral organs refer pain to their related dermatomal distributions.

Using this rule, let's consider the somatotopic map of referred pain for a few important organs. Draw the trunk and upper left arm. Indicate that innervation of the diaphragm comes from C3, C4, and C5, which cover the neck, shoulders, and upper lateral arm. We remember this innervation pattern by the mnemonic: C3, C4, C5 keeps the diaphragm alive! In accordance with the visceral-dermatomal rule we have established, diaphragmatic pain is felt in the neck and upper shoulder: the dermatomal distribution of these cervical levels. Next, let's consider the visceral map for the heart. Show that, generally, the T1 to T5 spinal nerves innervate this organ; the upper thoracic spinal nerves cover the chest and medial upper arm and forearm. Again, in accordance with the referred pain principle, myocardial ischemia is commonly felt along this upper thoracic dermatomal distribution: the left side of the chest and inside of the left arm. Note that classic cardiac pain does not extend into the fingers, which are supplied by the C6 to C8 spinal nerves. Finally, consider the appendix, which is innervated by T10. Appendicitis is first felt as a vague, painful sensation at the umbilicus—the dermatomal distribution of T10. Only later, when the appendicitis worsens, does the pain become somatic, at which time it moves to the right lower quadrant.[12]

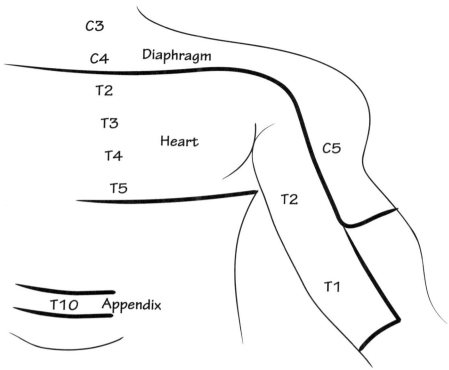

DRAWING 5-7 **Referred Pain**

References

1. Standring, S. & Gray, H. *Gray's anatomy: the anatomical basis of clinical practice,* 40th ed. (Churchill Livingstone/Elsevier, 2008).

2. Preston, D. C. & Shapiro, B. E. *Electromyography and neuromuscular disorders: clinical-electrophysiologic correlations,* 2nd ed. (Elsevier Butterworth-Heinemann, 2005).

3. Perotto, A. & Delagi, E. F. *Anatomical guide for the electromyographer: the limbs and trunk,* 4th ed. (Charles C Thomas, 2005).

4. Netter, F. H. & Dalley, A. F. *Atlas of human anatomy,* 2nd ed., Plates 4–7 (Novartis, 1997).

5. Furuya, H. Usefulness of manual muscle testing of pronator teres and supinator muscles in assessing cervical radiculopathy. *Fukuoka Acta Med.* 96, 319–325 (2005).

6. .Stevens, J. C. AAEM minimonograph #26: the electrodiagnosis of carpal tunnel syndrome. American Association of Electrodiagnostic Medicine. *Muscle Nerve* 20, 1477–1486 (1997).

7. Rathakrishnan, R., Therimadasamy, A. K., Chan, Y. H. & Wilder-Smith, E. P. The median palmar cutaneous nerve in normal subjects and CTS. *Clin Neurophysiol* 118, 776–780 (2007).

8. Haymaker, W. & Woodhall, B. *Peripheral nerve injuries; principles of diagnosis,* 2d ed. (Saunders, 1953).

9. Takakura, Y., Kitada, C., Sugimoto, K., Tanaka, Y. & Tamai, S. Tarsal tunnel syndrome. Causes and results of operative treatment. *J Bone Joint Surg Br* 73, 125–128 (1991).

10. Stewart, J. D. Foot drop: where, why and what to do? *Pract Neurol* 8, 158–169 (2008).

11. Brodal, P. *The central nervous system: structure and function,* 4th ed. (Oxford University Press, 2010).

12. Snell, R. S. *Clinical neuroanatomy,* 7th ed., Chapter 14 (Wolters Kluwer Lippincott Williams & Wilkins, 2010).

6

Peripheral Nervous System

Autonomic Nervous System

Know-It Points

Autonomic Fiber Arrangements

■ The parasympathetic nervous system originates within the cranial nerve nuclei and the sacral intermediolateral cell column from S2 to S4.
■ The sympathetic nervous system originates within the thoracolumbar intermediolateral cell column from T1 to L2.
■ Parasympathetic ganglia lie close to (or within) their target organ.
■ Sympathetic ganglia lie far from their target organ.

■ Preganglionic parasympathetic and sympathetic neurons release acetylcholine.
■ Postganglionic parasympathetic fibers release acetylcholine.
■ Postganglionic sympathetic fibers release norepinephrine (except for those fibers to the sweat glands and adrenal gland, which release acetylcholine and epinephrine, respectively).

Parasympathetic Nervous System

■ The Edinger-Westphal nucleus of cranial nerve 3 innervates the ciliary ganglion.
■ The superior salivatory nucleus of cranial nerve 7 innervates both the pterygopalatine and submandibular ganglia.
■ The inferior salivatory nucleus of cranial nerve 9 innervates the otic ganglion.
■ The dorsal motor nucleus of the vagus nerve of cranial nerve 10 innervates the ganglia of numerous

pharyngeal and thoracoabdominal glands and organs.
■ The nucleus ambiguus of cranial nerves 9 and 10 innervates ganglia related to the carotid body and carotid sinus and the cardiac ganglion.
■ Sacral nuclei of the intermediolateral cell column (S2–S4) project to abdomino-pelvic ganglia.

Sympathetic Nervous System

■ The paravertebral chain lies just lateral to the vertebral column.
■ Superior cervical ganglion fibers ascend the carotid artery to innervate the head and neck.
■ Loss of sympathetic tone to the face results in Horner's syndrome: ptosis, miosis, and anhidrosis.

■ Sympathetic splanchnic nerves innervate the four prevertebral ganglia.
■ Certain preganglionic sympathetic fibers synapse directly in adrenal medullary chromaffin cells.

The Urinary System (*Advanced*)

- The sympathetic and somatomotor efferents inhibit urination.
- The parasympathetic fibers activate urination.
- Parasympathetic fibers excite bladder wall contraction and inhibit internal urethral sphincter constriction.
- Sympathetic fibers inhibit bladder wall contraction, excite internal urethral sphincter constriction, and tonically inhibit the parasympathetic ganglion.
- Somatomotor efferents provide tonic activation of the external urethral sphincter.
- Male reproductive mnemonic: Parasympathetic—Point and Sympathetic—Shoot.

The Cardiac Reflex (*Advanced*)

- The glossopharyngeal nerve carries afferents from the carotid body and carotid sinus.
- The vagus nerve carries afferents from the aortic bodies and aortic arch baroreceptors.
- The glossopharyngeal and vagus nerves project to the solitary tract nucleus, which, via the nucleus ambiguus, induces heart rate deceleration.
- The rostral ventrolateral medulla provides tonic sympathetic stimulation to the intermediolateral cell column of the spinal cord to produce heart rate acceleration.

Autonomic Fiber Arrangements

Here, we will draw the motor fiber arrangements for the parasympathetic and sympathetic divisions of the autonomic nervous system. First, indicate that the parasympathetic nervous system brings the body into a rest state whereas the sympathetic nervous system is activated in states of physical and psychological stress: it produces the so-called "fight-or-flight" response. Next, draw representative preganglionic neurons for both the parasympathetic and sympathetic nervous systems. Indicate that the visceral neurons of the parasympathetic nervous system lie within cranial nerve nuclei and the sacral intermediolateral cell column of the spinal cord, from S2 to S4, and that the visceral neurons of the sympathetic nervous system lie within the thoracolumbar intermediolateral cell column, from T1 to L2. Next, in the parasympathetic arrangement show a long preganglionic axon synapse on a ganglion within its effector tissue: cranial and sacral parasympathetic ganglia lie either very close to or within the wall of their target organ. Then, show a postganglionic parasympathetic fiber project deep into the target organ.

Now, let's draw the axons of the sympathetic nervous system. Show a preganglionic sympathetic axon synapse on a nearby peripheral ganglion. Other than the preganglionic sympathetic fibers that travel to the adrenal gland, sympathetic preganglionic axons are short and synapse close to their site of origin: either in the paravertebral chain or one of the prevertebral ganglia. Next, show a postganglionic sympathetic fiber travel a long distance to its target organ and also to the body walls and limbs, where the sympathetic nervous system innervates sweat glands, hair fibers, and blood vessels of skeletal muscle and skin.

Now, let's label the relevant neurotransmitters involved in these autonomic fiber pathways. As a class, neurotransmitters are small molecules with transient effects. Indicate that both the preganglionic parasympathetic and sympathetic neurons release acetylcholine.

Then, indicate that all postganglionic parasympathetic fibers release acetylcholine and also that most postganglionic sympathetic fibers release norepinephrine (noradrenaline). The exceptions are the postganglionic sympathetic fibers to sweat glands, which release acetylcholine, and the adrenal medullary cells, which mostly release epinephrine (adrenaline).[1]

In addition to the neurotransmitters, neuropeptides also exist within autonomic neurons. In comparison to the neurotransmitters, neuropeptides are generally packaged into larger vesicles and have more wide-reaching and long-lasting effects. The neuropeptides are organized into many different classes, such as the calcitonin family, hypothalamic hormones, hypothalamic- releasing and -inhibiting hormones, neuropeptide Y family, opioid peptides, pituitary hormones, tachykinins, VIP-glucagon family, and additional peptides that do not fall into any of these categories.[2,3]

Lastly, consider that the digestive tract also contains its own autonomic system, called the enteric nervous system. The enteric nervous system comprises numerous neurons distributed in myenteric and submucosal plexuses. The enteric nervous system and the pacemaker cells of the digestive system wall (the interstitial cells of Cajal) generate and propagate patterns of depolarization that result in waves of peristaltic muscle contraction. Food ingestion triggers the peristaltic reflex, which propels food through the digestive tract, and the enteric neural circuits adjust intestinal blood flow and secretomotor activity for absorption. Notably, psychopharmacologic drugs often affect the neurotransmitters and neuromodulators of the enteric nervous system. For instance, acetylcholine is an important peristaltic promoter, so cholinesterase inhibitors, which increase circulating levels of acetylcholine, promote gastrointestinal activity and can result in diarrhea. In contrast, tricyclic antidepressants contain anticholinergic properties and, as a result, can cause constipation.[4-8]

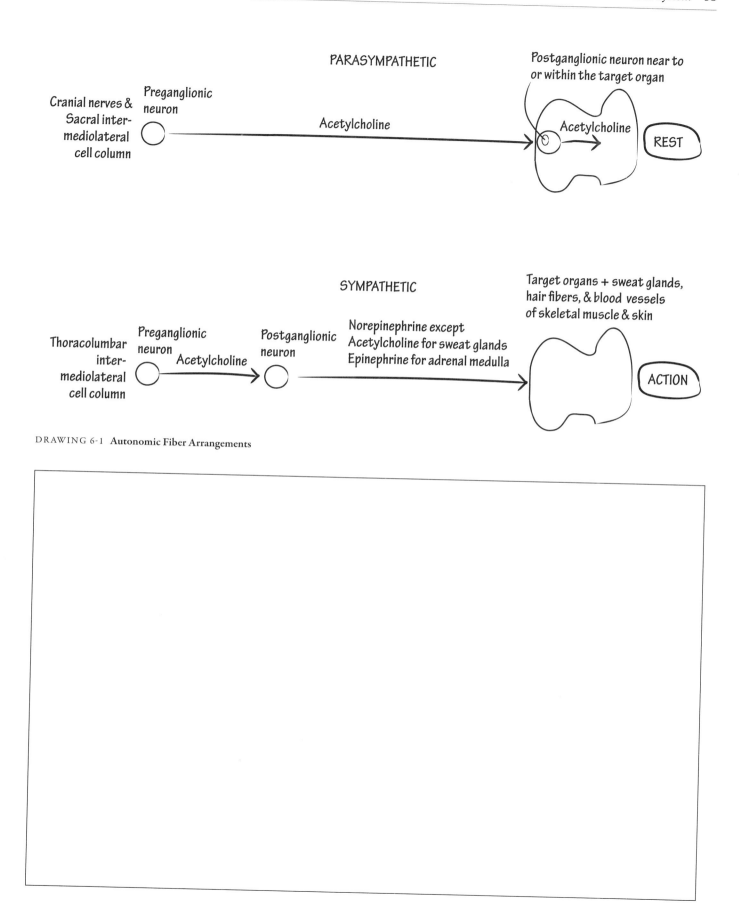

DRAWING 6-1 **Autonomic Fiber Arrangements**

Parasympathetic Nervous System

Here, will draw the motor division of the parasympathetic nervous system. First, draw a coronal view through the brainstem and label the midbrain, pons, and medulla; indicate that the brainstem contains the cranial component of the parasympathetic system. Then, draw a coronal view of the sacral spinal cord and label it as the sacral component.

In the midbrain, draw the Edinger-Westphal nucleus of cranial nerve 3. Show that it innervates the ciliary ganglion, which innervates the ciliary body and pupillary constrictor muscles.

Next, in the pons, draw the superior salivatory nucleus of cranial nerve 7, which innervates both the pterygopalatine and submandibular ganglia, which innervate the majority of the major glands of the face. Indicate that the pterygopalatine ganglion innervates the major glands of the upper face except for the parotid gland (which the otic ganglion innervates). Specifically, the pterygopalatine ganglion innervates the nasal, lacrimal, pharyngeal, and palatine glands. Then, show that the submandibular ganglion innervates the submandibular and sublingual glands.

Now, in the medulla, draw the inferior salivatory nucleus of cranial nerve 9. Show that it innervates the otic ganglion, which, as mentioned, innervates the parotid gland. Then, draw the dorsal motor nucleus of the vagus nerve of cranial nerve 10. Show that it innervates the ganglia of numerous pharyngeal and thoracoabdominal glands and organs. Notably, it innervates the abdominal foregut and midgut derivatives (but not the hindgut derivates: its innervation stops at the splenic flexure of the colon). The target organs of the dorsal motor nucleus of the vagus include the pharyngeal and laryngeal mucosa, lungs, esophagus, liver, pancreas, gallbladder, stomach, small intestine, and colon to the splenic flexure. It induces bronchoconstriction and increases gut peristalsis. As we will show in a moment, however, the dorsal motor nucleus of the vagus provides minimal, if any, innervation to the heart; nucleus ambiguus is responsible for that, instead.

Next, draw the nucleus ambiguus of cranial nerves 9 and 10. Show that through its glossopharyngeal nerve parasympathetic fibers, nucleus ambiguus innervates ganglia that lie within and act on the carotid body and carotid sinus, and then show that through its vagus nerve parasympathetic fibers, nucleus ambiguus innervates the cardiac ganglion, which induces heart rate deceleration. Note that although not drawn as such here, nucleus ambiguus and the dorsal motor nucleus of the vagus both lie at the same rostro-caudal level of the medulla (see Drawing 11-4, for details).

Now, let's turn our attention to the sacral component of the parasympathetic nervous system. Draw the sacral nuclei of the intermediolateral cell column for sacral levels 2–4. These nuclei reside in lamina 7 in the intermediate gray matter horn of the spinal cord. Show that the visceromotor axons from sacral levels 2–4 travel as pelvic splanchnic nerves, which relay in the ganglia of their target organs in the abdomen and pelvis. Their targets are the hindgut derivatives: the distal transverse colon, descending colon, sigmoid colon, and rectum; and also the anal canal, lower urinary tract, and reproductive organs. Sacral parasympathetic activation increases blood flow to the gut, increases gut peristalsis and secretion, provides urinary bladder detrusor muscle tone, and induces genital engorgement.[4-8]

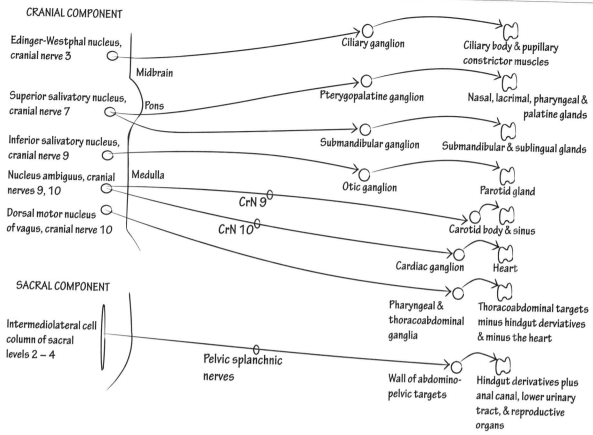

CRANIAL COMPONENT

Edinger-Westphal nucleus, cranial nerve 3

Midbrain

Ciliary ganglion

Ciliary body & pupillary constrictor muscles

Superior salivatory nucleus, cranial nerve 7

Pons

Pterygopalatine ganglion

Nasal, lacrimal, pharyngeal & palatine glands

Inferior salivatory nucleus, cranial nerve 9

Submandibular ganglion

Submandibular & sublingual glands

Nucleus ambiguus, cranial nerves 9, 10

Medulla

Otic ganglion

Parotid gland

Dorsal motor nucleus of vagus, cranial nerve 10

CrN 9

CrN 10

Carotid body & sinus

Cardiac ganglion

Heart

SACRAL COMPONENT

Intermediolateral cell column of sacral levels 2 – 4

Pelvic splanchnic nerves

Pharyngeal & thoracoabdominal ganglia

Thoracoabdominal targets minus hindgut derviatives & minus the heart

Wall of abdomino-pelvic targets

Hindgut derivatives plus anal canal, lower urinary tract, & reproductive organs

DRAWING 6-2 Parasympathetic Nervous System

Sympathetic Nervous System

Here, we will draw the motor division of the thoracolumbar sympathetic nervous system. Across the top of the page, write nucleus, ganglion, and effector tissue. Next, draw an outline of the spinal cord; show that the origins of the sympathetic nervous system lie in the intermediolateral cell column from T1 to L2. Now, draw the paravertebral chain; it resembles a string of pearls and lies just lateral to the vertebral column: we draw it as four circles and a long tail because only 4 of the roughly 24 sympathetic ganglia are worth specifying for our purposes, here. Label them now from superior to inferior as the superior cervical ganglion, the middle cervical ganglion, the inferior cervical ganglion, and, lastly, the first thoracic ganglion. The inferior cervical and first thoracic ganglia combine to form the stellate ganglion. Next, show that there are 10 additional thoracic paravertebral ganglia (for a total of 11), and 4 lumbar paravertebral ganglia, and 4 or 5 sacral paravertebral ganglia, and the ganglion impar, the most caudal paravertebral ganglion, which neighbors the coccyx.[9]

Now, let's divide the sympathetic motor innervation into its different anatomic segments. First, draw the innervation to the thorax and upper abdomen: show that preganglionic sympathetic fibers synapse in the paravertebral chain and then project the long distance to their thoracoabdominal targets. The targets within this anatomic segment include the lungs, trachea, heart, and esophagus; the preganglionic sympathetic fibers that innervate this segment originate in the intermediolateral cell column from T1 to T5.

Next, let's show the innervation pattern to the upper extremity. Indicate that it stems from postganglionic fibers of the middle cervical and stellate paravertebral ganglia. Then, also show that the stellate ganglion plays an important supplementary role in sympathetic innervation to the heart.

Now, in regards to the head and neck, show that the superior cervical ganglion receives innervation from the C8 to T2 spinal cord level: this region is called the cilisopinal center of Budge; and then, show that the cilisopinal center of Budge is innervated by the posterolateral hypothalamus via the hypothalamospinal pathway. Next, show that postganglionic superior cervical ganglion fibers ascend the carotid arteries to innervate the head and neck. Notable causes of injury along this sympathetic pathway are medullary brainstem strokes, paravertebral masses, such as Pancoast tumor (a form of apical lung tumor), and carotid dissection. Loss of sympathetic tone to the face results in Horner's syndrome: ptosis, miosis, and anhidrosis.

Next, we will draw the innervation to the rest of the abdomen and pelvis, which is derived from sympathetic splanchnic nerves, which generally originate from the T5 to L2 level of the spinal cord. Rather than relay in the paravertebral ganglia, show that these nerves, instead, synapse in the four prevertebral ganglia, which span from the lower thoracic to the sacral vertebral column. Indicate that the prevertebral ganglia are, from superior to inferior: the celiac, aorticorenal, superior mesenteric, and inferior mesenteric ganglia. Then, show that the celiac ganglion innervates the spleen and foregut derivatives; the aorticorenal ganglion innervates the renal vessels; the superior mesenteric ganglion innervates the midgut derivatives; and the inferior mesenteric ganglion innervates the hindgut derivatives, the lower urinary system, and the reproductive organs.[5]

As our last anatomic segment, show that preganglionic sympathetic fibers synapse directly in the adrenal gland, most commonly on adrenal medullary chromaffin cells, which predominantly release epinephrine (and to a much lesser extent norepinephrine).[1]

Finally, within the sympathetic nervous system, we need to show that both divergence and convergence of preganglionic sympathetic fibers occurs. Indicate that in divergence, fibers from one preganglionic axon form synapses on multiple postganglionic neurons, whereas in convergence, there is a confluence of fibers from different preganglionic axons onto a single postganglionic neuron.[4–8,10]

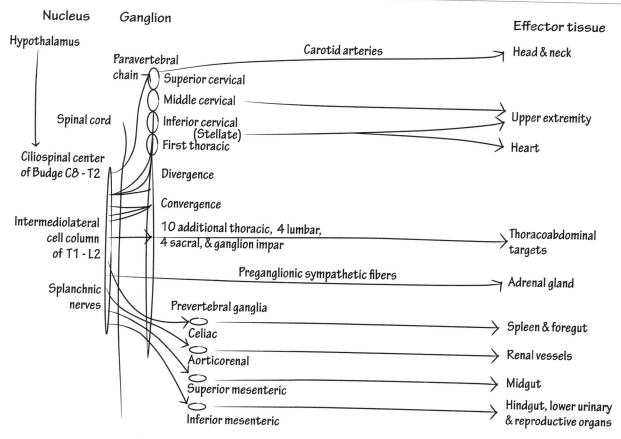

Nucleus   Ganglion   Effector tissue

Hypothalamus

Carotid arteries   Head & neck

Paravertebral
chain
                Superior cervical

                Middle cervical   Upper extremity

Spinal cord   Inferior cervical
                (Stellate)   Heart
                First thoracic

Ciliospinal center
of Budge C8 - T2   Divergence

                Convergence

Intermediolateral
cell column   10 additional thoracic, 4 lumbar,   Thoracoabdominal
of T1 - L2   4 sacral, & ganglion impar   targets

                Preganglionic sympathetic fibers   Adrenal gland

Splanchnic
nerves   Prevertebral ganglia

                Celiac   Spleen & foregut

                Aorticorenal   Renal vessels

                Superior mesenteric   Midgut

                Inferior mesenteric   Hindgut, lower urinary
                                                                        & reproductive organs

DRAWING 6-3 Sympathetic Nervous System

The Urinary System (*Advanced*)

Here, we will draw the innervation of the bladder and urethra, which are responsible for micturition (urination). We will address three classes of fiber circuitry: parasympathetic, sympathetic, and somatomotor. We will address the urinary system in detail, but quite simply, the sympathetic and somatomotor efferents inhibit urination and the parasympathetic fibers activate it. First, draw a bladder and urethra; then, label the bladder wall as the detrusor muscle; next, draw the internal and external urethral sphincters; and then, draw viscerosensory afferents from the bladder and urethra—afferents pass through the hypogastric, pelvic splanchnic, and pudendal nerves to innervate select spinal cord and supraspinal nervous system regions. Now, let's draw the efferent pathways of the lower urinary system; we will draw the pathways, first, and then label their function.[11]

First, indicate that S2 to S4 parasympathetic efferents project to the parasympathetic vesical ganglion. Then, show that postganglionic parasympathetic fibers innervate the bladder wall and also the internal urethral sphincter. Next, indicate that preganglionic sympathetic efferents from T12 to L2 synapse in the paravertebral chain and the inferior mesenteric prevertebral ganglion, and then show that postganglionic fibers from these ganglia project to three separate targets: the bladder wall, the parasympathetic ganglion, and the internal urethral sphincter. Finally, show that somatomotor neurons in Onuf's nucleus, a circumscribed region of the sacral ventral horn from S2 to S4, project to the external urethral sphincter.

Next, let's include the function of each of these fiber types (parasympathetic, sympathetic, and somatomotor), but again, we can reason out these functions if we remember that the sympathetic and somatomotor fibers inhibit urination and the parasympathetic fibers activate it. First, show that the parasympathetic fibers excite bladder wall contraction and inhibit internal urethral sphincter constriction. Then, show that the sympathetic fibers inhibit bladder wall contraction, excite internal urethral

sphincter constriction, and tonically inhibit the parasympathetic ganglion. Lastly, show that the somatomotor efferents provide tonic activation of the external urethral sphincter.

Now, we need to address the supraspinal control of urination. The command center for bladder emptying (micturition) and the command center for bladder filling (continence) lie within neighboring regions of the pons. The pontine micturition center lies in the medial (M) region of the dorsolateral pontine tegmentum and the pontine continence center lies ventro-lateral to it in the lateral (L) region. These regions receive afferents from many brain regions, including the periaqueductal gray area, the hypothalamus, cerebellum, and certain limbic system regions. Barrington first described the pontine micturition center, so it is often referred to as the Barrington nucleus.

Lastly, let's add to our diagram the peripheral nerves that carry the aforementioned autonomic and somatic fibers. Show that postganglionic thoracolumbar sympathetic fibers initially travel within the superior hypogastric plexus and then emerge as hypogastric nerves. Next, show that the sacral parasympathetic fibers travel via the pelvic splanchnic nerve. Then, indicate that both the hypogastric and pelvic splanchnic nerves join within the inferior hypogastric plexus (aka the pelvic plexus), which provides both sympathetic and parasympathetic innervation to the bladder and urethra. Finally, show that somatomotor efferent fibers travel as the pudendal nerve to provide somatomotor innervation to the external urethral sphincter.

Note that the inferior hypogastric plexus innervates the reproductive organs, as well. In regards to sexual function, the parasympathetic nervous system is responsible for penile and clitoral engorgement and the sympathetic nervous system is responsible for penile ejaculation. We remember this functional relationship with the mnemonic Parasympathetic—Point and Sympathetic—Shoot.[4–8,10,12–14]

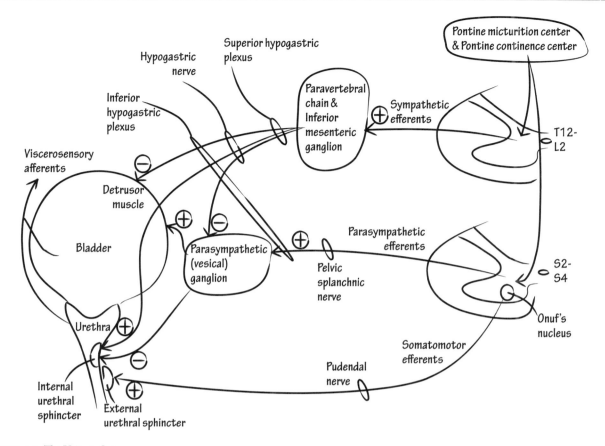

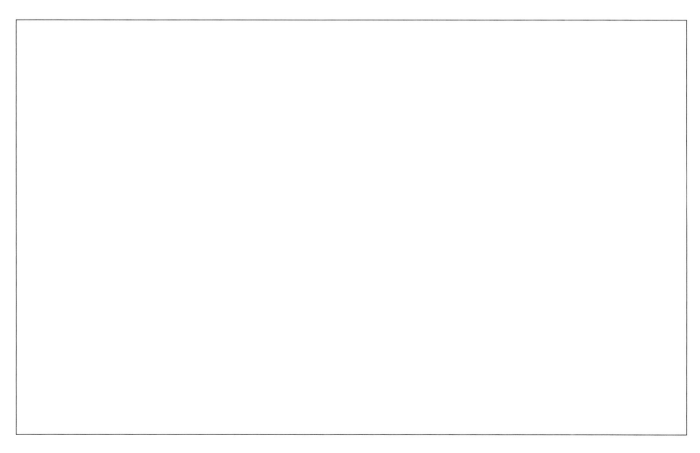

DRAWING 6-4 **The Urinary System**

The Cardiac Reflex *(Advanced)*

Here, we will draw the cardiovascular reflex, which maintains blood pressure and cardiac output. It involves a wide range of autonomic receptors, fibers, and nuclei, so we will limit our drawing to a few fundamental nuclei and fiber types. To begin, let's draw some of the key involved structures. First, draw the heart; aorta and aortic arch; and the common carotid artery—include its bifurcation into the internal carotid and external carotid arteries (denote the internal carotid artery, for reference). Next, draw the inferior ganglia of the glossopharyngeal and vagus nerves. Then, draw the medulla; then, the spinal cord; and lastly, the adjacent thoracic paravertebral ganglia.

Now, let's draw the specific components of the cardiovascular reflex. First, draw the carotid body at the bifurcation of the common carotid artery and then the aortic bodies below the arch of the aorta. Next, draw the carotid sinus in the proximal walls of the internal carotid artery and then the aortic arch baroreceptors in the aortic arch. The carotid body and aortic bodies are chemoreceptors that respond to arterial oxygen and carbon dioxide levels and blood acidity. The carotid sinus and aortic arch baroreceptors are baroreceptors, which respond to stretch changes in the arterial vasculature due to changes in blood pressure. Now, show that the glossopharyngeal nerve carries afferents from the carotid body and carotid sinus and that the vagus nerve carries afferents from the aortic bodies and aortic arch baroreceptors.

Next, within the lateral dorsal medulla, label the solitary tract nucleus, and within the central medulla, label the nucleus ambiguus. Then, draw a coronal view through the ventrolateral medullary reticular formation, called simply the ventrolateral medulla. Divide the ventrolateral medulla into rostral and caudal segments for reasons we will show soon. Now, indicate that the glossopharyngeal and vagus nerves project their central processes to the solitary tract nucleus. Then, show that the solitary tract nucleus innervates the nucleus ambiguus, which

projects to the parasympathetic cardiac ganglion and induces heart rate deceleration. Note that the dorsal motor nucleus of the vagus may play a parallel but very minor role to that of nucleus ambiguus in cardiac innervation. Now, show that the rostral ventrolateral medulla provides tonic sympathetic stimulation to the intermediolateral cell column of the spinal cord, which produces heart rate acceleration. Then, indicate that the solitary tract nucleus excites the caudal ventrolateral medulla, which inhibits the rostral segment of the ventrolateral medulla, which provides further means for heart rate deceleration. Note that we have left out some of the nuclei and regions involved in this reflex for simplicity; they are the parabrachial pontine nucleus, sensorimotor cortex, amygdala, and hypothalamus.

A simple way to test the cardiovascular response is by varying your pulse. Take your pulse and get a good sense of your heart rate. Then, take a deep breath and hold it for 5 or 6 seconds. Your heart rate should speed up because when you inhale deeply, you open up lung tissue and shunt blood into the lung capillaries, which reduces your effective circulating blood volume (ie, your stroke volume). Cardiac output is stroke volume multiplied by heart rate; therefore, to compensate for a decreased stroke volume, your heart rate increases (typically by 8 beats per minute).

An additional, slower response to a reduced stroke volume is to increase the effective circulating blood volume, itself. For instance, when we stand, blood pools in our veins, so after we stand upright for a full minute, T5 sympathetic splanchnic fibers command our abdominal vessels to shunt roughly 1.5 units of blood from our abdomen into our peripheral vasculature. Because there is a delay in the shunting of blood between systems, when we check orthostatic blood pressure, we must wait at least a few minutes in between measuring supine and standing blood pressure (and possibly longer, even).[4–9,15–17]

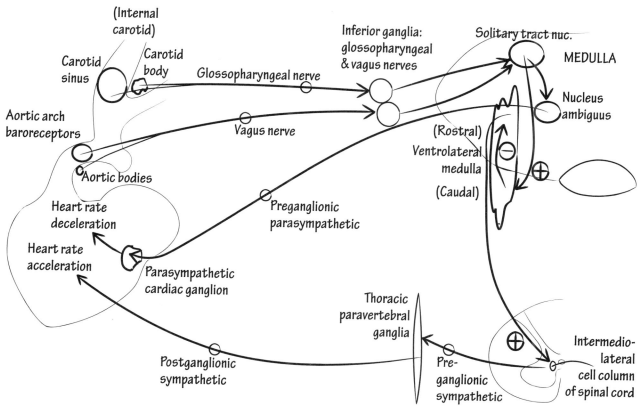

Carotid sinus

(Internal carotid)

Carotid body

Aortic arch baroreceptors

Aortic bodies

Glossopharyngeal nerve

Vagus nerve

Inferior ganglia: glossopharyngeal & vagus nerves

Solitary tract nuc.

MEDULLA

Nucleus ambiguus

(Rostral)

Ventrolateral medulla

(Caudal)

Heart rate deceleration

Heart rate acceleration

Preganglionic parasympathetic

Parasympathetic cardiac ganglion

Thoracic paravertebral ganglia

Postganglionic sympathetic

Pre-ganglionic sympathetic

Intermedio-lateral cell column of spinal cord

DRAWING 6-5 **The Cardiac Reflex**

References

1. Sherwood, L. *Fundamentals of physiology: a human perspective,* 3rd ed. (Brooks/Cole; Thomson Learning distributor, 2006).

2. Nestler, E. J., Hyman, S. E. & Malenka, R. C. *Molecular neuropharmacology: a foundation for clinical neuroscience,* pp. 183–184 (McGraw-Hill, Medical Publishing Division, 2001).

3. Perry, E. K., Ashton, H. & Young, A. H. *Neurochemistry of consciousness: neurotransmitters in mind* (J. Benjamins Pub. Co., 2002).

4. Afifi, A. K. & Bergman, R. A. *Functional neuroanatomy: text and atlas,* 2nd ed. (Lange Medical Books/McGraw-Hill, 2005).

5. Haines, D. E. & Ard, M. D. *Fundamental neuroscience: for basic and clinical applications,* 3rd ed. (Churchill Livingstone Elsevier, 2006).

6. Netter, F. H. & Dalley, A. F. *Atlas of human anatomy,* 2nd ed., Plates 4–7 (Novartis, 1997).

7. Snell, R. S. *Clinical neuroanatomy,* 7th ed., Chapter 14 (Wolters Kluwer Lippincott Williams & Wilkins, 2010).

8. Standring, S. & Gray, H. *Gray's anatomy: the anatomical basis of clinical practice,* 40th ed. (Churchill Livingstone/Elsevier, 2008).

9. Robertson, D. *Primer on the autonomic nervous system,* 2nd ed. (Elsevier Academic Press, 2004).

10. Cohen, H. S. *Neuroscience for rehabilitation,* 2nd ed. (Lippincott; Williams & Wilkins, 1999).

11. Ostergard, D. R., Bent, A. E., Cundiff, G. W. & Swift, S. E. *Ostergard's urogynecology and pelvic floor dysfunction,* 6th ed., Chapter 4 (Wolters Kluwer/Lippincott Williams & Wilkins, 2008).

12. Siegel, A. & Sapru, H. N. *Essential neuroscience,* 2nd ed. (Wolters Kluwer Health/Lippincott Williams & Wilkins, 2011).

13. Stoker, J., Taylor, S. A. & DeLancey, J. O. L. *Imaging pelvic floor disorders,* 2nd rev. ed. (Springer, 2008).

14. Yamada, S. & American Association of Neurological Surgeons. *Tethered cord syndrome in children and adults,* 2nd ed., pp. 12–13 (Thieme; American Association of Neurosurgeons, 2010).

15. Kiernan, J. A. & Barr, M. L. *Barr's the human nervous system: an anatomical viewpoint,* 9th ed. (Wolters Kluwer/Lippincott, Williams & Wilkins, 2009).

16. Posner, J. B. & Plum, F. *Plum and Posner's diagnosis of stupor and coma,* 4th ed. (Oxford University Press, 2007).

17. Loewy, A. D. & Spyer, K. M. *Central regulation of autonomic functions,* Chapter 9 (Oxford University Press, 1990).

7

Spinal Cord

Know-It Points

Spinal Cord Overview

- The posterior, middle, and anterior white matter form the posterior, lateral, and anterior funiculi, respectively.
- The gray matter of the spinal cord divides into the posterior horn, intermediate zone, and anterior horn.
- The gray matter of the spinal cord comprises Rexed laminae, which are numbered I to X.
- Laminae I–VI are the sensory laminae.
- Lamina VII is the spinocerebellar and autonomic lamina.
- Laminae VIII and IX are the motor laminae.
- Lamina X surrounds the central canal.
- In the lumbosacral cord, white matter is small and gray matter is large.
- In the thoracic cord, white matter is moderately large and gray matter is small.
- In the cervical spinal cord, both the gray and white matter regions are large.

Ascending Pathways

- The posterior column pathway comprises large sensory fibers, which carry vibration, two-point discrimination, and joint position sensory information.
- The gracile fasciculus carries large fiber sensory information from the lower body.
- The cuneate fasciculus carries large fiber sensory information from the upper body.
- The anterolateral system comprises small fiber sensory pathways, which carry pain, itch, and thermal sensory information.
- The anterolateral system includes the spinothalamic tract and the spinal-hypothalamic and spinal-brainstem pathways.
- The spinocerebellar tracts comprise large sensory fibers, which carry joint proprioception to the cerebellum for the coordination of movement.

Descending Pathways *(Advanced)*

- The anterior corticospinal tract innervates proximal musculature for gross motor movements.
- The lateral corticospinal tract innervates distal musculature for fine motor movements.
- The hypothalamospinal tract carries hypothalamic control of autonomic function.
- The rubrospinal tract innervates the upper cervical spinal cord to produce arm flexion.
- The tectospinal tract innervates the upper cervical spinal segments to produce contralateral head turn.
- The reticulospinal tracts and vestibulospinal tracts maintain posture through the activation of antigravity muscles.

Major Ascending & Descending Tracts

- Posterior column fibers ascend the spinal cord ipsilateral to their side of origin.
- Anterolateral system fibers ascend the spinal cord contralateral to their side of origin.
- Lateral corticospinal tract fibers descend the spinal cord contralateral to their side of origin.
- Posterior column pathway: 1st order neuron in the dorsal root ganglion, 2nd order neuron in the gracile and cuneate nuclei, 3rd order neuron in the ventrolateral posterior nucleus of the thalamus.
- Anterolateral system: 1st order neuron in the dorsal root ganglion, 2nd order neuron in the dorsal horn of the spinal cord, 3rd order neuron in the ventrolateral posterior nucleus of the thalamus.
- Corticospinal tract: 1st order neuron in the motor cortices (primarily), 2nd order neuron in the anterior horn of the spinal cord.

Spinocerebellar Pathways (Advanced)

- The posterior spinocerebellar tract originates from afferents of the lower trunk and lower limb, synapses in the dorsal nucleus of Clarke, and enters the cerebellum via the ipsilateral inferior cerebellar peduncle.
- The anterior spinocerebellar tract originates from afferents of the lower limb and enters the cerebellum via the superior cerebellar peduncle.
- The cuneocerebellar tract originates in the upper limb and upper trunk and enters the cerebellum via the ipsilateral inferior cerebellar peduncle.
- The rostral spinocerebellar tract originates in the upper limb and enters the cerebellum via the ipsilateral inferior cerebellar peduncle.

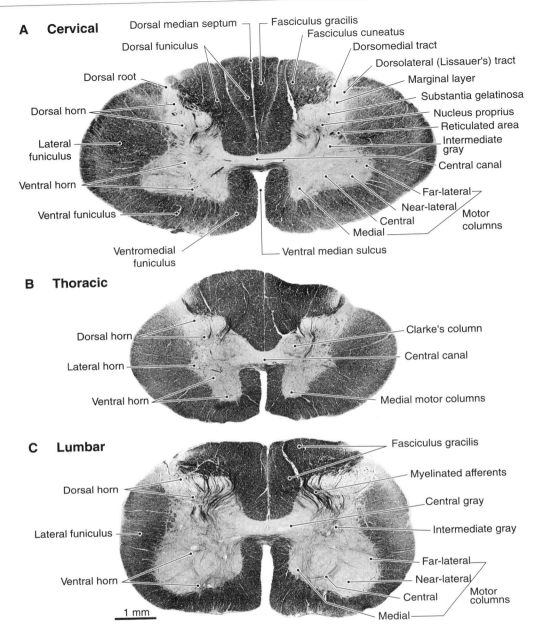

FIGURE 7-1   Histologic axial sections through cervical, thoracic, and lumbosacral spinal cord. Used with permission from Altman, Joseph, and Shirley A. Bayer. *Development of the Human Spinal Cord: An Interpretation Based on Experimental Studies in Animals.* Oxford ; New York: Oxford University Press, 2001.

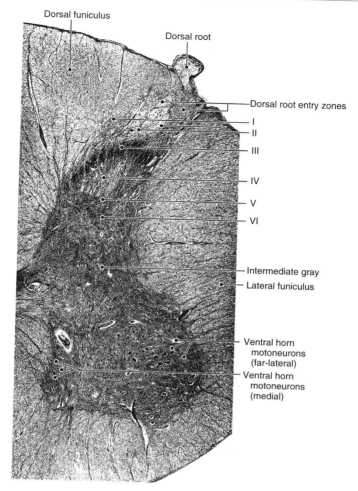

FIGURE 7-2 **Gray matter horns. Used with permission from the estate of Dr. William DeMyer.**

Spinal Cord Overview

Here, we will draw the spinal cord in axial cross-section. Show that the spinal cord is ovoid and has a thin fissure on its anterior surface. Next, draw the internal gray matter, which resembles a butterfly. Then, draw the central canal in the center of the gray matter; it is mostly obliterated by the second decade of life. The white matter of the spinal cord is segmented into posterior, lateral, and anterior funiculi (aka columns). Label the posterior white matter as the posterior funiculus, the middle white matter as the lateral funiculus, and the anterior white matter as the anterior funiculus. Lastly, show that interspinal rostro-caudal white matter projections travel via the proprius fasciculus, which surrounds the gray matter horns. Next, introduce the posterior median septum, which divides the posterior white matter into two halves, and label the anterior median fissure in parallel along the anterior surface of the spinal cord.

The gray matter of the spinal cord divides into three different regions, which are further classified as Rexed laminae. First, label the regions from posterior to anterior as the posterior horn, intermediate zone, and anterior horn. Then, label the Rexed laminae, which are numbered from I to X. In the posterior horn, label laminae I–VI: they are the sensory laminae; then, in the intermediate zone, label lamina VII, which is the spinocerebellar and autonomic lamina; next, in the anterior horn, label laminae VIII and IX, which are the motor laminae; and finally, label lamina X around the central canal.

Now, let's address a few neuroanatomic highlights of the Rexed laminae. Lamina I is the marginal nucleus (aka posteromarginal nucleus); lamina II is the substantia gelatinosa—so named because its lack of myelinated fibers gives it a gelatinous appearance on myelin staining; and laminae III and IV comprise nucleus proprius (the proper sensory nucleus). Laminae I through V receive the central processes of sensory fibers in a complicated way; generally, laminae I, II, and V receive small, poorly myelinated or unmyelinated fibers, which carry pain and temperature sensation, and laminae III and IV receive large cutaneous sensory fibers—note, however, that the majority of large fibers do not synapse within the Rexed laminae at all but instead directly ascend the posterior columns.[1]

Laminae V and VI receive descending motor fibers and assist in sensorimotor integration. Lamina VII contains the dorsal nucleus of Clarke, a key spinocerebellar nuclear column, and the intermediolateral column, a key autonomic nuclear column. Laminae VIII and IX contain motor neurons. Lamina X surrounds the central canal.[2,3]

Now, let's illustrate the relative size of the white and gray matter regions of the spinal cord at different anatomic heights. Show that in the lumbosacral cord, the amount of white matter is small, because the ascending fibers have yet to coalesce and the descending motor fibers have already terminated on their anterior horn cells. Indicate that the amount of gray matter is large because of the numerous neurons needed to innervate the lower limbs. Then, show that in the thoracic cord, the amount of white matter is moderately large because of the presence of the lumbosacral afferents and efferents, and then show that the amount of gray matter is small, because thoracic innervation to the trunk requires far fewer neurons than lumbosacral or cervical innervation to the limbs. Finally, in the cervical spinal cord, indicate that both the gray and white matter regions are large: the white matter bundles are dense with ascending and descending fibers from throughout the spinal cord and the gray matter horns are large because of the large populations of neurons required to innervate the upper limbs.[2,4–12]

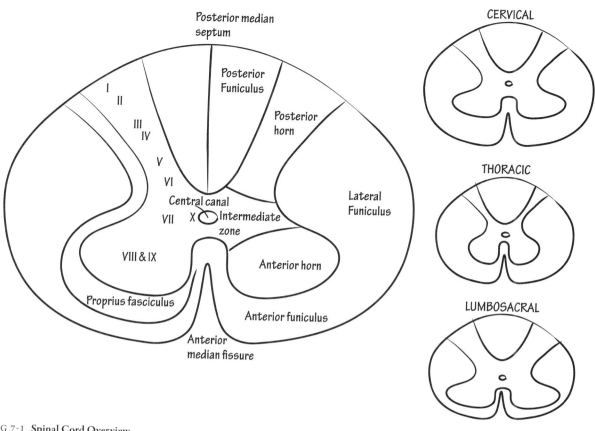

DRAWING 7-1 **Spinal Cord Overview**

Ascending Pathways

Here, we will draw the ascending spinal cord pathways in axial cross-section. Draw an outline of a spinal cord in axial cross-section and include the gray matter horns. We start with the posterior column pathway, which comprises large sensory fibers that carry vibration, two-point discrimination, and joint position sensory information. Within the posterior column, draw the posterior median septum, which divides the posterior white matter into right and left posterior columns. Then, label the posterior intermediate septum, which further subdivides each posterior column into medial and lateral segments. Label the medial segment as the gracile fasciculus and the lateral segment as the cuneate fasciculus. Write thoracic level 6 (T6) over the posterior intermediate septum to indicate that the gracile fasciculus carries large fiber sensory information from the lower body (from below T6) and the cuneate fasciculus carries sensory information from the upper body (from T6 and above).[4] Sensory afferents from the face travel via the trigeminal sensory system. A mnemonic to remember the function of the *gracile* fasciculus is that ballerinas must have good sensory input from their feet to twirl *grace*fully.

Now, label the anterolateral system as a long pathway that lies just outside of the anterior gray matter horn and extends between the anterior and lateral white matter funiculi. It comprises small fiber sensory pathways that carry pain, itch, and thermal sensory information. The anterolateral system includes the spinothalamic tract and the spinal-hypothalamic and spinal-brainstem pathways. In regards to the anterolateral system's somatotopic organization, the lower-most spinal levels comprise its outermost somatotopic layer and the upper-most spinal levels comprise its innermost somatotopic layer; thus, indicate that the arms lie along the inner aspect of the anterolateral system and the legs lie along the outer aspect. As a helpful mnemonic, consider that in cervical syringomyelia, a fluid-filled cavity within the central cord (see Drawing 7-8), there is often a suspended sensory level wherein small fiber sensation is lost in a cape-like distribution in the arms and upper trunk but is preserved in the legs. We can imagine that as the central fluid collection expands outward, it affects the arms and upper trunk first, and only later the legs. In regards to the sensory information carried by the anterolateral system, the lateral regions subserve pain and temperature and the anterior regions subserve tactile and pressure sensation. Indeed, texts often further subdivide the anterolateral system into separate ventral and lateral pathways. Next, label the ventral commissure, which lies in between the anterior horns; it is the white matter pathway through which the anterolateral system fibers decussate.

Lastly, along the posterior lateral wall of the spinal cord, label the posterior spinocerebellar tract, and along the anterior lateral wall, label the anterior spinocerebellar tract. These tracts comprise large sensory fibers that carry joint proprioception to the cerebellum for the coordination of movement; we address the spinocerebellar pathways in Drawing 7-5.

Now, show that the cell bodies for spinal sensory fibers lie within dorsal root ganglia, which are situated just proximal to where the anterior and posterior roots merge, within the intervertebral foramina. Indicate that spinal sensory axons are pseudo-unipolar, meaning they contain a single short axon that emanates from the cell body and divides into processes that extend peripherally (eg, to the skin's surface) and centrally (eg, to the spinal cord).

Finally, let's draw the anterolateral system and posterior column projections. Label Lissauer's tract along the dorsal edge of the dorsal horn. Indicate that the central processes of the anterolateral system pass through Lissauer's tract, synapse within the ipsilateral dorsal horn, and cross within the ventral commissure to ascend the spinal cord within the anterolateral system. Then, indicate that the posterior column pathway fibers enter the spinal cord medial to Lissauer's tract and directly ascend the spinal cord within the ipsilateral posterior column.[2,4–12]

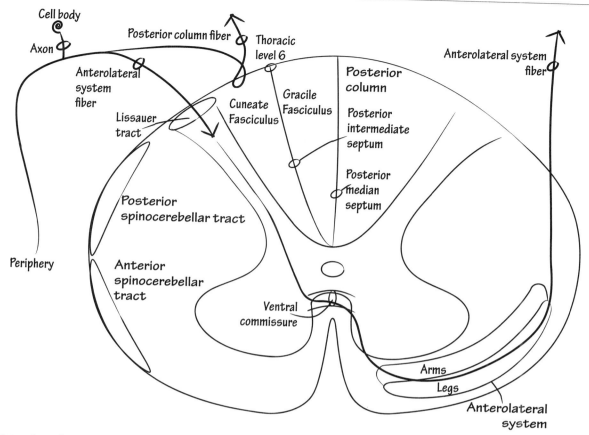

DRAWING 7-2 **Ascending Pathways**

Descending Pathways *(Advanced)*

Here, we will draw the descending spinal cord pathways in axial cross-section. First, draw one half of an outline of an axial cross-section of the spinal cord and include a gray matter horn. Then, label the following terms across the top of the page: tract, origin, termination, and function. Next, label the lateral corticospinal tract in the lateral funiculus and then the anterior corticospinal tract along the anterior median fissure. Indicate that the anterior corticospinal tract fibers originate in the motor cortices (most notably), terminate in contralateral spinal motor neurons, and innervate proximal musculature for gross motor movements. Next, outside of our table, make a notation that the lateral corticospinal tract fibers innervate distal musculature for fine motor movements (we draw this pathway in Drawing 7-4). Then, label the somatotopic organization of the lateral corticospinal tract: indicate that the medial aspect of the lateral corticospinal tract carries the arm fibers and the lateral aspect carries the leg fibers.

Next, label the hypothalamospinal tract alongside the lateral corticospinal tract in the lateral funiculus. Indicate that this tract originates in the hypothalamus, descends ipsilaterally, and carries hypothalamic control of autonomic function. Now, label the rubrospinal tract near to the lateral corticospinal tract. Indicate that it originates from the red nucleus in the midbrain, crosses in the ventral tegmental area of the brainstem, and innervates the upper cervical spinal cord to produce arm flexion. Next, label the tectospinal tract in the anterior-medial spinal cord. Indicate that it originates in the superior colliculus of the midbrain, decussates in the dorsal midbrain tegmentum, and innervates the upper cervical spinal segments to produce contralateral head turn.

Now, let's address the reticulospinal tracts and vestibulospinal tracts, both of which maintain posture through the activation of antigravity muscles. In our axial cross-section, label the medial reticulospinal tract and medial vestibulospinal tract in the anterior-medial spinal cord and label the lateral reticulospinal tract and lateral vestibulospinal tract in the lateral funiculus (the lateral vestibulospinal tract borders the anterior funiculus). Next, indicate that the medial reticulospinal tract originates in the medial zone of the pontine reticular formation and passes predominantly ipsilaterally to *activate* the axial and proximal limb extensors. Then, indicate that the lateral reticulospinal tract originates in the medial zone of the medullary reticular formation and passes predominantly ipsilaterally to *inhibit* the axial and proximal limb extensors (and to a lesser degree it also excites axial and proximal limb flexors). Now, make a notation that the vestibulospinal tracts excite the axial and proximal limb extensors. Specifically, the medial vestibulospinal tract acts on the cervical spinal cord to excite neck extensor musculature and the lateral vestibulospinal tract projects along the height of the spinal cord to excite paravertebral and proximal limb extensor muscles.[7,9,13,14]

Next, consider that normally the cerebral cortex inhibits the rubrospinal and reticulo- and vestibulospinal tracts, but when cortical inhibition is lost, these three tracts are left unchecked, which results in upper extremity flexion and lower extremity extension, referred to as decorticate posturing. Then, consider that a lesion that cuts off both the cortical and rubrospinal tracts (ie, a lesion below the level of the midbrain) leaves the reticulo- and vestibulospinal tracts unchecked, which results in neck and limb extension, referred to as decerebrate posturing.

Finally, in regards to the somatotopy of the anterior gray matter horns, show that the posterior nuclei innervate the flexor muscles and the anterior nuclei innervate the extensor muscles, and then show that the medial nuclei innervate the proximal muscles and the lateral nuclei innervate the distal muscles. Notice how the somatotopic organization of the gray matter parallels the positions of the functionally-related white matter pathways.[2,4–12]

TRACT	ORIGIN	TERMINATION	FUNCTION
Anterior corticospinal	Motor cortices (mostly)	Contralateral	Proximal muscle activation
Hypothalamospinal	Hypothalamus	Ipsilateral	Autonomic function
Rubrospinal	Red nucleus	Contralateral	Activates upper limb flexion
Tectospinal	Superior colliculus	Contralateral	Neck movement - head turn
Medial reticulospinal	Pontine reticular formation	Ipsilateral (mostly)	Activates limb extension
Lateral reticulospinal	Medullary reticular formation	Ipsilateral (mostly)	Inhibits limb extension

*Lateral corticospinal - innervate distal muscles

*Vestibulospinal - activate axial & proximal limb extensors

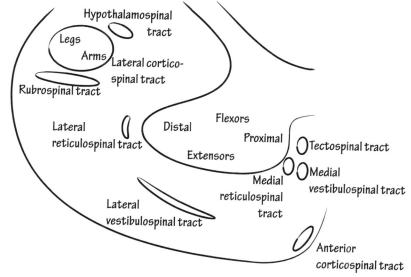

*Further details drawn elsewhere

DRAWING 7-3 **Descending Pathways**

Major Ascending & Descending Tracts

Here, we will draw the posterior column pathway, the anterolateral system (which includes, most notably, the spinothalamic tract), and the lateral corticospinal tract. First, draw an axial cross-section through the spinal cord. Next, label the origin and termination points of our pathway; label the right peripheral nerve and the left cerebral hemisphere's primary motor cortex and primary sensory cortex.

Now, label the posterior column of the right side of the posterior white matter. Posterior column fibers ascend the spinal cord ipsilateral to their side of origin. Next, label the anterolateral system bundle on the left side of the spinal cord—the anterolateral system fibers ascend the spinal cord contralateral to their side of origin. Finally, draw the lateral corticospinal tract on the right side of the spinal cord—the lateral corticospinal tract fibers descend the spinal cord contralateral to their side of origin.

Next, let's label cell bodies for each pathway and then draw each pathway's course. We will abbreviate the cell bodies for each pathway as follows: posterior column pathway cell body as PCP, anterolateral system cell body as ALS, and lateral corticospinal tract cell body as CST. Show that the first cell body (the first-order sensory neuron) for the posterior column pathway lies in the dorsal root ganglion. This cell body is pseudo-unipolar: indicate that it projects a single axon bundle over a very short distance, which divides into a peripheral process (the peripheral nerve) and a central process (the posterior nerve root). Next, show that the second-order sensory neurons lie in the gracile and cuneate nuclei in the medulla. Then, draw the third-order sensory neuron in the contralateral thalamus. Now, draw the posterior column pathway, itself. Indicate that the central process enters and ascends the posterior column without forming a synapse in the spinal cord and that it instead first synapses in the gracile and cuneate nuclei in the medulla. Next, show that the gracile and cuneate nuclei send decussating fibers across the medulla via the internal arcuate fasciculus; these fibers ascend the brainstem via

the medial lemniscus and synapse in the third-order neuron in the ventroposterior lateral nucleus of the thalamus. Finally, indicate that the thalamus projects to the sensory cortex.

Now, let's draw the cell bodies and fiber pathway for the anterolateral system. Indicate that the first-order neuron lies within the dorsal root ganglion; then, show that the second-order neuron lies within the dorsal horn of the spinal cord; and finally, show that the third-order neuron lies within the contralateral thalamus (also within the ventroposterior lateral nucleus). Now, draw the anterolateral system pathway, itself. Show that anterolateral system central processes project from the dorsal root ganglion to the dorsal horn. These inputs ascend and descend a variable number of spinal cord levels before synapsing in the spinal cord. Then, show that at or near their level of entry into the spinal cord, the anterolateral system fibers decussate via the ventral commissure and bundle in the anterolateral spinal cord, where they ascend the spinal cord and brainstem to synapse in the thalamus. Finally, show that the thalamus projects to the sensory cortex. Note that whereas the posterior column pathway ascends the spinal cord ipsilateral to its side of origin, the anterolateral system ascends the spinal cord contralateral to its side of origin.

Lastly, let's draw the cell bodies and pathway for the lateral corticospinal tract. Indicate that the first-order neuron lies in the motor cortex, most notably, but also in the premotor and sensory cortices, and then that the second-order neuron lies within the contralateral anterior gray matter horn of the spinal cord. Now, show that lateral corticospinal fibers descend from the motor cortex through the ipsilateral brainstem, decussate within the medullary pyramids at the cervicomedullary junction, and then descend through the spinal cord in the lateral corticospinal tract to synapse in spinal motor neurons. Then, show that motor neurons project nerve fibers via the anterior nerve root, which joins the posterior nerve root to form a mixed spinal nerve.[2,4-12]

Posterior column pathway - PCP
Anterolateral system - ALS
Lateral corticospinal tract - CST

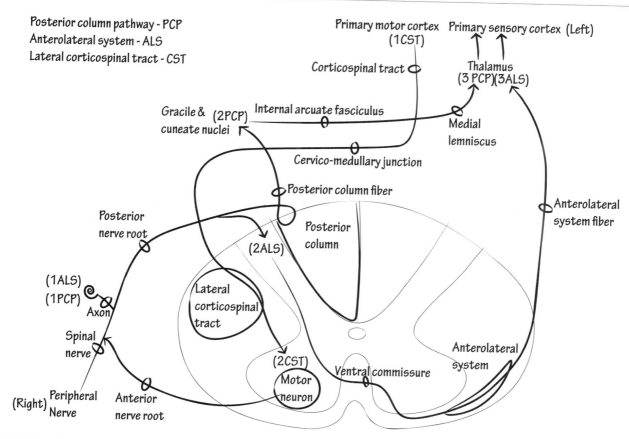

DRAWING 7-4 Major Ascending & Descending Tracts

Spinocerebellar Pathways *(Advanced)*

Here we will draw the spinocerebellar pathways, which carry proprioceptive sensory information to the cerebellum for the coordination of movement and the maintenance of posture. The spinocerebellar pathways comprise the posterior, anterior, and rostral spinocerebellar tracts, and the cuneocerebellar tract. Except for the cuneocerebellar tract, all of the spinocerebellar tracts synapse within the spinal cord (generally within the intermediate zone of the gray matter) prior to reaching the cerebellum. The posterior and anterior spinocerebellar pathways are the best understood of these pathways; we will draw them first.

Draw an axial cross-section through the spinal cord. In the corner of the diagram, write the words "tract" and "origin." We will list the origin of each spinocerebellar pathway as we complete our diagram. First, indicate that the posterior spinocerebellar tract originates from afferents of the lower trunk and lower limb. Now, to draw the posterior spinocerebellar tract course, draw a peripheral nerve and show its central process synapse in the intermediate zone of the spinal cord from T1 to L2 in a region called the dorsal nucleus of Clarke. The majority of the posterior spinocerebellar tract afferent fibers arise from below the L2 spinal level, ascend in the posterior funiculus, and then make their synapse in the dorsal nucleus of Clarke. Now, show that the dorsal nucleus of Clarke projects via the ipsilateral inferior cerebellar peduncle to enter the cerebellum.

Next, let's draw the anterior spinocerebellar tract. Indicate that it originates from afferents of the lower limb. Then, to draw the anterior spinocerebellar tract course, show the central process of a peripheral nerve fiber synapse at the L3 to L5 levels of the spinal cord. The course of the anterior spinocerebellar tract is quite long and involves a double decussation. Indicate that the anterior spinocerebellar tract projects from L3 to L5 across midline within the ventral commissure, ascends the spinal cord and brainstem within the anterior spinocerebellar tract, enters the cerebellum within the superior cerebellar peduncle, and then decussates again within the cerebellum to terminate on its side of origin (although a small portion of fibers terminate in the contralateral cerebellum and do not make this last decussation). Thus, through this double decussation, the anterior spinocerebellar tract remains ipsilateral to its side of origin. Note that, generally, the inferior and middle cerebellar peduncles are the inflow pathways into the cerebellum and the superior cerebellar peduncle is the outflow pathway for fibers from the cerebellum—the anterior spinocerebellar pathway is an important exception to this rule.

Now, let's draw the cuneocerebellar tract. Indicate that the cuneocerebellar tract originates in the upper limb and upper trunk. Then, just beneath the inferior cerebellar peduncle, label the lateral cuneate nucleus (aka accessory cuneate nucleus)—the first synapse of the cuneocerebellar tract. Next, to draw the cuneocerebellar tract course, show the central process of a peripheral nerve fiber enter the posterior column and directly ascend the spinal cord to the lateral cuneate nucleus. Then, indicate that the cuneocerebellar fibers project from the lateral cuneate nucleus through the ipsilateral inferior cerebellar peduncle to enter the cerebellum.

Finally, let's draw our last pathway, the rostral spinocerebellar tract. Indicate that it originates in the upper limb. Then, to draw the rostral spinocerebellar tract course, show the central process of a peripheral nerve synapse at the C4 to C8 spinal levels. Indicate that along a poorly described course, fibers project from the C4 to C8 spinal levels to the cerebellum via the ipsilateral inferior cerebellar peduncle.[2,4-12]

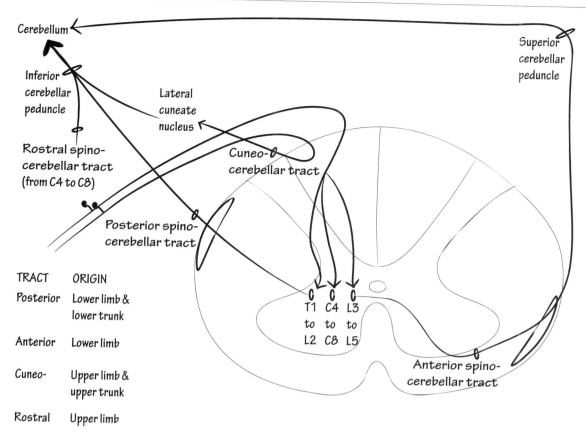

Cerebellum

Inferior
cerebellar
peduncle

Lateral
cuneate
nucleus

Superior
cerebellar
peduncle

Rostral spino-
cerebellar tract
(from C4 to C8)

Cuneo-
cerebellar tract

Posterior spino-
cerebellar tract

T1   C4   L3
to   to   to
L2   C8   L5

Anterior spino-
cerebellar tract

TRACT	ORIGIN
Posterior	Lower limb & lower trunk
Anterior	Lower limb
Cuneo-	Upper limb & upper trunk
Rostral	Upper limb

DRAWING 7-5 **Spinocerebellar Pathways**

Spinal Cord Disorders

Case I

Patient presents with years of progressive "lightning-like" pain in the lower extremities. Exam reveals profound lower extremity loss of vibration/proprioception sensation with preserved pain/temperature sensation and preserved strength in the lower extremities. There is areflexia in the lower extremities. The upper extremities are normal.

Show that the loss of vibration/proprioception sensation with preserved pain/temperature sensation and preserved motor function suggests posterior column spinal cord involvement. The lower extremity areflexia suggests lower motor neuron involvement, so also show that there is dorsal root involvement. The dorsal root involvement causes the lancinating pain—presumably from irritation of the pain/temperature fibers.

Indicate that this constellation of deficits suggests a diagnosis of tabes dorsalis (aka syphilitic myelopathy), in which the posterior columns and dorsal roots are affected.[15-21]

Case II

Patient presents with an abrupt onset of interscapular pain, lower extremity weakness, sensory disturbance, and bowel and bladder incontinence. Exam reveals areflexia of the lower extremities; paraparesis; loss of pain/temperature sensation with preserved vibration/proprioception sensation in the lower extremities; anal sphincter atonia; and a normal motor, sensory, and reflex exam in the upper extremities.

Show that the sudden weakness and areflexia suggests bilateral anterior motor horn cell involvement, and that the longitudinal loss of pain/temperature sensation suggests involvement of the anterolateral system with preservation of the posterior columns.

Indicate that this constellation of deficits suggests anterior spinal artery ischemia, in which the anterior two thirds of the spinal cord are affected. Note that this syndrome variably affects the lateral corticospinal tracts. The most common site of anterior spinal artery ischemia is at the T4 level.[18-22]

Case III

Patient presents with sudden weakness on the right side of the body and sensory disturbance. Exam reveals right-side weakness, right-side loss of vibration/proprioception sensation, and left-side loss of pain/temperature sensation. Reflexes are absent on the right side and normal on the left.

Show that the right-side hemi-body weakness suggests right-side corticospinal tract involvement; that the right-side loss of vibration/proprioception suggests right-side posterior column tract involvement; that the left-side loss of pain/temperature sensation suggests right-side anterolateral system involvement; and that the right-side areflexia suggests right-side lower motor neuron involvement, which could occur from either anterior or posterior horn injury.

Indicate that this constellation of deficits suggests a hemi-cord syndrome involving the right half of the spinal cord, called Brown-Séquard syndrome.[18-21]

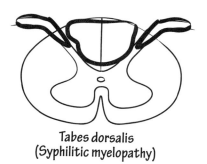

Tabes dorsalis
(Syphilitic myelopathy)

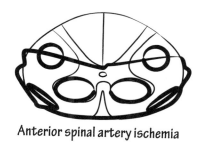

Anterior spinal artery ischemia

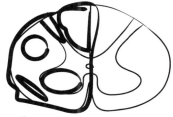

Brown Sequard syndrome

DRAWING 7-6 **Spinal Cord Disorders—Partial**

Spinal Cord Disorders (Cont.)

Case IV

Patient presents with a few-month course of progressive burning pain across the shoulders. Exam reveals weakness of the upper extremities; absent biceps reflexes with hyperreflexia of lower extremities; pathologic (ie, positive) Babinski's; absent pain/temperature sensation across the upper chest and limbs with preserved vibration/proprioception sensation.

Show that the dissociation of loss of pain/temperature sensation with preserved vibration/proprioception sensation in a suspended sensory level suggests damage to the crossing anterolateral system fibers. Show that the loss of strength and areflexia of the upper limbs in that same segment suggests bilateral anterior motor horn damage.

Indicate that this constellation of deficits suggests a central cord syndrome, often a syringomyelia.

Syringomyelia is a fluid-filled cavity within the spinal cord, which may be limited to a dilatation of the central canal, may extend outside of the central canal, or may be separate from the central canal, entirely. It causes lower motor neuron signs at the level of the lesion, impaired pain/temperature sensation but preserved vibration/proprioception in a segmental distribution (classically, in a cape-like distribution across the arms and upper trunk): a so-called suspended sensory level, and upper motor neuron signs below the level of the lesion.[18–21]

Case V

Patient presents with a few-month course of trunk and lower limb sensory dysesthesias. Exam reveals hyperreflexia throughout except for absent ankle jerks; pathologic (ie, positive) Babinski's; loss of vibration/proprioception sensation in the lower extremities with preserved pain/temperature sensation; and mild, diffuse lower extremity weakness.

Show that the loss of vibration/proprioception sensation with preserved pain/temperature sensation suggests posterior column involvement. Then, show that the diffuse motor weakness is due to corticospinal tract involvement.

Indicate that this combination of deficits is often found in subacute combined degeneration due to vitamin B12 deficiency. Subacute combined degeneration affects the posterior and lateral columns. Although not mentioned, gait ataxia is often present in this disorder and may be due to the profound vibration/proprioception sensory loss or due to posterior spinocerebellar tract involvement from lateral column pathology. B12 deficiency also often causes a superimposed neuropathy, which explains the absent ankle jerks.[18–21,23,24]

Case VI (*Advanced*)

Patient presents with longstanding gait disturbance and weakness. Exam shows lower extremity areflexia with preserved upper extremity reflexes; pathologic (ie, positive) Babinski's; profound ataxia; vibration/proprioception sensory loss out of proportion to pain/temperature sensory loss; and motor weakness of the upper and lower extremities.

First, show that the mixed reflex pattern in the presence of pathologic Babinski's suggests a mixed upper and lower motor neuron disease pattern with pathology of the dorsal nerve roots and dorsal horns. Then, show that

the vibration/proprioception sensory loss with preserved pain/temperature sensation suggests posterior column involvement. Next, show that the profound ataxia suggests spinocerebellar tract involvement. And finally, indicate that the motor weakness suggests corticospinal tract involvement.

Indicate that this constellation of deficits is found in Friedreich's ataxia, an inherited progressive ataxia with pathology that first appears in the dorsal roots. Spinocerebellar tract involvement is an important distinguishing feature of this disorder.[18–21]

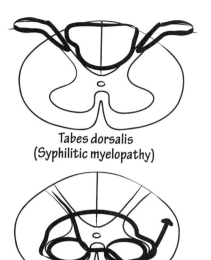

**Tabes dorsalis
(Syphilitic myelopathy)**

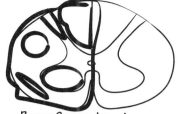

Anterior spinal artery ischemia

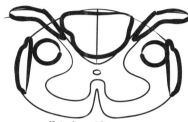

Brown Sequard syndrome

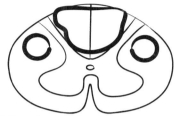

**Central cord syndrome
(often Syringomyelia)**

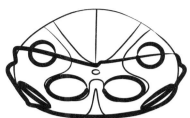

**Subacute combined degeneration
(Vitamin B12 deficiency)**

Friedreich's ataxia

DRAWING 7-7 **Spinal Cord Disorders—Partial**

Spinal Cord Disorders (Cont.)

Case VII

Patient presents with a several-month course of weakness that began in the left arm and has since spread to both arms and legs. Exam reveals asymmetric but diffuse upper and lower extremity weakness. There is mixed hyperreflexia and areflexia throughout the bilateral upper and lower extremities. There are bilateral pathologic (ie, positive) Babinski's. Sensory exam is normal.

Show that the presence of motor weakness in conjunction with mixed hyperreflexia and areflexia with bilateral pathologic Babinski's and a normal sensory exam suggests both corticospinal tract and anterior motor horn involvement.

Indicate that this constellation of deficits is often found in amyotrophic lateral sclerosis (aka ALS or Lou Gehrig's disease).[18-21]

Case VIII (*Advanced*)

Patient presents with muscle pains and slowly progressive muscle wasting. Exam reveals asymmetric lower extremity weakness; hyporeflexia in the lower extremities; the absence of pathologic Babinski's (ie, negative Babinski's); and normal sensation.

Show that the weakness in conjunction with hyporeflexia and a normal sensory exam suggests anterior motor horn involvement, only.

Many illnesses cause select anterior horn cell loss. Indicate that two common illnesses that cause this pathology are polio syndrome and spinal muscular atrophy.[18-21]

Case IX (*Advanced*)

Patient presents with slowly progressive lower extremity weakness. Exam reveals spastic weakness of the lower extremities more so than the upper extremities; hyperreflexia; bilateral pathologic (ie, positive) Babinski's; gait ataxia; and a normal sensory exam.

Show that the weakness in conjunction with spasticity, hyperreflexia, bilateral pathologic Babinski's, and a normal sensory exam suggests corticospinal tract involvement.

Indicate that select corticospinal tract involvement suggests a diagnosis of primary lateral sclerosis.[18-21]

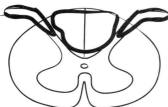

Tabes dorsalis
(Syphilitic myelopathy)

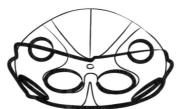

Anterior spinal artery ischemia

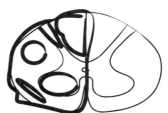

Brown Sequard syndrome

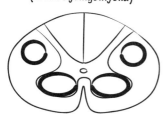

Central cord syndrome
(often Syringomyelia)

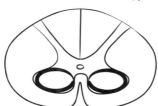

Subacute combined degeneration
(Vitamin B12 deficiency)

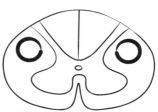

Friedreich's ataxia

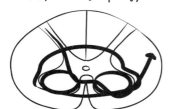

Amyotrophic lateral sclerosis
(aka ALS or Lou Gehrig's disease)

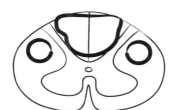

Spinal muscular atrophy,
Polio syndrome

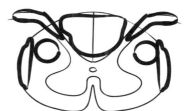

Primary lateral sclerosis

DRAWING 7-8 Spinal Cord Disorders—Complete

References

1. Siegel, A. & Sapru, H. N. *Essential neuroscience* (Lippincott Williams & Wilkins, 2006).
2. Siegel, A. & Sapru, H. N. *Essential neuroscience,* 2nd ed. (Wolters Kluwer Health/Lippincott Williams & Wilkins, 2011).
3. Shimoji, K. O. & Willis, W. D. *Evoked spinal cord potentials: an illustrated guide to physiology, pharmacology, and recording techniques* (Springer, 2006).
4. Watson, C., Paxinos, G., Kayalioglu, G. & Christopher & Dana Reeve Foundation. *The spinal cord: a Christopher and Dana Reeve Foundation text and atlas,* 1st ed. (Elsevier/Academic Press, 2009).
5. Standring, S. & Gray, H. *Gray's anatomy: the anatomical basis of clinical practice,* 40th ed. (Churchill Livingstone/Elsevier, 2008).
6. Pierrot-Deseilligny, E. & Burke, D. J. *The circuitry of the human spinal cord: its role in motor control and movement disorders* (Cambridge University Press, 2005).
7. Patestas, M. A. & Gartner, L. P. *A textbook of neuroanatomy* (Blackwell Pub., 2006).
8. Netter, F. H. & Dalley, A. F. *Atlas of human anatomy,* 2nd ed., Plates 4–7 (Novartis, 1997).
9. Haines, D. E. & Ard, M. D. *Fundamental neuroscience: for basic and clinical applications,* 3rd ed. (Churchill Livingstone Elsevier, 2006).
10. DeMyer, W. *Neuroanatomy,* 2nd ed. (Williams & Wilkins, 1998).
11. Baehr, M., Frotscher, M. & Duus, P. *Duus' topical diagnosis in neurology: anatomy, physiology, signs, symptoms,* 4th completely rev. ed., Chapter 3 (Thieme, 2005).
12. Altman, J. & Bayer, S. A. *Development of the human spinal cord: an interpretation based on experimental studies in animals* (Oxford University Press, 2001).
13. Campbell, W. W., DeJong, R. N. & Haerer, A. F. *DeJong's the neurologic examination: incorporating the fundamentals of neuroanatomy and neurophysiology,* 6th ed. (Lippincott Williams & Wilkins, 2005).
14. Benarroch, E. E. *Basic neurosciences with clinical applications* (Butterworth Heinemann Elsevier, 2006).
15. Larner, A. J. *A dictionary of neurological signs,* 2nd ed. (Springer, 2006).
16. Chilver-Stainer, L., Fischer, U., Hauf, M., Fux, C. A. & Sturzenegger, M. Syphilitic myelitis: rare, nonspecific, but treatable. *Neurology* 72, 673–675 (2009).
17. Berger, J. R. & Sabet, A. Infectious myelopathies. *Semin Neurol* 22, 133–142 (2002).
18. Samuels, M. A., Feske, S. & Daffner, K. R. *Office practice of neurology,* 2nd ed. (Churchill Livingstone, 2003).
19. Rowland, L. P., Pedley, T. A. & Kneass, W. *Merritt's neurology,* 12th ed. (Wolters Kluwer Lippincott Williams & Wilkins, 2010).
20. Ropper, A. H., Adams, R. D., Victor, M. & Samuels, M. A. *Adams and Victor's principles of neurology,* 9th ed. (McGraw-Hill Medical, 2009).
21. Merritt, H. H. & Rowland, L. P. *Merritt's neurology,* 10th ed. (Lippincott Williams & Wilkins, 2000).
22. Takahashi, S. O. *Neurovascular imaging: MRI & microangiography* (Springer, 2010).
23. Paul, I. & Reichard, R. R. Subacute combined degeneration mimicking traumatic spinal cord injury. *Am J Forensic Med Pathol* 30, 47–48 (2009).
24. Kumar, A. & Singh, A. K. Teaching NeuroImage: Inverted V sign in subacute combined degeneration of spinal cord. *Neurology* 72, e4 (2009).

8

Spinal Canal and Muscle–Nerve Physiology

Know-It Points

The Spinal Canal

- The vertebral column contains 33 vertebrae and 31 spinal nerves.
- The spinal cord ends at the L1–L2 vertebral column level.
- Motor and sensory roots combine within an intervertebral neural foramen at each level to form a mixed spinal nerve.
- Only the C1 through C7 nerve roots exit above their related vertebral bodies, the rest exit beneath them.

- The collection of nerve fibers in the caudal spinal canal is the cauda equina.
- The distal, bulbous region of the spinal cord is the conus medullaris.
- The site of fluid collection during a lumbar puncture is the lumbar cistern, which is the subarachnoid space below the level of the spinal cord.

The Muscle Stretch Reflex

- The muscle spindle sends an excitatory volley along the type Ia sensory afferent, which directly innervates the motor neuron.
- Through the inhibitory neurotransmitter glycine, Renshaw cells inhibit the antagonist reflex from firing.
- Muscle spindle fibers have a lower threshold to fire than Golgi tendon organs, which is the

basis for the termination of the muscle stretch reflex.
- The biceps reflex involves C5, C6.
- The triceps reflex involves C7, C8.
- The patellar reflex involves L2–L4.
- The Achilles reflex involves S1, S2.

Muscle–Nerve Physiology (*Advanced*)

- Aγ motor neurons project to the muscle spindles to stimulate muscle tone.
- Initially, when supraspinal input to the Aγ motor neurons is disrupted, muscle tone becomes flaccid; days or weeks later, spasticity develops.
- Skeletal muscle fibers outside of the capsule are extrafusal fibers and are innervated by the Aα motor nerves.
- Intrafusal fibers lie within the muscle spindle and are innervated by the Aγ motor nerves.

- The largest peripheral nerve fibers are 12 to 22 micrometers in diameter and conduct at 70 to 120 meters per second.
- The smallest peripheral nerve fibers are less than 1 micrometer in diameter and conduct at less than 2 meters per second.
- Saltatory conduction is the firing of impulses in the interspaces between segments of myelin: the nodes of Ranvier.

Nerve Roots & Rami

- The ventral root carries motor fibers and the dorsal root carries sensory fibers.
- The dorsal root ganglion lies within the intervertebral foramen along the posterior nerve root; it houses the cell bodies of sensory nerves.
- Sensory cell bodies are pseudo-unipolar: they contain a short axon with bipolar processes that pass both centrally and peripherally.
- Just distal to the dorsal root ganglion, the anterior and posterior roots join to form a mixed spinal nerve, which then separates into dorsal and ventral rami.

- Dorsal rami innervate the paraspinal muscles and provide sensory coverage to the back of the head and posterior trunk.
- Ventral rami provide motor and sensory innervation to a widespread group of muscles and sensory areas, including the anterior trunk and upper and lower limbs.
- Impulses travel up the white ramus (myelinated) to the paravertebral sympathetic ganglion and then down the gray ramus (unmyelinated) back to the ventral ramus.

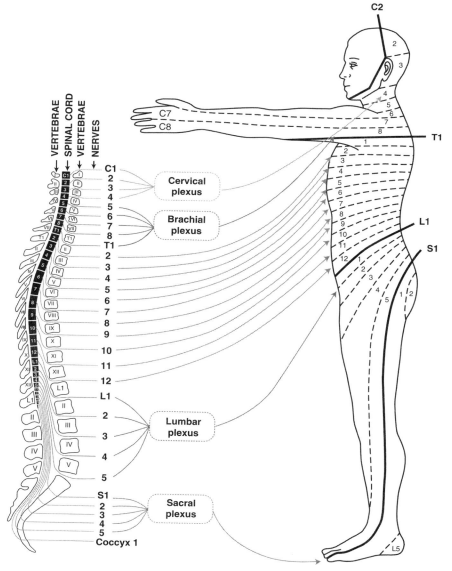

FIGURE 8-1 Segmental organization of the spinal canal and the peripheral nerves. Used with permission from Altman, Joseph, and Shirley A. Bayer. *Development of the Human Spinal Cord: An Interpretation Based on Experimental Studies in Animals.* Oxford; New York: Oxford University Press, 2001.

The Spinal Canal

Here, we will draw a sagittal view of the spinal canal, which encases the spinal cord and spinal nerve roots. To begin, draw a sagittal section through the brainstem and then the spinal cord. Indicate that the cervical segment of the spinal cord angles anteriorly; the thoracic segment angles posteriorly; and the lumbosacral and coccygeal segments angle anteriorly, again.

The vertebral column contains 33 vertebrae: 7 cervical, 12 thoracic, and 5 lumbar vertebrae, and then the vertebral fusions that constitute the sacrum and coccyx. The spinal cord ends at the L1–L2 vertebral column level; thus the spinal cord is shorter than the spinal canal, and therefore, at any vertical height, the spinal cord level is lower than the surrounding vertebral level. Now, show the following vertebral bodies: C1, C2, C7, T1, T12, and L1; then, show that there is hyperflexion of the sacral column at the clinically important L5–S1 junction, a common site of nerve root compression; then, show that S5 angles further posteriorly; and finally show that the coccyx angles back anteriorly.[1]

A pair of motor and sensory roots exit the spinal cord at each level and combine within an intervertebral neural foramen to form a spinal nerve. There are a total of 31 spinal nerves: 8 cervical, 12 thoracic, 5 lumbar, 5 sacral, and 1 coccygeal. Show that the first cervical spinal nerve, C1, exits below the skull (beneath the foramen magnum) and above the first cervical vertebra. Then, indicate that C2 exits above its vertebra, and so on—show that C7 exits above the C7 vertebra, which is the lowermost cervical vertebra. As mentioned, however, there are 8 cervical spinal nerves, so show that C8 exits underneath the C7 vertebra and above the T1 vertebra. Where, then, must the T1 nerve exit? Show that the T1 spinal nerve exits below its corresponding vertebra because C8 fills the space above it. Then, show that T12 exits beneath the T12 body, L1 beneath L1, L5 under L5, S1 under S1, S5 under S5, and the coccygeal nerve exits underneath the coccyx. Only C1 through C7 exit above their related vertebral bodies; the rest exit beneath them.

Now, let's label a few important caudal spinal canal structures. Indicate that the collection of nerve fibers that traverses the caudal spinal canal is the cauda equina, which is the Latin term "tail of the horse." Then, indicate that the anatomically related, threadlike fibrous tissue that extends from the distal tip of the spinal cord through the caudal spinal canal is the filum terminale. Finally, label the most distal, bulbous region of the spinal cord as the conus medullaris. The cauda equina and conus medullaris each have related syndromes, which are self-named. Cauda equina syndrome is a lower motor neuron syndrome, whereas conus medullaris syndrome is an upper motor neuron syndrome. Injury to both the cauda equina and conus medullaris causes mixed upper and lower motor neuron disease.

Next, let's label the meningeal coverings of the spinal canal. First, label the surface of the spinal cord as the pia mater. Then, draw a combined layer of dura and underlying arachnoid mater. Show that there is plenty of separation between these meningeal coverings and the underlying pia mater. Label the naturally occurring space between the arachnoid and pia mater layers as the subarachnoid space. Then, show that the site of fluid collection during a lumbar puncture is in the lumbar cistern, the subarachnoid space below the level of the spinal cord. Finally, draw the vertebral arch (the posterior portion of the vertebral column), and between it and the dura mater, label the epidural space. Note that although we have only labeled the posterior aspect of the epidural space, here, throughout the spinal canal, the spinal epidural space exists superficial to the dura mater and internal to the periosteal lining of the vertebral canal. The spinal epidural space is a common site for hematoma, infection, and spread of neoplastic disease.[2–4]

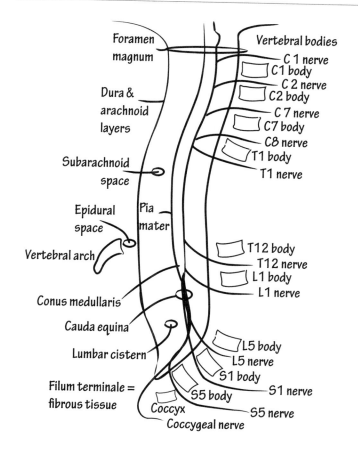

Foramen magnum

Vertebral bodies

Dura & arachnoid layers

Subarachnoid space

Epidural space

Pia mater

Vertebral arch

Conus medullaris

Cauda equina

Lumbar cistern

Filum terminale = fibrous tissue

Coccyx

C 1 nerve
C1 body
C 2 nerve
C2 body
C 7 nerve
C7 body
C8 nerve
T1 body
T1 nerve

T12 body
T12 nerve
L1 body
L1 nerve

L5 body
L5 nerve
S1 body
S5 body   S1 nerve
S5 nerve
Coccygeal nerve

DRAWING 8-1 The Spinal Canal

The Muscle Stretch Reflex

Here, we will draw a muscle stretch reflex (aka myotatic or deep tendon reflex). First, draw an axial cross-section through the spinal cord. Then, draw a lower extremity that is flexed at the knee and show a knee extensor muscle fiber of the quadriceps muscle group at the top of the thigh and a knee flexor fiber of the hamstrings muscle group at the bottom of the thigh: we use the knee extensor reflex as our example, here. Next, denote the location of the related motor neurons within the anterior horn of the spinal cord. Now, draw a muscle spindle and show a type Ia sensory fiber project from it to the extensor motor neuron. Then, draw an Aα motor fiber projection from the extensor motor neuron to the representative extrafusal extensor fiber. In large muscle groups, such as the quadriceps, a single motor neuron commands as many as 1,000 extrafusal muscle fibers, whereas in small muscle groups, such as the extraocular muscles, a motor neuron commands as few as 10 extrafusal muscle fibers. Show that when the patellar tendon is stretched with the tap of a reflex hammer, the muscle spindle sends an excitatory volley along the type Ia sensory afferent, which excites the extensor motor neuron and nerve, and the muscle extensor contracts so the knee extends.[5,6]

If the hamstrings were also activated (meaning, if the extensor and flexors shortened simultaneously), the thigh would only stiffen and not move. So, now, draw a Renshaw cell (an interneuron) in the anterior horn of the gray matter of the spinal cord, and show that through the inhibitory neurotransmitter glycine, the Renshaw cell inhibits the flexor motor neuron from firing.

Interneurons are the lynchpins to more complicated spinal reflexes, as well, such as the triple flexor reflex, which has the following sequential mechanics: a painful stimulus to the bottom of the foot causes reflex upward flexion of the affected foot (aka foot dorsiflexion) with simultaneous flexion of the knee and the hip. In order for us to remain upright when we undergo the triple flexor reflex, our opposite leg must bear our weight. Thus, through a simultaneous but opposing reflex in our opposite leg, the crossed extension reflex, our non-affected foot flexes downward and our non-affected hip and knee extend.

Now, let's show how to terminate the muscle stretch reflex; bear in mind that there are a number of neurobiological influences on the relaxation of muscle contraction, which include myosin ATPase and calcium re-accumulation into the endoplasmic reticulum, which we will not draw, here. Delay in the relaxation phase of the muscle stretch reflex (aka Woltman's sign) is observed in symptomatic hypothyroidism. Re-draw our muscle stretch reflex arrangement but exclude the flexor neuron and its motor fiber. Then, label a Golgi tendon organ where the quadriceps tendon inserts into the patella. Next, show that a type Ib fiber projects from the Golgi tendon organ to the Renshaw interneuron. Now, show an inhibitory fiber project from the interneuron to the quadriceps (extensor) motor neuron. The type Ia and Ib fibers fire at the same rate, but muscle spindle fibers have a much lower threshold to fire than Golgi tendon organs. Thus, the muscle spindle fires first, and then later the Golgi tendon organ fires, which terminates the muscle stretch reflex. This completes our diagram.

For reference, the commonly tested muscle stretch reflexes are the biceps, which involves the C5, C6 nerve roots; the triceps, which involves the C7, C8 nerve roots; the patella (drawn here), which involves the L2 to L4 nerve roots; and the Achilles, which involves the S1, S2 nerve roots.[2,4,7–10]

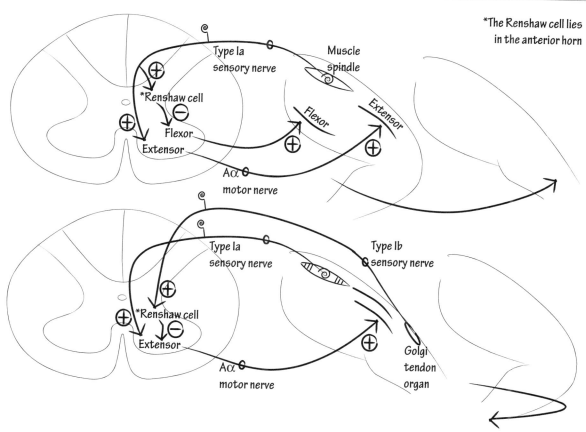

*The Renshaw cell lies in the anterior horn

DRAWING 8-2 **The Muscle Stretch Reflex**

Muscle–Nerve Physiology (*Advanced*)

Here, let's address muscle tone, the muscle spindle, and peripheral nerve classification. We begin with muscle tone. Re-draw our Aα motor reflex loop: draw the spinal cord and lower extremity and then show the muscle spindle project via a type Ia sensory afferent to excite the motoneuron, which projects via an Aα motor nerve to excite the extrafusal muscle fiber. Next, label an Aγ motor neuron in the anterior gray matter and show that it projects to the muscle spindle. The Aγ motor neurons stimulate muscle tone. Finally, draw a supraspinal projection to the Aγ motor neuron to show that supraspinal centers send descending excitatory inputs to the Aγ motor neurons. Initially, when supraspinal input to the Aγ motor neurons is disrupted, muscle tone becomes flaccid; it is not until days or weeks later that spasticity develops.

Now, let's draw the muscle spindle anatomy. Begin with the connective tissue-enclosed muscle spindle capsule. Next, label the skeletal muscle fibers outside of the capsule as extrafusal fibers; these fibers produce limb movement and they are innervated by the Aα motor nerves. Now, draw several intrafusal fibers within the muscle spindle; they are innervated by the Aγ motor nerves. Then, within the central, non-contractile portion of the muscle spindle, draw nuclei clustered together like marbles in a bag and label this as the nuclear bag fiber; next, draw a row of nuclei like pearls on a chain and label this as the nuclear chain fiber. Both fiber types exist within the muscle spindle and they each are attuned to different aspects of muscle tone.

Next, let's address the type Ia and type II sensory afferents of the muscle spindle. Show an annulospiral sensory nerve ending around the non-contractile, central portion of both the nuclear bag and nuclear chain fibers; the annulospiral nerve ending connects to the type Ia sensory afferent fiber. Then, show that flower spray sensory nerve endings connect the type II fibers to the nuclear chain fibers. However, to complicate matters, two forms of nuclear bag fiber actually exist, bag$_1$

and bag$_2$—the latter shares many similarities with nuclear chain fibers. Indicate, now, that in addition to attaching to chain fibers, the type II sensory afferents also attach to bag$_2$ fibers.

Now, let's address the efferent innervation of the muscle spindle. The Aγ motor nerves terminate in either plate or trail endings in the polar region of the muscle spindle along the intrafusal muscle fibers. Indicate that, generally, plate endings lie along nuclear bag fibers and trail endings lie along nuclear chain fibers and bag$_2$ fibers. The bag$_1$ fibers act when there is a change in muscle fiber length, during the dynamic phase, whereas the chain fibers and bag$_2$ fibers act when muscle length is unchanged, during the static phase.

Lastly, let's address the classification of peripheral nerves. Two classification schemes are commonly used: the Gasser scheme, which applies to all nerve types—motor, sensory, and autonomic, and the Lloyd scheme, which applies to sensory nerves, only. The two schemes are fairly redundant, however, and can be learned together. We will only list the largest and smallest fibers, here, but the table in Drawing 8-3 is complete for reference. Label the top row of our table as the Gasser nerve class, Lloyd nerve class, diameter, and speed (ie, conduction velocity). Make a notation that the diameter units are micrometers and the speed units are meters per second. List the largest fiber type as Gasser class Aα and Lloyd class Ia and Ib; indicate that they are 12 to 22 micrometers (μm) in diameter and conduct at 70 to 120 meters per second (m/s). Then, label the smallest fibers as Gasser class C and Lloyd class IV, and show that they are less than 1 μm in diameter and conduct at less than 2 m/s. Impulses slowly ascend the small unmyelinated nerve axons, whereas they quickly ascend the large, heavily myelinated nerve fibers because impulses of myelinated fibers fire only in the interspaces between segments of myelin—the nodes of Ranvier; this pattern of firing is called saltatory conduction.[1,2,4,5,9–16]

MUSCLE TONE

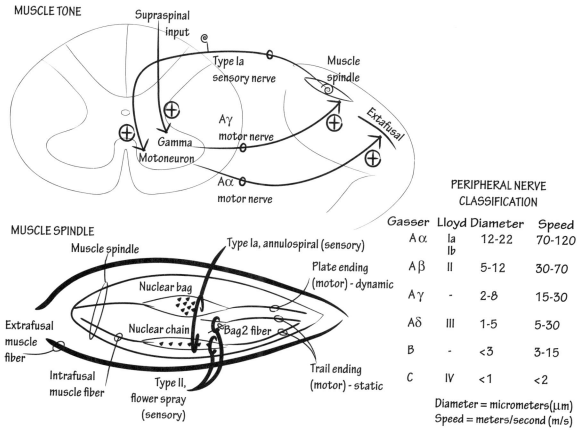

MUSCLE SPINDLE

PERIPHERAL NERVE CLASSIFICATION

Gasser	Lloyd	Diameter	Speed
A α	Ia Ib	12-22	70-120
A β	II	5-12	30-70
A γ	-	2-8	15-30
A δ	III	1-5	5-30
B	-	<3	3-15
C	IV	<1	<2

Diameter = micrometers(μm)
Speed = meters/second (m/s)

DRAWING 8-3 **Muscle–Nerve Physiology**

Nerve Roots & Rami

To draw the anatomy of the nerve roots and rami, first draw an outline of an axial cross-section through the spinal cord. Then, draw the spinal cord dorsal and ventral gray matter horns. Next, draw the anterior-lying vertebral body. Then, draw the pedicle on the right side of the page but leave out the pedicle on the left; otherwise we would obstruct our view of the dorsal root ganglion, which sits in the intervertebral foramen, underneath the pedicle. Next, draw the transverse processes, then the laminae, and finally the spinous process. We leave out the articular processes, which form facet joints between the vertebral arches.

Now, draw an anterior horn cell on the right side of the spinal cord (the left side of the page) and show a ventral root emerge from it. The ventral root carries motor fibers. Next, show a dorsal root enter the dorsal horn: it carries sensory fibers. As mentioned, underlying the pedicle is the intervertebral foramen. Within the intervertebral foramen, attach a dorsal root ganglion to the posterior nerve root. The dorsal root ganglion houses the cell bodies of sensory nerves. Sensory cell bodies are pseudo-unipolar because they contain a short axon with bipolar processes that pass both centrally and peripherally. Next, just distal to the dorsal root ganglion, indicate that the anterior and posterior roots join to form a mixed spinal nerve, which then separates into dorsal and ventral rami.

In brief, dorsal rami innervate the paraspinal muscles and provide sensory coverage to the back of the head and posterior trunk, whereas the ventral rami provide motor and sensory innervation to a far more widespread group of muscles and sensory areas, including the anterior trunk and upper and lower limbs.

Show a representative thoracic nerve originate from the anterior ramus and pass along the chest wall to form an intercostal nerve. Now, turn your attention back to where the rami split to draw the sympathetic ganglion and related autonomic rami. Along the ventral ramus, attach the white ramus, so named because it is myelinated. Then, more proximally, just past the takeoff of the dorsal ramus, attach the gray ramus, which is unmyelinated. Indicate that the gray and white rami meet in a paravertebral sympathetic ganglion. Sympathetic ganglia form two long chains that flank the vertebral column; the sympathetic cell bodies lie within the intermediolateral cell column of the spinal cord and project to the paravertebral sympathetic chains.

Finally, show an impulse travel along the ventral ramus and then up the white ramus to the paravertebral sympathetic ganglion. Then, show it pass down the gray ramus back to the ventral ramus. From there, the impulse disseminates along either the dorsal ramus or the ventral ramus.[2,4,7,17]

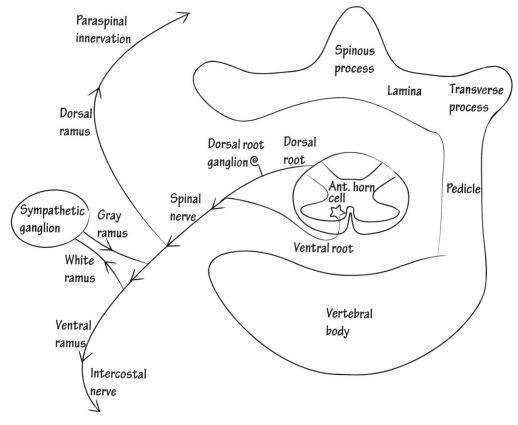

DRAWING 8-4 **Nerve Roots & Rami**

References

1. Bruni, J. E. & Montemurro, D. G. *Human neuroanatomy: a text, brain atlas, and laboratory dissection guide* (Oxford University Press, 2009).

2. Standring, S. & Gray, H. *Gray's anatomy: the anatomical basis of clinical practice,* 40th ed. (Churchill Livingstone/Elsevier, 2008).

3. Netter, F. H. & Dalley, A. F. *Atlas of human anatomy,* 2nd ed., Plates 4–7 (Novartis, 1997).

4. Haines, D. E. & Ard, M. D. *Fundamental neuroscience: for basic and clinical applications,* 3rd ed. (Churchill Livingstone Elsevier, 2006).

5. MacIntosh, B. R., Gardiner, P. F. & McComas, A. J. *Skeletal muscle: form and function,* 2nd ed. (Human Kinetics, 2006).

6. Conn, P. M. *Neuroscience in medicine,* 3rd ed. (Humana Press, 2008).

7. Preston, D. C. & Shapiro, B. E. *Electromyography and neuromuscular disorders: clinical-electrophysiologic correlations,* 2nd ed. (Elsevier Butterworth-Heinemann, 2005).

8. Perotto, A. & Delagi, E. F. *Anatomical guide for the electromyographer: the limbs and trunk,* 4th ed. (Charles C Thomas, 2005).

9. Mendell, J. R., Kissel, J. T. & Cornblath, D. R. *Diagnosis and management of peripheral nerve disorders* (Oxford University Press, 2001).

10. Nielsen, J. B., Crone, C. & Hultborn, H. The spinal pathophysiology of spasticity—from a basic science point of view. *Acta Physiol (Oxf)* 189, 171–180 (2007).

11. Siegel, A. & Sapru, H. N. *Essential neuroscience,* 2nd ed. (Wolters Kluwer Health/Lippincott Williams & Wilkins, 2011).

12. Robinson, A. J. & Snyder-Mackler, L. *Clinical electrophysiology: electrotherapy and electrophysiologic testing,* 3rd ed. (Wolters Kluwer/Lippincott Williams & Wilkins, 2008).

13. Pierrot-Deseilligny, E. & Burke, D. J. *The circuitry of the human spinal cord: its role in motor control and movement disorders* (Cambridge University Press, 2005).

14. Khurana, I. *Textbook of medical physiology* (Elsevier, 2006).

15. Enoka, R. M. *Neuromechanics of human movement,* 4th ed. (Human Kinetics, 2008).

16. DiGiovanna, E. L., Schiowitz, S. & Dowling, D. J. *An osteopathic approach to diagnosis and treatment,* 3rd ed. (Lippincott Williams and Wilkins, 2005).

17. DeMyer, W. *Neuroanatomy,* 2nd ed. (Williams & Wilkins, 1998).

9

Brainstem

Part One

Know-It Points

Brainstem Composite—Axial View

- The axial plane of the brainstem divides from anterior to posterior into a basis, tegmentum, and tectum.
- Within the basis lie the corticopontine, corticonuclear, and corticospinal tracts, and most of the supplementary motor nuclei.
- In the anterior tegmentum lie the medial lemniscus, anterolateral system, and trigeminothalamic tracts.
- In the posterior tegmentum lie the cranial nerve nuclei and neurobehavioral cells.
- Additional tegmental structures are the reticular formation, supplementary motor and sensory tracts, and the brainstem auditory components.
- The tectum is the roof of the brainstem and includes the superior and inferior colliculi.

The Midbrain

- The substantia nigra contains dopaminergic nuclei; it lies within the basis just posterior to the white matter pathways.
- The superior cerebellar peduncle decussates in the central midbrain tegmentum in the inferior midbrain.
- The periaqueductal gray area contains opioids, which function in pain suppression.
- The reticular formation divides into lateral, medial, and median zones.
- The raphe nuclei populate the median zone of the reticular formation and are primarily serotinergic.
- The central tegmental tract carries ascending reticular fibers to the rostral intralaminar nuclei of the thalamus as part of the ascending arousal system and descending fibers from the red nucleus to the inferior olive as part of the triangle of Guillain-Mollaret.
- The superior colliculi lie in the upper midbrain and are involved in visual function.
- The inferior colliculi lie in the lower midbrain and are involved in auditory function.

The Pons

- The pontine nuclei send pontocerebellar tracts into the cerebellum via the middle cerebellar peduncle as part of the corticopontocerebellar pathway.
- Corticospinal tract fibers descend through the pontine basis.
- The cerebrospinal fluid space of the pons is the fourth ventricle and the central gray area surrounds it.
- Locus coeruleus nuclei are most heavily concentrated in the pons and they are nearly entirely noradrenergic.

The Medulla

- The descending corticospinal tract fibers populate the medullary pyramids.
- In the lower medulla, internal arcuate fibers originate from the gracile and cuneate nuclei and form the great sensory decussation.
- The inferior olive receives tracts from the spinal cord (from below) and from the red nucleus (from above).
- The olivary nuclei send climbing fibers to the contralateral dentate nucleus of the cerebellum, which projects back to the contralateral red nucleus to complete the triangle of Guillain-Mollaret.
- Along the anterior border of the fourth ventricle (in its inferior floor) lies the area postrema.

Brain Stem, Thalamus, and Striatum (1.5X)— Anterior Aspect

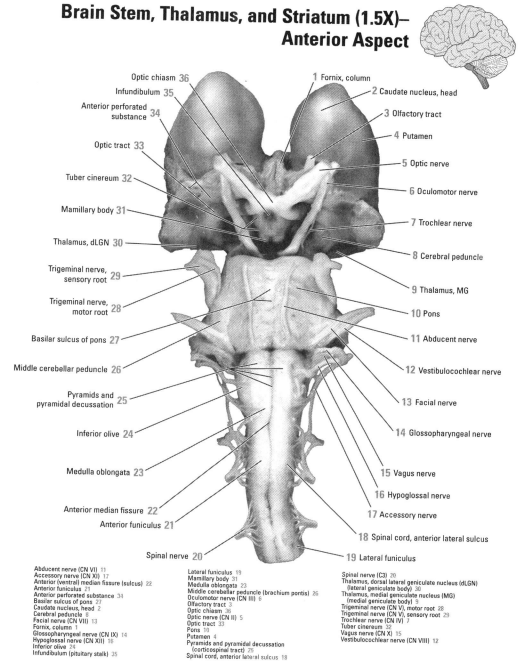

Optic chiasm 36
Infundibulum 35
Anterior perforated substance 34
Optic tract 33
Tuber cinereum 32
Mamillary body 31
Thalamus, dLGN 30
Trigeminal nerve, sensory root 29
Trigeminal nerve, motor root 28
Basilar sulcus of pons 27
Middle cerebellar peduncle 26
Pyramids and pyramidal decussation 25
Inferior olive 24
Medulla oblongata 23
Anterior median fissure 22
Anterior funiculus 21
Spinal nerve 20

1 Fornix, column
2 Caudate nucleus, head
3 Olfactory tract
4 Putamen
5 Optic nerve
6 Oculomotor nerve
7 Trochlear nerve
8 Cerebral peduncle
9 Thalamus, MG
10 Pons
11 Abducent nerve
12 Vestibulocochlear nerve
13 Facial nerve
14 Glossopharyngeal nerve
15 Vagus nerve
16 Hypoglossal nerve
17 Accessory nerve
18 Spinal cord, anterior lateral sulcus
19 Lateral funiculus

Abducent nerve (CN VI) 11
Accessory nerve (CN XI) 17
Anterior (ventral) median fissure (sulcus) 22
Anterior funiculus 21
Anterior perforated substance 34
Basilar sulcus of pons 27
Caudate nucleus, head 2
Cerebral peduncle 8
Facial nerve (CN VII) 13
Fornix, column 1
Glossopharyngeal nerve (CN IX) 14
Hypoglossal nerve (CN XII) 16
Inferior olive 24
Infundibulum (pituitary stalk) 35

Lateral funiculus 19
Mamillary body 31
Medulla oblongata 23
Middle cerebellar peduncle (brachium pontis) 26
Oculomotor nerve (CN III) 6
Olfactory tract 3
Optic chiasm 36
Optic nerve (CN II) 5
Optic tract 33
Pons 10
Putamen 4
Pyramids and pyramidal decussation (corticospinal tract) 25
Spinal cord, anterior lateral sulcus 18

Spinal nerve (C3) 20
Thalamus, dorsal lateral geniculate nucleus (dLGN) (lateral geniculate body) 30
Thalamus, medial geniculate nucleus (MG) (medial geniculate body) 9
Trigeminal nerve (CN V), motor root 28
Trigeminal nerve (CN V), sensory root 29
Trochlear nerve (CN IV) 7
Tuber cinereum 32
Vagus nerve (CN X) 15
Vestibulocochlear nerve (CN VIII) 12

FIGURE 9-1 Anterior aspect of brainstem, thalamus, and striatum. Used with permission from Woolsey, Thomas A., Joseph Hanaway, and Mokhtar H. Gado. *The Brain Atlas: A Visual Guide to the Human Central Nervous System*, 3rd ed. Hoboken, NJ: Wiley, 2008.

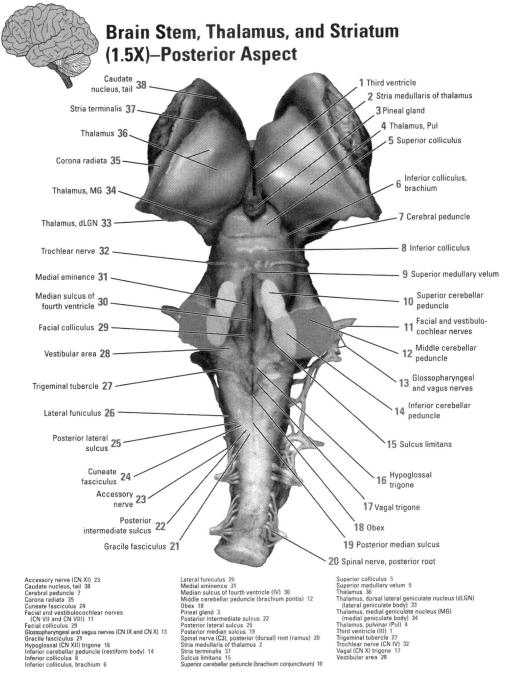

Brain Stem, Thalamus, and Striatum (1.5X)–Posterior Aspect

Caudate nucleus, tail **38**
Stria terminalis **37**
Thalamus **36**
Corona radiata **35**
Thalamus, MG **34**
Thalamus, dLGN **33**
Trochlear nerve **32**
Medial eminence **31**
Median sulcus of fourth ventricle **30**
Facial colliculus **29**
Vestibular area **28**
Trigeminal tubercle **27**
Lateral funiculus **26**
Posterior lateral sulcus **25**
Cuneate fasciculus **24**
Accessory nerve **23**
Posterior intermediate sulcus **22**
Gracile fasciculus **21**

1 Third ventricle
2 Stria medullaris of thalamus
3 Pineal gland
4 Thalamus, Pul
5 Superior colliculus
6 Inferior colliculus, brachium
7 Cerebral peduncle
8 Inferior colliculus
9 Superior medullary velum
10 Superior cerebellar peduncle
11 Facial and vestibulo-cochlear nerves
12 Middle cerebellar peduncle
13 Glossopharyngeal and vagus nerves
14 Inferior cerebellar peduncle
15 Sulcus limitans
16 Hypoglossal trigone
17 Vagal trigone
18 Obex
19 Posterior median sulcus
20 Spinal nerve, posterior root

Accessory nerve (CN XI) 23
Caudate nucleus, tail 38
Cerebral peduncle 7
Corona radiata 35
Cuneate fasciculus 24
Facial and vestibulocochlear nerves (CN VII and CN VIII) 11
Facial colliculus 29
Glossopharyngeal and vagus nerves (CN IX and CN X) 13
Gracile fasciculus 21
Hypoglossal (CN XII) trigone 16
Inferior cerebellar peduncle (restiform body) 14
Inferior colliculus 8
Inferior colliculus, brachium 6

Lateral funiculus 26
Medial eminence 31
Median sulcus of fourth ventricle (IV) 30
Middle cerebellar peduncle (brachium pontis) 12
Obex 18
Pineal gland 3
Posterior intermediate sulcus 22
Posterior lateral sulcus 25
Posterior median sulcus 19
Spinal nerve (C3), posterior (dorsal) root (ramus) 20
Stria medullaris of thalamus 2
Stria terminalis 37
Sulcus limitans 15
Superior cerebellar peduncle (brachium conjunctivum) 10

Superior colliculus 5
Superior medullary velum 9
Thalamus 36
Thalamus, dorsal lateral geniculate nucleus (dLGN) (lateral geniculate body) 33
Thalamus, medial geniculate nucleus (MG) (medial geniculate body) 34
Thalamus, pulvinar (Pul) 4
Third ventricle (III) 1
Trigeminal tubercle 27
Trochlear nerve (CN IV) 32
Vagal (CN X) trigone 17
Vestibular area 28

FIGURE 9-2 **Posterior aspect of brainstem, thalamus, and striatum.** Used with permission from Woolsey, Thomas A., Joseph Hanaway, and Mokhtar H. Gado. *The Brain Atlas: A Visual Guide to the Human Central Nervous System,* 3rd ed. Hoboken, NJ: Wiley, 2008.

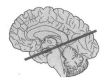

Transverse Section Through Superior Colliculus (3X) with Vessel Territories

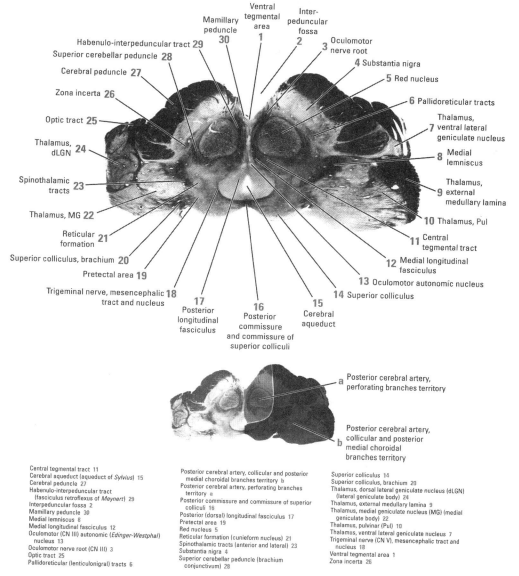

Mamillary peduncle **30**
Ventral tegmental area **1**
Inter-peduncular fossa **2**
3 Oculomotor nerve root
Habenulo-interpeduncular tract **29**
Superior cerebellar peduncle **28**
Cerebral peduncle **27**
Zona incerta **26**
Optic tract **25**
Thalamus, dLGN **24**
Spinothalamic tracts **23**
Thalamus, MG **22**
Reticular formation **21**
Superior colliculus, brachium **20**
Pretectal area **19**
Trigeminal nerve, mesencephalic tract and nucleus **18**
17 Posterior longitudinal fasciculus
16 Posterior commissure and commissure of superior colliculi
15 Cerebral aqueduct
14 Superior colliculus
13 Oculomotor autonomic nucleus
12 Medial longitudinal fasciculus
11 Central tegmental tract
10 Thalamus, Pul
9 Thalamus, external medullary lamina
8 Medial lemniscus
7 Thalamus, ventral lateral geniculate nucleus
6 Pallidoreticular tracts
5 Red nucleus
4 Substantia nigra

a Posterior cerebral artery, perforating branches territory

b Posterior cerebral artery, collicular and posterior medial choroidal branches territory

Central tegmental tract 11
Cerebral aqueduct (aqueduct of *Sylvius*) 15
Cerebral peduncle 27
Habenulo-interpeduncular tract (fasciculus retroflexus of *Meynert*) 29
Interpeduncular fossa 2
Mamillary peduncle 30
Medial lemniscus 8
Medial longitudinal fasciculus 12
Oculomotor (CN III) autonomic (*Edinger-Westphal*) nucleus 13
Oculomotor nerve root (CN III) 3
Optic tract 25
Pallidoreticular (lenticulonigral) tracts 6

Posterior cerebral artery, collicular and posterior medial choroidal branches territory b
Posterior cerebral artery, perforating branches territory a
Posterior commissure and commissure of superior colliculi 16
Posterior (dorsal) longitudinal fasciculus 17
Pretectal area 19
Red nucleus 5
Reticular formation (cunieform nucleus) 21
Spinothalamic tracts (anterior and lateral) 23
Substantia nigra 4
Superior cerebellar peduncle (brachium conjunctivum) 28

Superior colliculus 14
Superior colliculus, brachium 20
Thalamus, dorsal lateral geniculate nucleus (dLGN) (lateral geniculate body) 24
Thalamus, external medullary lamina 9
Thalamus, medial geniculate nucleus (MG) (medial geniculate body) 22
Thalamus, pulvinar (Pul) 10
Thalamus, ventral lateral geniculate nucleus 7
Trigeminal nerve (CN V), mesencephalic tract and nucleus 18
Ventral tegmental area 1
Zona incerta 26

FIGURE 9-3 Axial section through the midbrain: the sections are in radiographic orientation. Used with permission from Woolsey, Thomas A., Joseph Hanaway, and Mokhtar H. Gado. *The Brain Atlas: A Visual Guide to the Human Central Nervous System*, 3rd ed. Hoboken, NJ: Wiley, 2008.

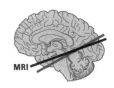

Transverse Section Through Superior Pons and Isthmus (4X) with MRI (0.7X)

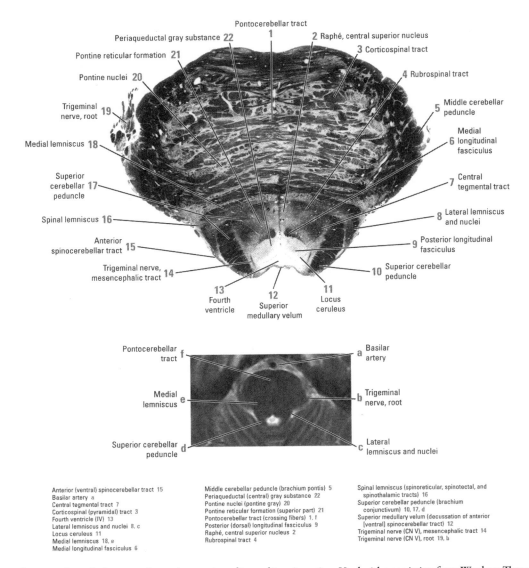

Pontocerebellar tract **1**

Periaqueductal gray substance **22**

Pontine reticular formation **21**

Pontine nuclei **20**

Trigeminal nerve, root **19**

Medial lemniscus **18**

Superior cerebellar peduncle **17**

Spinal lemniscus **16**

Anterior spinocerebellar tract **15**

Trigeminal nerve, mesencephalic tract **14**

13 Fourth ventricle

12 Superior medullary velum

11 Locus ceruleus

2 Raphé, central superior nucleus

3 Corticospinal tract

4 Rubrospinal tract

5 Middle cerebellar peduncle

6 Medial longitudinal fasciculus

7 Central tegmental tract

8 Lateral lemniscus and nuclei

9 Posterior longitudinal fasciculus

10 Superior cerebellar peduncle

Pontocerebellar tract **f**

Medial lemniscus **e**

Superior cerebellar peduncle **d**

a Basilar artery

b Trigeminal nerve, root

c Lateral lemniscus and nuclei

Anterior (ventral) spinocerebellar tract 15
Basilar artery a
Central tegmental tract 7
Corticospinal (pyramidal) tract 3
Fourth ventricle (IV) 13
Lateral lemniscus and nuclei 8, c
Locus ceruleus 11
Medial lemniscus 18, e
Medial longitudinal fasciculus 6

Middle cerebellar peduncle (brachium pontis) 5
Periaqueductal (central) gray substance 22
Pontine nuclei (pontine gray) 20
Pontine reticular formation (superior part) 21
Pontocerebellar tract (crossing fibers) 1, f
Posterior (dorsal) longitudinal fasciculus 9
Raphé, central superior nucleus 2
Rubrospinal tract 4

Spinal lemniscus (spinoreticular, spinotectal, and spinothalamic tracts) 16
Superior cerebellar peduncle (brachium conjunctivum) 10, 17, d
Superior medullary velum (decussation of anterior [ventral] spinocerebellar tract) 12
Trigeminal nerve (CN V), mesencephalic tract 14
Trigeminal nerve (CN V), root 19, b

FIGURE 9-4 **Axial section through the pons: the sections are in radiographic orientation.** Used with permission from Woolsey, Thomas A., Joseph Hanaway, and Mokhtar H. Gado. *The Brain Atlas: A Visual Guide to the Human Central Nervous System,* 3rd ed. Hoboken, NJ: Wiley, 2008.

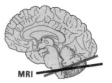

Transverse Section Through Hypoglossal Nucleus (5X) with MRI (0.7X)

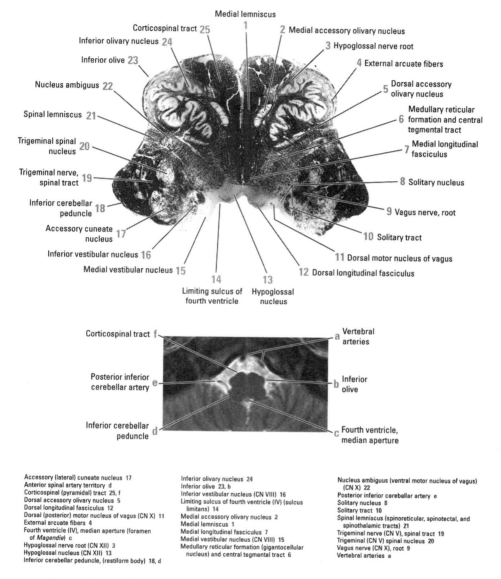

Medial lemniscus **1**
Corticospinal tract **25**
2 Medial accessory olivary nucleus
Inferior olivary nucleus **24**
3 Hypoglossal nerve root
Inferior olive **23**
4 External arcuate fibers
Nucleus ambiguus **22**
5 Dorsal accessory olivary nucleus
Spinal lemniscus **21**
6 Medullary reticular formation and central tegmental tract
Trigeminal spinal nucleus **20**
7 Medial longitudinal fasciculus
Trigeminal nerve, spinal tract **19**
8 Solitary nucleus
Inferior cerebellar peduncle **18**
9 Vagus nerve, root
Accessory cuneate nucleus **17**
10 Solitary tract
Inferior vestibular nucleus **16**
11 Dorsal motor nucleus of vagus
Medial vestibular nucleus **15**
12 Dorsal longitudinal fasciculus
14 Limiting sulcus of fourth ventricle
13 Hypoglossal nucleus

Corticospinal tract **f**
a Vertebral arteries
Posterior inferior cerebellar artery **e**
b Inferior olive
Inferior cerebellar peduncle **d**
c Fourth ventricle, median aperture

Accessory (lateral) cuneate nucleus 17
Anterior spinal artery territory d
Corticospinal (pyramidal) tract 25, f
Dorsal accessory olivary nucleus 5
Dorsal longitudinal fasciculus 12
Dorsal (posterior) motor nucleus of vagus (CN X) 11
External arcuate fibers 4
Fourth ventricle (IV), median aperture (foramen of *Magendie*) c
Hypoglossal nerve root (CN XII) 3
Hypoglossal nucleus (CN XII) 13
Inferior cerebellar peduncle, (restiform body) 18, d

Inferior olivary nucleus 24
Inferior olive 23, b
Inferior vestibular nucleus (CN VIII) 16
Limiting sulcus of fourth ventricle (IV) (sulcus limitans) 14
Medial accessory olivary nucleus 2
Medial lemniscus 1
Medial longitudinal fasciculus 7
Medial vestibular nucleus (CN VIII) 15
Medullary reticular formation (gigantocellular nucleus) and central tegmental tract 6

Nucleus ambiguus (ventral motor nucleus of vagus) (CN X) 22
Posterior inferior cerebellar artery e
Solitary nucleus 8
Solitary tract 10
Spinal lemniscus (spinoreticular, spinotectal, and spinothalamic tracts) 21
Trigeminal nerve (CN V), spinal tract 19
Trigeminal (CN V) spinal nucleus 20
Vagus nerve (CN X), root 9
Vertebral arteries a

FIGURE 9-5 **Axial section through the medulla: the sections are in radiographic orientation. Used with permission from Woolsey, Thomas A., Joseph Hanaway, and Mokhtar H. Gado.** *The Brain Atlas: A Visual Guide to the Human Central Nervous System,* **3rd ed. Hoboken, NJ: Wiley, 2008.**

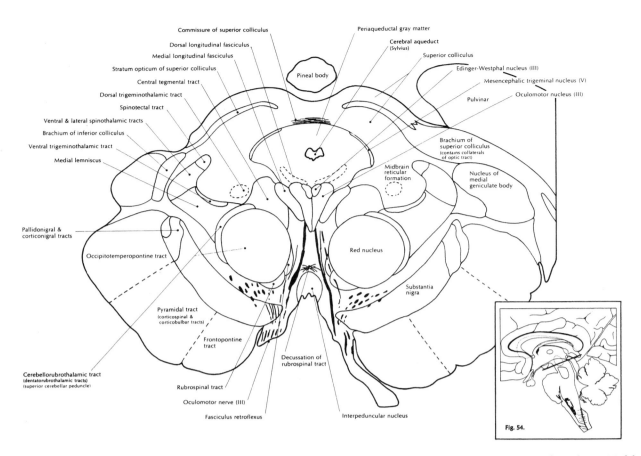

FIGURE 9-6 **Axial section through the midbrain: the section is in anatomic orientation.** Used with permission from DeArmond, Stephen J., Madeline M. Fusco, and Maynard M. Dewey. *Structure of the Human Brain: A Photographic Atlas,* 3rd ed. New York: Oxford University Press, 1989.

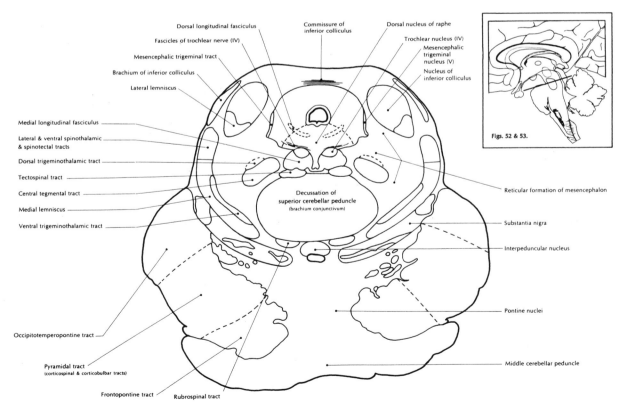

FIGURE 9-7 **Axial section through the inferior midbrain and high pons: the section is in anatomic orientation.** Used with permission from DeArmond, Stephen J., Madeline M. Fusco, and Maynard M. Dewey. *Structure of the Human Brain: A Photographic Atlas,* 3rd ed. New York: Oxford University Press, 1989.

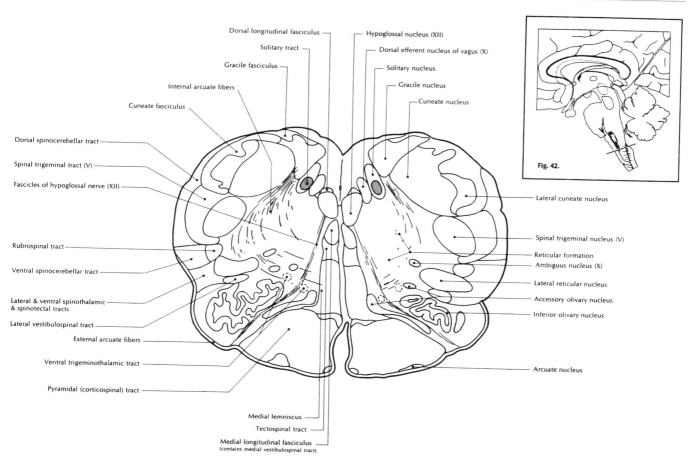

FIGURE 9-8 **Axial section through the medulla: the section is in anatomic orientation.** Used with permission from DeArmond, Stephen J., Madeline M. Fusco, and Maynard M. Dewey. *Structure of the Human Brain: A Photographic Atlas,* 3rd ed. New York: Oxford University Press, 1989.

Brainstem Composite—Axial View

Here, we will draw an axial composite of the brainstem: a consolidation of the different brainstem levels into a single general organizational pattern. First, draw an ovoid outline of the brainstem. Then, show the axes of our diagram: indicate that the anterior pole is at the bottom of the page and that the posterior pole is at the top and then show the anatomic left–right orientational plane. Next, label the left side of the page as nuclei and the right side of the page as tracts.

Now, divide the brainstem from anterior to posterior into its basis, tegmentum, and tectum. The basis comprises descending white matter tracts and certain supplementary motor nuclei. The tegmentum is the central bulk of the brainstem; it contains the cranial nerve nuclei, neurobehavioral cells, ascending sensory tracts, additional supplementary motor nuclei, and the supplementary motor and sensory tracts. The tectum is the roof of the brainstem. In the midbrain, the tectum is the quadrigeminal plate, whereas in the pons and medulla, by at least one commonly held definition, the tectum is limited to the nonfunctioning medullary velum. Note, however, that select authors include the superior cerebellar peduncles as part of the pontine tectum, as well.[1–3]

Within the basis, show the ventral-lying corticofugal tracts, which comprise the efferent fiber tracts from the cerebral cortex; they include the corticopontine, corticonuclear (aka corticobulbar), and corticospinal tracts. The corticonuclear tracts peel off and synapse in target nuclei as they descend the brainstem; the corticopontine tracts synapse in the pontine basis; and the corticospinal tracts pass through the medullary pyramids to reach their targets in the spinal cord.

Moving posteriorly, label the supplementary motor nuclei, which in the midbrain include the substantia nigra and red nucleus; in the pons, the pontine nuclei; and in the medulla, the inferior olive. Next, in the anterior tegmentum, label the medial lemniscus pathway—the major large fiber sensory pathway from the body. Then, lateral to it, label the anterolateral system pathway, which, most notably, carries the spinothalamic tract—the major small fiber sensory pathway from the body. Next, posterior to the anterolateral system, label the trigeminothalamic tracts, which carry sensory information from the face.

Now, in the posterior tegmentum, label the cranial nerve nuclei. The cell bodies for cranial nerves 3–10 and cranial nerve 12 lie within the brainstem (cranial nerve 11 lies in the upper cervical spinal cord). Next, label the neurobehavioral cells, which include the periaqueductal gray area in the midbrain; the locus coeruleus in the pons; and the raphe nuclei, which span much of the height of the midline brainstem. Then, label the broad reticular formation in the tegmentum.

Now, label the supplementary motor and sensory tracts, which include the medial longitudinal fasciculus and tectospinal tracts, which run the midline height of the brainstem, and the central tegmental and rubrospinal tracts. Next, label the brainstem auditory components, which are the cochlear nucleus, superior olivary nucleus, trapezoid body, inferior colliculus, and lateral lemniscus. We address these components in detail in Drawing 14-4. Now, label the cerebrospinal fluid space, which in the midbrain is the cerebral aqueduct and in the pons and medulla is the fourth ventricle. Lastly, label the cerebellar peduncles: superior, middle, and inferior.[1–11]

NUCLEI

TRACTS

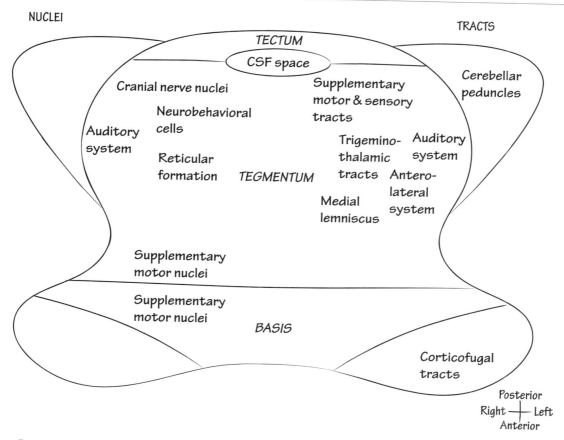

TECTUM

CSF space

Cranial nerve nuclei

Supplementary motor & sensory tracts

Cerebellar peduncles

Auditory system

Neurobehavioral cells

Trigemino-thalamic tracts

Auditory system

Reticular formation

TEGMENTUM

Medial lemniscus

Antero-lateral system

Supplementary motor nuclei

Supplementary motor nuclei

BASIS

Corticofugal tracts

Posterior
Right — Left
Anterior

DRAWING 9-1 **Brainstem Composite—Axial View**

The Midbrain

Here, we will draw an anatomic, axial cross-section through the midbrain. First, show the anterior–posterior and left–right axes of our diagram and then label the left side of the page as nuclei and the right side as tracts. Then, label the basis, tegmentum, and tectum. Next, anteriorly, draw the bilateral crus cerebri. Divide the center of the crus into the corticonuclear tracts (aka corticobulbar tracts), medially, and the corticospinal tracts, laterally. Next, in the most medial portion of the crus, draw the frontopontine tracts, and in the most lateral portion, draw the additional corticopontine tracts, which emanate from the occipital, parietal, and temporal cortices.

Now, label the substantia nigra as the long stretch of dopaminergic nuclei just posterior to the white matter pathways in the base of the midbrain. Loss of dopaminergic cells in the dark, melanin-rich pars compacta division of the substantia nigra results in Parkinson's disease. The reddish, iron-rich, pars reticulata division of the substantia nigra plays an important role in the direct and indirect basal ganglia pathways (see Drawing 18-4). The substantia nigra helps initiate movement, and pathology to it, either from degeneration or injury, produces bradykinesia, a slowness and stiffness of movement.

Next, in the anterior aspect of the midbrain tegmentum, draw the circular red nucleus just off midline. The red nuclei receive fibers from both the motor cortex and cerebellum. Each red nucleus connects with the ipsilateral inferior olive as part of the triangle of Guillain-Mollaret (via the central tegmental tract), and each red nucleus also sends rubrospinal tract fibers down the brainstem and spinal cord to produce flexion movements of the upper extremities (see Drawing 7-3). Make a notation that the red nuclei span the mid and upper midbrain. Injury in the vicinity of the red nucleus can produce a low-frequency, coarse postural and action tremor on the contralateral side of the body, called a rubral tremor. Despite its name, which suggests a close relationship to the red nucleus, rubral tremor can occur from injury to other brainstem areas, as well, and also from injury to the cerebellum and thalamus.

Now, show that fibers from the superior cerebellar peduncle (the major outflow tract of the cerebellum) decussate in the central midbrain tegmentum, and indicate that this decussation occurs in the inferior midbrain (below the level of the red nuclei). Injury to these crossing fibers produces cerebellar ataxia on the side of the body that the fibers originated from (regardless of where they are injured along their path). For instance, whether it happens pre- or post-decussation, injury to superior cerebellar fibers from the right cerebellum produces ataxia on the right side of the body.

Next, draw a red nucleus on the opposite side of the midbrain so we can see how its presence forces the ascending sensory pathways out laterally. Immediately lateral to the red nuclei, draw the medial lemniscus, and posterolateral to it, draw the anterolateral system. Next, along the posterior wall of the medial lemniscus, label the anterior trigeminothalamic tract (we draw the posterior trigeminothalamic tract later). Then, along the posterolateral wall of the anterolateral system, label the lateral lemniscus.

Now, label the cerebral aqueduct as the small cerebrospinal fluid space in the dorsum of the midbrain. Then, label the surrounding periaqueductal gray area. The periaqueductal gray area is packed with neuropeptides, monoamines, and amino acids, but it most notably contains opioids, which help in pain suppression. Electrical stimulation of the periaqueductal gray area to produce analgesia was first attempted in the 1970s but has had mixed results. Of note, the periaqueductal gray area receives ascending spinomesencephalic fibers via the anterolateral system, which play a role in the emotional aspect of pain, and it receives descending fibers from the hypothalamus via the dorsal longitudinal fasciculus.

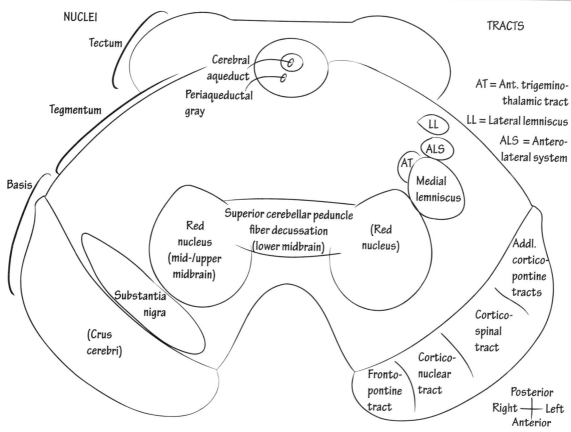

NUCLEI

Tectum

Tegmentum

Basis

Cerebral
aqueduct

Periaqueductal
gray

Red
nucleus
(mid-/upper
midbrain)

Substantia
nigra

(Crus
cerebri)

Superior cerebellar peduncle
fiber decussation
(lower midbrain)

(Red
nucleus)

TRACTS

AT = Ant. trigemino-
thalamic tract

LL = Lateral lemniscus

ALS = Antero-
lateral system

LL

ALS

AT

Medial
lemniscus

Addl.
cortico-
pontine
tracts

Cortico-
spinal
tract

Cortico-
nuclear
tract

Fronto-
pontine
tract

Posterior
Right — Left
Anterior

DRAWING 9-2 **The Midbrain—Partial**

The Midbrain (Cont.)

Periaqueductal gray area functions include far-reaching modulation of sympathetic responses (ie, pupillary dilation and cardiovascular responses); parasympathetic-induced micturition; modulation of reproductive behavior; and even affect locomotion and vocalization. However, its most widely recognized function is in pain modulation.

Next, in front of the periaqueductal gray area, label the reticular formation. Initially, the indistinct histology of the reticular formation led people to believe it was simply a "diffuse arousal network," but now the functional specialization of the reticular formation is well recognized. The reticular formation divides into lateral, medial, and median zones, and the raphe nuclei populate the last—the median zone. The raphe nuclei are primarily serotinergic and are heavily modulated by psychotropic medications. They affect sleep–wake cycles, pain management, and motor activity but are most commonly referenced for their role in mood disorders and the hallucinatory effects of illicit drugs. The raphe nuclei lie along much of the height of the midline brainstem as six separate subnuclei, which divide into rostral and caudal nuclear groups based on whether they lie above or below the mid-pons. The rostral raphe group (aka oral raphe group) comprises the upper pontine and midbrain raphe nuclei: the caudal linear, dorsal raphe, and median raphe nuclei. The caudal raphe group comprises the lower pontine and medullary raphe nuclei: the raphe magnus, raphe obscurus, and raphe pallidus nuclei. Note that additional serotinergic reticular formation areas are also categorized as part of the raphe nuclei. Efferent projections from the rostral raphe group mostly ascend into the upper brainstem and forebrain, whereas projections from the caudal raphe group primarily descend into the lower brainstem and spinal cord. Afferents to the raphe nuclei also exist, which generally originate from behavioral brain areas.[7]

Now, label the presence of the cranial nerve 3 and 4 nuclei and also a portion of the cranial nerve 5 nuclei— subnuclei of cranial nerve 5 lie along the height of the brainstem. Note that although we show cranial nerves 3 and 4 in the lateral midbrain, here, this is only because of the constraints of our diagram; they actually lie in the midline midbrain, as shown more accurately in Chapters 11 and 12.

Next, let's address the supplementary motor and sensory fiber tracts. In midline, just in front of the periaqueductal gray area, label the medial longitudinal fasciculus, which plays an important role in conjugate horizontal eye movements (see Drawing 23-1). Then, in the central, dorsal tegmentum, label the central tegmental tract. It carries ascending reticular fibers to the rostral intralaminar nuclei of the thalamus as part of the ascending arousal system and descending fibers from the red nucleus to the inferior olive as part of the triangle of Guillain-Mollaret. Along the posterior wall of the central tegmental tract, label the posterior trigeminothalamic pathway: it originates in the upper pons and ascends through the midbrain.

Now, let's draw the key contents of the tectum. First, draw the colliculi, which divide into paired bilateral superior and inferior colliculi. The superior colliculi lie in the upper midbrain and are involved in visual function and the inferior colliculi lie in the lower midbrain and are involved in auditory function. Then, draw the posterior commissure. The pathway for the pupillary light reflex passes through the posterior commissure and the nucleus of the posterior commissure helps control vertical eye movements.

Next, label the tectospinal tract just anterior to the medial longitudinal fasciculus. The tectospinal tract originates in the superior colliculus and decussates in the midbrain tegmentum and descends in front of the medial longitudinal fasciculus. Both the medial longitudinal fasciculus and the tectospinal tract maintain their posterior, midline position throughout the height of the brainstem. Regional stimulation of the superior colliculus stimulates efferent impulses through the tectobulbar tract to the brainstem for eye movements and through the tectospinal tract to the upper cervical nuclei for visually directed neck and head movements.[1–11]

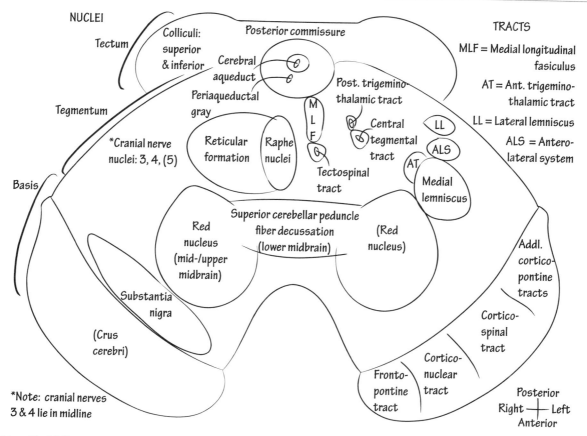

NUCLEI

Tectum

Colliculi:
superior
& inferior

Tegmentum

Basis

*Cranial nerve
nuclei: 3, 4, (5)

Periaqueductal
gray

Cerebral
aqueduct

Posterior commissure

Reticular
formation

Raphe
nuclei

Red
nucleus
(mid-/upper
midbrain)

Substantia
nigra

(Crus
cerebri)

Superior cerebellar peduncle
fiber decussation
(lower midbrain)

Tectospinal
tract

Post. trigemino-
thalamic tract

Central
tegmental
tract

(Red
nucleus)

Medial
lemniscus

MLF

LL

ALS

AT

TRACTS

MLF = Medial longitudinal
fasiculus

AT = Ant. trigemino-
thalamic tract

LL = Lateral lemniscus

ALS = Antero-
lateral system

Addl.
cortico-
pontine
tracts

Cortico-
spinal
tract

Cortico-
nuclear
tract

Fronto-
pontine
tract

Posterior
Right — Left
Anterior

*Note: cranial nerves
3 & 4 lie in midline

DRAWING 9-3 The Midbrain—Complete

The Pons

Here, we will draw an anatomic, axial cross-section of the pons. First, show the axes of our diagram: indicate that the anterior pole is at the bottom of the page and that the posterior pole is at the top and then show the anatomic left–right orientational plane. Next, in the opposite corner, draw a small axial pons section and separate the large basis from the comparatively small tegmentum. For our main diagram, exclude the bulk of the basis to make room for the complexity of the tegmentum. Next, label the left side of the page as nuclei and the right side as tracts.

First, in the basis, draw the corticofugal tracts, which we pare down to the corticospinal and corticonuclear tracts because the corticopontine fibers synapse within the pons, itself. Draw the pontine nuclei within the pontine basis; the frontopontine and additional corticopontine fibers synapse within these nuclei. Next, show that the pontine nuclei send pontocerebellar tracts into the cerebellum via the middle cerebellar peduncle (aka brachium pontis) as part of the corticopontocerebellar pathway.

Now, draw the inferior cerebellar peduncle, which comprises the restiform and juxtarestiform bodies. Spinocerebellar, reticulocerebellar, and olivocerebellar fibers pass through the restiform body, whereas the juxtarestiform body is primarily reserved for fibers that pass between the vestibular nucleus and vestibulocerebellum.[8] Next, show that the superior cerebellar peduncle (aka brachium conjunctivum) lies posterior to the inferior cerebellar peduncle. The middle and inferior cerebellar peduncles are the main inflow pathways into the cerebellum and the superior cerebellar peduncle is the main outflow pathway. The superior cerebellar peduncle attaches to the upper pons and midbrain; the middle cerebellar peduncle attaches to the pons and extends to the pontomedullary junction; and the inferior cerebellar peduncle attaches to the lower pons and medulla. Now, draw the anterior spinocerebellar fibers in the posterolateral pons; the other spinocerebellar pathways enter the cerebellum below the pons through the inferior cerebellar peduncle (see Drawing 7-5).

Next, show that in the pons, the medial lemniscus lies medially—unlike in the midbrain, where the red nuclei push the medial lemniscus out laterally. Then, lateral to the medial lemniscus, draw the anterolateral system, and along the posterior wall of the medial lemniscus, draw the anterior trigeminothalamic tract.

Now, let's show the supplementary motor and sensory tracts of the pontine tegmentum. Indicate that the medial longitudinal fasciculus and the tectospinal tract continue to descend through the dorsal midline tegmentum and that the central tegmental tract descends through the dorsal, central tegmentum. Also, include the rubrospinal tract just posterior to the anterolateral system. Now, label the cerebrospinal fluid space of the pons as the fourth ventricle and show that the central gray area surrounds it. Next, label the locus coeruleus in the posterior tegmentum, just in front of the central gray area.

Although technically the locus coeruleus spans from the caudal end of the periaqueductal gray area in the lower midbrain to the facial nucleus in the mid-pons, locus coeruleus nuclei are most heavily concentrated in the pons. The locus coeruleus nuclei are nearly entirely noradrenergic and, thus, are far more uniform in their neurotransmitter makeup than the periaqueductal gray area and even more uniform than the raphe nuclei, which are mostly serotinergic.

Next, label the reticular formation and raphe nuclei and then label the nuclei of cranial nerves 5, 6, 7, and 8 in the dorsal pontine tegmentum. Cranial nerves 6 and 7 lie within the mid to low pons; cranial nerve 8 lies within both the pons and medulla; and portions of cranial nerve 5 lie along the height of the brainstem. Again, note that our diagram does not reflect the medial-lateral position of the cranial nerve nuclei. Next, draw the pontine components of the auditory system: the lateral lemniscus in the lateral tegmentum and the trapezoid body and superior olivary nucleus in the anterolateral tegmentum.[1-11]

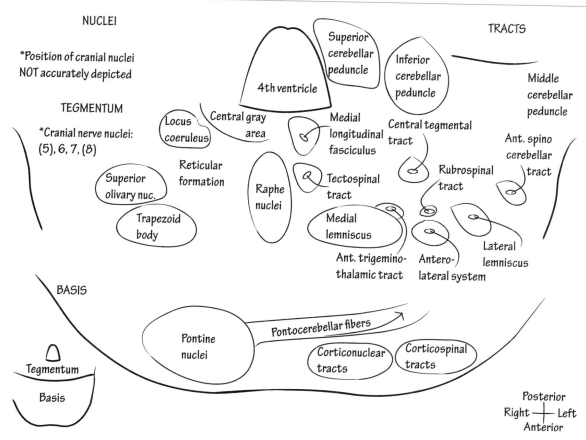

NUCLEI

*Position of cranial nuclei NOT accurately depicted

TEGMENTUM

*Cranial nerve nuclei: (5), 6, 7, (8)

Superior olivary nuc.

Trapezoid body

Locus coeruleus

Central gray area

Reticular formation

Raphe nuclei

4th ventricle

Superior cerebellar peduncle

Medial longitudinal fasciculus

Tectospinal tract

Medial lemniscus

Ant. trigemino-thalamic tract

Antero-lateral system

Inferior cerebellar peduncle

Central tegmental tract

Rubrospinal tract

Lateral lemniscus

TRACTS

Middle cerebellar peduncle

Ant. spino cerebellar tract

BASIS

Pontine nuclei

Pontocerebellar fibers

Corticonuclear tracts

Corticospinal tracts

Tegmentum

Basis

Posterior
Right ┼ Left
Anterior

DRAWING 9-4 **The Pons**

The Medulla

Here, we will draw an anatomic, axial cross-section of the medulla. First, show the axes of our diagram: indicate that the anterior pole is at the bottom of the page and that the posterior pole is at the top and then show the anatomic left–right orientational plane. Next, on one side, label the nuclei and, on the other, the tracts. Now, draw an outline of the medulla. Show that the bulk of the medulla is tegmentum and that the basis is reserved for the descending corticospinal tract fibers, which populate the medullary pyramids. Most of the classes of corticofugal fibers (corticonuclear and corticopontine) synapse above or at the level of the medulla; the only corticofugal pathway within the medulla is the corticospinal tract.

Now, let's draw the large fiber sensory system. In the dorsal medulla, label the gracile nucleus, medially, and the cuneate nucleus, laterally; they receive the ascending gracile and cuneate posterior column tracts from the spinal cord. Then, draw the medial lemniscus tract along the midline of the medulla and indicate that in the lower medulla, internal arcuate fibers decussate from the gracile and cuneate nuclei to the opposite side of the medulla in what is referred to as the great sensory decussation (see Drawing 10-1). Next, along the outside of the medial lemniscus, label the anterior trigeminothalamic tract. We find anterior trigeminothalamic projections throughout the brainstem because the anterior trigeminothalamic tract is formed from fibers of the spinal trigeminal nucleus, which extends inferiorly into the upper cervical spinal cord. On the contrary, fibers from the posterior trigeminothalamic tracts originate and ascend from the principal sensory nucleus in the pons, so no posterior trigeminothalamic tract fibers are found within the medulla.

Next, label the inferior olive (aka inferior olivary complex), which comprises the main inferior olivary nucleus and the accessory olivary nuclei. The inferior olive receives many different fiber pathways, including tracts from the spinal cord (from below) and from the red nucleus (from above). The inferior olive sends climbing fibers to the contralateral dentate nucleus of the cerebellum, which projects back to the contralateral red nucleus to complete the triangle of Guillain-Mollaret.

Now, let's focus on the lateral wall of the medulla. First, posterior to the inferior olive, draw the anterolateral system. At the medullary level, the anterolateral system contains many ascending sensory pathways in addition to the spinothalamic fibers, including the spinoreticular, spinomesencephalic, and spinotectal pathways. It also carries spino-olivary and spinovestibular fibers, which disperse within the medulla, itself. Next, posterior to the anterolateral system, draw the spinocerebellar tracts: both the anterior and posterior spinocerebellar pathways are found within the medulla. Then, medial to the anterolateral system and spinocerebellar tracts, label the rubrospinal tract.

Now, draw the other main supplementary pathways: the medial longitudinal fasciculus in the posterior midline and the tectospinal tract anterior to it (the anterior-posterior and medial-lateral positions of these pathways remain roughly unchanged throughout their course through the brainstem). Next, along the outer, posterior wall of the medulla, label the inferior cerebellar peduncle. Now, indicate that the fourth ventricle is the cerebrospinal fluid space of most of the medulla. A small tissue fold, called the obex, exists where the fourth ventricle funnels inferiorly into the central canal. At the rostral–caudal level of the obex lies the gracile tubercle—the swelling formed by the gracile nucleus in the posterior wall of the medulla. Along the anterior border of fourth ventricle (in its inferior floor) label the area postrema, which is an important chemoreceptor trigger zone for emesis (vomiting). Next, indicate that the central gray area surrounds the fourth ventricle. Then, show that within the central medullary tegmentum lies the reticular formation, in the median zone of which lies the raphe nuclei.

Lastly, label the nuclei of cranial nerves 5, 8, 9, 10, and 12 in the dorsal medulla. Again, note that our diagram does not reflect the medial-lateral position of the cranial nerve nuclei. The cochlear nucleus of cranial nerve 8 represents the medulla's contribution to the auditory system.[1–11]

NUCLEI

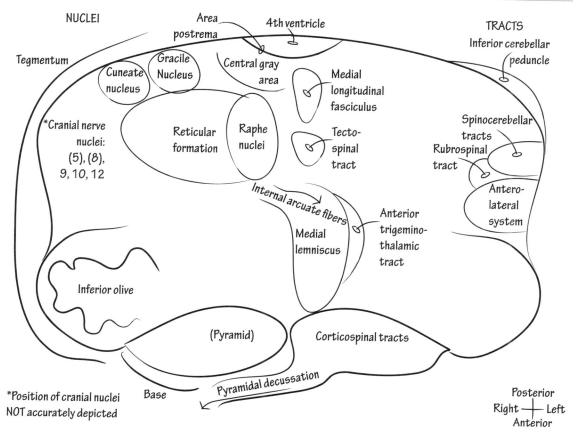

Tegmentum

Cuneate nucleus

Gracile Nucleus

Area postrema

4th ventricle

Central gray area

Medial longitudinal fasciculus

Tecto-spinal tract

*Cranial nerve nuclei:
(5), (8),
9, 10, 12

Reticular formation

Raphe nuclei

TRACTS

Inferior cerebellar peduncle

Spinocerebellar tracts

Rubrospinal tract

Antero-lateral system

Internal arcuate fibers

Medial lemniscus

Anterior trigemino-thalamic tract

Inferior olive

(Pyramid)

Corticospinal tracts

*Position of cranial nuclei NOT accurately depicted

Base

Pyramidal decussation

Posterior
Right —— Left
Anterior

DRAWING 9-5 **The Medulla**

References

1. Campbell, William, W., DeJong, Russell N., Haerer, Armin F. *DeJong's The Neurologic Examination*, 6th ed., Chapter 11 (Lippincott, Williams, & Wilkins, 2005).

2. Jinkins, J. R. *Atlas of Neuroradiologic Embryology, Anatomy, & Variants*, Chapter 2H (Lippincott, Williams, & Wilkins, 2000).

3. Arslan, O. *Neuroanatomical Basis of Clinical Neurology*, Chapter 4 (Parthenon Publishing, 2001).

4. Baehr, M., Frotscher, M. & Duus, P. *Duus' topical diagnosis in neurology: anatomy, physiology, signs, symptoms,* 4th completely rev. ed., Chapter 3 (Thieme, 2005).

5. Bogousslavsky, J. & Caplan, L. R. *Stroke syndromes*, 2nd ed. (Cambridge University Press, 2001).

6. DeMyer, W. *Neuroanatomy,* 2nd ed. (Williams & Wilkins, 1998).

7. Haines, D. E. & Ard, M. D. *Fundamental neuroscience: for basic and clinical applications,* 3rd ed. (Churchill Livingstone Elsevier, 2006).

8. Jacobson, S. & Marcus, E. M. *Neuroanatomy for the neuroscientist* (Springer, 2008).

9. Naidich, T. P. & Duvernoy, H. M. *Duvernoy's atlas of the human brain stem and cerebellum: high-field MRI: surface anatomy, internal structure, vascularization and 3D sectional anatomy* (Springer, 2009).

10. Paxinos, G. & Mai, J. K. *The human nervous system,* 2nd ed. (Elsevier Academic Press, 2004).

11. Noback, C. R. *The human nervous system: structure and function,* 6th ed. (Humana Press, 2005).

10

Brainstem

Part Two

Know-It Points

Major Sensory Projections

- The leg fibers of the medial lemniscus originate in the gracile nucleus of the medulla.
- The arm fibers of the medial lemniscus originate in the cuneate nucleus of the medulla.
- The gracile nucleus lies medial to the cuneate nucleus.
- Within the internal arcuate decussation, the leg fibers shift anterior to the arm fibers.
- As the medial lemniscus ascends the brainstem, the arm fibers shift medial to the leg fibers.

- The arm and leg fibers project to the ventroposterior lateral thalamic nucleus.
- The facial fibers project to the ventroposterior medial thalamic nucleus.
- The leg, arm, and face fibers project from medial to lateral along the posterior paracentral gyrus and postcentral gyrus.

Major Motor Projections

- The leg, arm, and face fibers originate from medial to lateral along the anterior paracentral gyrus and precentral gyrus.
- The descending fibers bundle in the internal capsule from anterior to posterior as face, arm, and leg fibers.

- The motor fiber arrangement in the brainstem, from medial to lateral, is the face, arm, and leg fibers.
- During the corticospinal tract decussation at the medullo-cervical junction, the arm and leg fibers shift so that despite the decussation, the arm fibers remain medial to the leg fibers.

Midbrain Syndromes (*Advanced*)

- Weber's syndrome results from injury to the paramedian midbrain.
- Weber's syndrome is a syndrome of ipsilateral third nerve palsy and contralateral face and body weakness.
- Benedikt's syndrome results from injury to the red nucleus and neighboring third nerve fibers.

- Benedikt's syndrome is a syndrome of ipsilateral third nerve palsy and contralateral choreiform movements.
- Claude's syndrome results from injury to the post-decussation superior cerebellar fibers and neighboring third nerve fibers.
- Claude's syndrome is a syndrome of ipsilateral third nerve palsy and contralateral ataxia.

Pontine Syndromes (*Advanced*)

- Locked-in syndrome results from injury to the pontine basis and ventral paramedian pontine tegmentum.
- In locked-in syndrome, there is:
  - Damage to the descending corticospinal and corticonuclear tracts
  - Preservation of most of the reticular formation
  - Destruction of the exiting facial motor nerve fibers

  - Destruction of the paramedian pontine reticular formation (the PPRF)
  - Spared third nerve innervation of the levator palpebrae
- Dysarthria-clumsy hand syndrome is due to restricted paramedian pontine injury.
- Dysarthria-clumsy hand syndrome is a syndrome of contralateral face and upper extremity weakness with preserved lower extremity strength.

Medullary Syndromes (*Advanced*)

- Wallenberg's syndrome results from lateral medullary injury; it most commonly occurs from a posterior inferior cerebellar artery territory infarct.
- In Wallenberg's syndrome, there is injury to:
  - The inferior cerebellar peduncle
  - The spinal trigeminal tract and nucleus
  - The anterolateral system (spinothalamic tract)
  - The nucleus ambiguus
  - The hypothalamospinal tract
  - The vestibular nucleus
- Dejerine's syndrome results from injury to the midline medulla.
- In Dejerine's syndrome, there is injury to the hypoglossal nucleus, medial lemniscus tract, and medullary pyramid.

Major Sensory Projections

There are three main somatosensory pathways within the brainstem: the medial lemniscus tract, the spinothalamic tract of the anterolateral system, and the trigeminothalamic tract. The medial lemniscus carries input from the large sensory fibers from the body, which transmit vibration, two-point discrimination, and joint position sensory information. The spinothalamic tract carries input from the small sensory fibers from the body, which transmit pain, itch, and thermal sensory information. The trigeminothalamic tract projects sensory information from the face. All three pathways ascend the brainstem separately and then bundle within the ventroposterior thalamus before they project to the somatosensory cortex. The position of the spinothalamic tract is largely unchanged throughout its spinal cord and brainstem ascent, so we will not draw it here, and we draw the trigeminothalamic tracts in detail where we discuss the trigeminal nucleus, itself (see Drawing 13-3), so we will not draw them here either. Here, we will focus on the medial lemniscus tract; specifically, we will draw the origins of the medial lemniscus tract in the gracile and cuneate nuclei, the internal arcuate decussation of the gracile and cuneate projection fibers, the medial lemniscus brainstem ascent, and the thalamocortical projections to the parietal lobe.

First, draw the lower medulla and show that the leg fibers of the medial lemniscus tract originate in the gracile nucleus in the posteromedial medulla and, then, that the arm fibers of the medial lemniscus tract originate in the cuneate nucleus in the posterolateral medulla. The gracile nucleus receives afferents from the spinal cord posterior column gracile tract and the cuneate nucleus receives afferents from the posterior column cuneate tract. Next, indicate that the gracile and cuneate fibers decussate (ie, cross midline) as internal arcuate fibers in the lower medulla; in the process, they rotate their somatotopic orientation from medial–lateral to anterior–posterior: the leg fibers go from medial to anterior and the arm fibers go from lateral to posterior. Postdecussation, these fibers bundle as the medial lemniscus tract.

Next, show that as the medial lemniscus ascends the pons and midbrain, it flips back to medial–lateral orientation but with the arm fibers medial, leg fibers lateral. Indicate that within the thalamus, the body fibers (arms and legs) project to the ventroposterior lateral nucleus and the facial fibers project to the ventroposterior medial nucleus. Next, draw the twisting thalamocortical sensory projections to the cerebral cortex. In their ascent, the sensory fibers again reverse their orientation: the leg fibers project medially to terminate in the posterior paracentral gyrus, the arm fibers project lateral to the legs and terminate in the upper convexity of the postcentral gyrus, and the facial fibers project lateral to both of them and terminate in the lower lateral postcentral gyrus.

Now, demonstrate this multi-step rotational ascent with your hand for easy reference. Place your right hand in front of you, palm down, with your fingers pointing to your right. Your thumb represents the leg fibers and your little finger represents the arm fibers. To demonstrate the decussation of the internal arcuate fibers, move your hand across midline and bring it in towards you. In the process, rotate your hand into anterior–posterior orientation with your little finger behind your thumb: arm fibers posterior to leg fibers. Next, to demonstrate the orientation reversal that occurs during the medial lemniscus ascent to the thalamus, rotate your hand back into medial–lateral orientation (the little finger [the arm] is medial and the thumb [the leg] is lateral) and simultaneously raise it. Then, to demonstrate the thalamocortical projection to the somatosensory cortex, twist your hand over so that the thumb (the leg) is medial and the little finger (the arm) is lateral.[1-6]

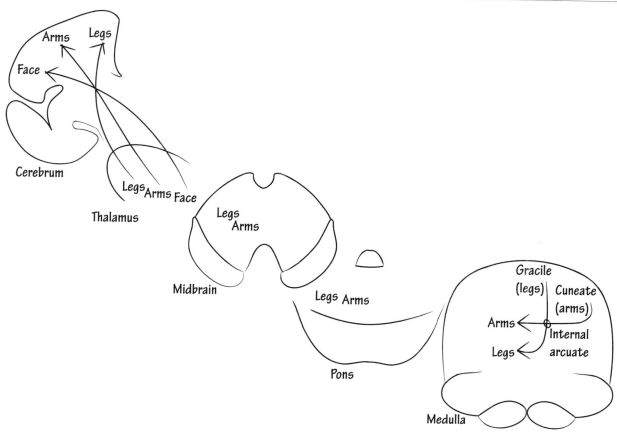

DRAWING 10-1 **Major Sensory Projections**

Major Motor Projections

Here, let's draw the corticonuclear and corticospinal motor fiber descent through the brainstem. Most of the motor fibers originate in parallel to the sensory fibers just in front of the central sulcus in the precentral gyrus and anterior paracentral gyrus, from lateral to medial as the face, arm, and leg fibers. Show the origins of the different somatomotor fibers: the facial fibers in the lateral cortex, the arm fibers in the upper convexity, and the leg fibers in the paracentral frontal lobe. Draw the twisting descent of each fiber group through the subcortical white matter. The facial fibers descend medially, the leg fibers descend laterally, and the arm fibers descend in between the two. Show these descending fibers bundle in the internal capsule and pass into the ipsilateral cerebral peduncle in the midbrain.

Next, show that the motor fiber arrangement in the midbrain, from medial to lateral, is as follows: face, arm, and leg. The facial fibers are called corticonuclear fibers (aka corticobulbar fibers) and they synapse on different cranial nerve nuclei throughout their descent. The arm and leg fibers form the corticospinal tract. In the pons, as the motor fibers descend through the pontine nuclei, the face, arm, and leg fibers maintain their same orientation. Show that they are positioned as follows, from medial to lateral: face, arm, and leg. At the most inferior level of the medulla, by definition, the corticonuclear fibers have completed their descent, so only the arm and leg corticospinal fibers are found; they descend through the base of the medulla in the ipsilateral medullary pyramid: indicate that the arms are still medial to the legs.

As the corticospinal tract descends through the medullo-cervical junction, show it decussate and shift posterolaterally to enter the lateral funiculus of the cervical spinal cord. Indicate that during the decussation, the arm and leg fibers twist so that the arms remain medial to the legs. Seventy-five to ninety percent of the corticospinal fibers undergo the aforementioned decussation;

they are called lateral corticospinal tract fibers due to their position in the lateral spinal cord. The remaining fibers travel ipsilaterally through the anteromedial spinal cord as the anterior corticospinal tract and remain uncrossed as they leave the brainstem. These fibers descend the spinal cord through the anterior funiculus, and when they reach the level of their target neuron, they cross within the anterior commissure.[1] Generally, lateral corticospinal tract fibers innervate distal musculature for fine motor movements, whereas anterior corticospinal tract fibers innervate proximal musculature for gross motor movements.

With our drawing complete, let's demonstrate the rotation and descent of the motor fibers with our hand. During the sensory fiber demonstration, we used our thumb as the leg fibers and our little finger as the arm fibers; let's use the same representation here. We begin where we ended our sensory fiber rotation—in the cerebral cortex with our hand turned palm towards us and our arm across our body. To demonstrate the twist and bundling of the motor fibers as they descend through the subcortical white matter and into the internal capsule, lower your hand and turn it over (palm away from you) as you bring your fingers together. Your pinky (the arm fibers) should be medial to your thumb (the leg fibers). To demonstrate the motor fiber descent through the brainstem, simply continue to drop your hand. Now, we need to demonstrate the pyramidal decussation at the medullo-cervical junction and the second twist of the corticospinal fibers. This rotation is important because it keeps the leg fibers lateral to the arm fibers when the corticospinal tract crosses midline in the upper cervical cord. For this step, bring your hand across midline and turn your palm back towards you so that your thumb is lateral and your little finger is medial when your hand crosses midline.[1–6]

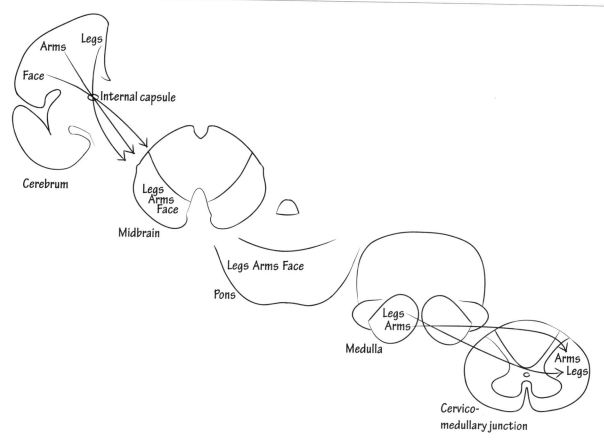

Arms
Legs
Face
Internal capsule
Cerebrum
Legs
Arms
Face
Midbrain
Legs Arms Face
Pons
Medulla
Legs
Arms
Arms
Legs
Cervico-
medullary junction

DRAWING 10-2 **Major Motor Projections**

Midbrain Syndromes (*Advanced*)

Case I

Patient presents with sudden onset of double vision and right-side weakness. Exam reveals left eye third nerve ophthalmoplegia with impaired pupillary constriction and also right face, arm, and leg weakness.

Draw an axial section through the midbrain. Then, draw the left-side oculomotor nucleus and its exiting third nerve. Next, label the left-side crus cerebri: it encompasses the corticonuclear and corticospinal tracts responsible for face, arm, and leg strength on the opposite side of the body (the right side). Now, encircle the paramedian midbrain, which is involved in Weber's syndrome: a syndrome of ipsilateral third nerve palsy and contralateral face and body weakness.[2,3,5,7,8]

Case II

Patient presents with sudden onset of double vision and right-side involuntary movements. Exam reveals left eye third nerve ophthalmoplegia with impaired pupillary constriction and also right-side choreiform movements.

Draw an axial section through the midbrain. Next, draw the left-side oculomotor nucleus and its exiting third nerve. Then, label the left red nucleus. Label the superior colliculus to show that this axial section is through the rostral midbrain. To keep track of the rostral–caudal plane, draw a sagittal brainstem and include the superior colliculus in the rostral midbrain and also the red nucleus.

Now, in the axial diagram, encircle the red nucleus and neighboring third nerve. Show that both are involved in Benedikt's syndrome: a syndrome of ipsilateral third nerve palsy and contralateral choreiform movements.[2,3,5,7–9]

Case III

Patient presents with double vision and right-side inco-ordination. Exam reveals left eye third nerve ophthalmoplegia with impaired pupillary constriction and also right-side ataxia.

Draw an axial section through the midbrain. Next, draw the left-side oculomotor nucleus and its exiting third nerve. Then, show that the superior cerebellar peduncle fibers exit the right cerebellum and decussate in the midbrain. Now, label the inferior colliculus in the axial diagram to establish that our section is in the caudal midbrain, and also do so in the sagittal brainstem diagram, as well. In the sagittal diagram, show that the superior cerebellar fibers exit the pons, ascend the brainstem, and decussate in the caudal midbrain beneath the red nuclei.

Now, encircle the post-decussation superior cerebellar fibers and neighboring third nerve. Injury to these two structures produces Claude's syndrome: a syndrome of ipsilateral third nerve palsy and contralateral ataxia. Note that the superior cerebellar peduncle fibers form a compact bundle along the dorsolateral wall of the fourth ventricle in the pons, and then decussate at the level of the inferior colliculus. We discuss the superior cerebellar decussation again as part of the corticopontocerebellar pathway in Drawing 15-7.[2,3,5,7,8,10–13]

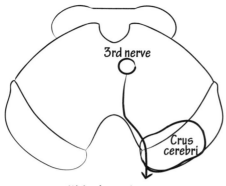

Weber's syndrome

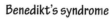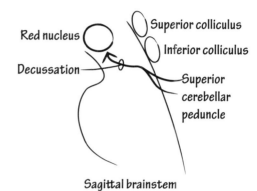

Benedikt's syndrome

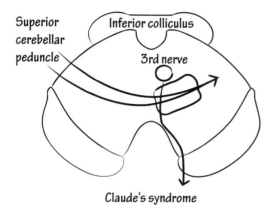

Claude's syndrome

Sagittal brainstem

DRAWING 10-3 **Midbrain Syndromes**

Pontine Syndromes (*Advanced*)

Case I

Patient is found in an apparent comatose state. Exam reveals normal pupil reactivity, normal vertical eye movements, volitional blinks, complete bilateral face and body paralysis, normal sleep–wake states, and an absent gag reflex.

First, draw an axial section through the pons and establish the anterior–posterior plane of orientation; this is an axial, anatomic view of the pons, with the anterior surface of the brainstem at the bottom of the page and the posterior surface at the top. Then, separate the basis from the tegmentum. Next, in the basis, draw the scattered descending corticonuclear (aka corticobulbar) and corticospinal tracts. Paralysis of the body and of the lower cranial nerves (tongue movements, gag, and swallow) results from damage to the descending corticospinal and corticonuclear tracts.

Next, draw the reticular formation in the pontine tegmentum; the normal sleep–wake states are maintained because the majority of the reticular formation is spared.

Now, draw the abducens nucleus of cranial nerve 6. And then draw the facial nucleus of cranial nerve 7 and show that cranial nerve 7 forms an internal genu around the abducens nucleus, which creates a bump in the floor of the fourth ventricle, called the facial colliculus. Paralysis of the face results from destruction of the exiting facial motor nerve fibers. The facial nucleus, itself, lies within the dorsal pons and is spared.

Next, show the pontine circuitry for horizontal eye movements. First draw the paramedian pontine reticular formation (PPRF) in the paramedian ventral pontine tegmentum. Then, show the medial longitudinal fasciculus (MLF) in the contralateral dorsal tegmentum. Indicate that the PPRF stimulates the abducens nucleus, which sends efferent nerve fibers through the medial pons to produce ipsilateral eye abduction. Then, also show that the abducens nucleus sends ascending interneuronal fibers up the contralateral MLF, which innervate the oculomotor nucleus and cause the ipsilateral eye (the eye contralateral to the abducens nucleus) to adduct. Paralysis of horizontal eye movements in this case results from destruction of the PPRF; note that although most of the reticular formation is spared, this small portion is injured. Volitional vertical eye movements are spared because the center for volitional vertical eye movements lies within the midbrain (above the level of the lesion).

The patient's ability to blink results from the ability to elevate and retract the upper eyelids through spared third nerve innervation of the levator palpebrae and through third nerve relaxation, which passively closes the eyelids. Orbicularis oculi is required for forced eyelid closure; it is innervated by the facial nerve, which is injured in this syndrome.

Finally, encircle the pontine basis and ventral paramedian pontine tegmentum and indicate that injury here produces the aforementioned constellation of symptoms, called locked-in syndrome. In locked-in syndrome, the pontine basis and ventral tegmentum are injured, causing devastating paralysis, which is often misperceived as coma when in reality consciousness is preserved.[2,3,5,7,8,14–16]

Case II

Patient presents with slurred speech and clumsiness of the right hand. Exam reveals impaired smile on the right; dysarthria; dysphagia; loss of fine motor movements in the right hand; and mild weakness of the right arm with normal right leg strength.

Draw another axial section through the pons and establish the anatomic right–left planes of orientation. Now, separate the basis from the tegmentum. Indicate that within the basis of the pons, from medial to lateral, lie the face, arm, and leg fibers. Encircle the face and arm fibers and show that injury here results in dysarthria-clumsy hand syndrome: a syndrome of contralateral face and upper extremity weakness with preserved lower extremity strength due to restricted paramedian pontine injury.[2,3,5,7,8,12,15,17]

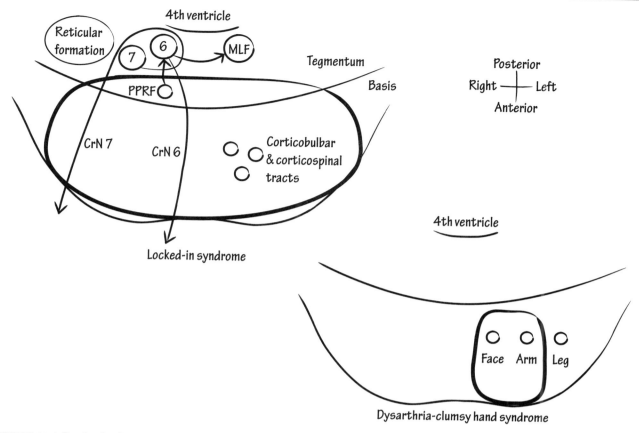

DRAWING 10-4 **Pontine Syndromes**

Medullary Syndromes (*Advanced*)

Case I

Patient presents with dizziness, incoordination, double vision, trouble swallowing, sensory disturbance, and pupillary asymmetry. Exam reveals left-side cerebellar ataxia; loss of pain and temperature sensation in the left face; loss of pain and temperature sensation on the right side of the body; left-side Horner's syndrome (ptosis, anhidrosis, and miosis); dysarthria and impaired gag reflex; ocular skew with the left eye lower than the right; and right-beating nystagmus (slow phase to the left, fast phase to the right).

Draw the left half of the medulla and define the planes of the diagram. This is an axial, anatomic view of the medulla with the anterior surface of the brainstem at the bottom of the page and the posterior surface at the top. First, show that the left cerebellar ataxia results from injury to the left inferior cerebellar peduncle. Next, show that the loss of sensation on the left side of the face results from spinal trigeminal tract and nucleus involvement. Then, show that the loss of pain and temperature sensation on the right side of the body is from injury to the anterolateral system bundle (spinothalamic fibers) on the left. Note that this case represents the classic pattern of sensory loss for this injury type but depending on the rostral-caudal level of the lesion, variation in sensory loss exists; most notably, the facial sensory loss can occur contralaterally or bilaterally rather than ipsilaterally (as shown here).

Now, show that the hoarseness and dysphagia is mostly from involvement of the left nucleus ambiguus. Next, show that the left-side Horner's syndrome is from injury to descending hypothalamospinal tract fibers on the left. Indicate that the descending hypothalamospinal fibers are believed to lie ventral to the solitary tract; injury to the solitary tract, itself, produces taste disturbance.

Next, show that the ocular skew deviation—the left eye being more inferior that the right, and the right-beating nystagmus (slow phase to the left)—results from injury to the left vestibular nucleus and cerebellar system. To understand the nystagmus, point your index fingers toward midline to demonstrate the tonic drive that each side of the medulla places on the eyes. Then drop your left hand to indicate a left medullary lesion: the right side now forces the eyes to the left, which is the slow phase. The direction of the nystagmus, itself, refers to the fast phase: the right-beating compensatory mechanisms that respond to the slow phase.

Encircle the aforementioned structures; injury to this lateral medullary region is called Wallenberg's syndrome. Wallenberg's syndrome most commonly occurs from a posterior inferior cerebellar artery territory infarct caused by a branch occlusion of a vertebral artery. As a final note, through not fully determined pathophysiologic mechanisms, hiccups are also commonly encountered in Wallenberg's syndrome.[2,3,5,7,8,18–23]

Case II

Patient presents with dysarthria, right-side weakness, and sensory disturbance. Exam reveals dysarthric speech; right hemibody loss of vibration and proprioception sensation; and right arm and leg weakness. And with tongue protrusion, there is tongue deviation to the left. Facial sensation and facial strength is spared.

Show that the dysarthria and tongue deviation result from injury to the left hypoglossal nucleus; that the right side large fiber sensory deficit is from injury to the left medial lemniscus tract; and that the right side weakness is from injury to the left medullary pyramid. Encircle these structures and label this syndrome as Dejerine's syndrome, which results from injury to the medial medulla.[2,3,5,7,8,24–26]

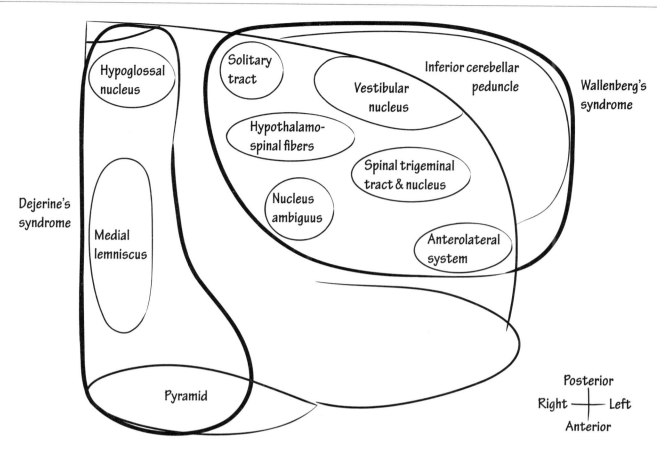

Hypoglossal
nucleus

Solitary
tract

Vestibular
nucleus

Inferior cerebellar
peduncle

Wallenberg's
syndrome

Hypothalamo-
spinal fibers

Spinal trigeminal
tract & nucleus

Dejerine's
syndrome

Nucleus
ambiguus

Medial
lemniscus

Anterolateral
system

Pyramid

Posterior
Right —+— Left
Anterior

DRAWING 10-5 **Medullary Syndromes**

References

1. Baehr, M., Frotscher, M. & Duus, P. *Duus' topical diagnosis in neurology: anatomy, physiology, signs, symptoms,* 4th completely rev. ed., Chapter 3 (Thieme, 2005).
2. DeMyer, W. *Neuroanatomy,* 2nd ed. (Williams & Wilkins, 1998).
3. Haines, D. E. & Ard, M. D. *Fundamental neuroscience: for basic and clinical applications,* 3rd ed. (Churchill Livingstone Elsevier, 2006).
4. Jacobson, S. & Marcus, E. M. *Neuroanatomy for the neuroscientist* (Springer, 2008).
5. Naidich, T. P. & Duvernoy, H. M. *Duvernoy's atlas of the human brain stem and cerebellum: high-field MRI: surface anatomy, internal structure, vascularization and 3D sectional anatomy* (Springer, 2009).
6. Paxinos, G. & Mai, J. K. *The human nervous system,* 2nd ed. (Elsevier Academic Press, 2004).
7. Bogousslavsky, J. & Caplan, L. R. *Stroke syndromes,* 2nd ed. (Cambridge University Press, 2001).
8. Roach, E. S., Toole, J. F., Bettermann, K. & Biller, J. *Toole's cerebrovascular disorders,* 6th ed. (Cambridge University Press, 2010).
9. Vidailhet, M., et al. Dopaminergic dysfunction in midbrain dystonia: anatomoclinical study using 3-dimensional magnetic resonance imaging and fluorodopa F 18 positron emission tomography. *Arch Neurol* 56, 982–989 (1999).
10. Coppola, R. J. Localization of Claude's syndrome. *Neurology* 58, 1707; author reply 1707-1708 (2002).
11. Seo, S. W., et al. Localization of Claude's syndrome. *Neurology* 57, 2304–2307 (2001).
12. Querol-Pascual, M. R. Clinical approach to brainstem lesions. *Semin Ultrasound CT MR* 31, 220–229 (2010).
13. Afifi, A. K. & Bergman, R. A. *Functional neuroanatomy: text and atlas,* 2nd ed. (Lange Medical Books/McGraw-Hill, 2005).
14. Lim, H. S. & Tong, H. I. Locked-in syndrome—a report of three cases. *Singapore Med J* 19, 166–168 (1978).
15. Schmahmann, J. D., Ko, R. & MacMore, J. The human basis pontis: motor syndromes and topographic organization. *Brain* 127, 1269–1291 (2004).
16. Al-Sardar, H. & Grabau, W. Locked-in syndrome caused by basilar artery ectasia. *Age Ageing* 31, 481–482 (2002).
17. Arboix, A., et al. Clinical study of 35 patients with dysarthria-clumsy hand syndrome. *J Neurol Neurosurg Psychiatry* 75, 231–234 (2004).
18. Furman, J. M. a. C., Stephen P. *Vestibular disorders: a case-study approach,* 2nd ed. (Oxford University Press, 2003).
19. Walsh, F. B., Hoyt, W. F. & Miller, N. R. *Walsh and Hoyt's clinical neuro-ophthalmology: the essentials,* 2nd ed. (Lippincott Williams & Wilkins, 2008).
20. Brodsky, M. C., Donahue, S. P., Vaphiades, M. & Brandt, T. Skew deviation revisited. *Surv Ophthalmol* 51, 105–128 (2006).
21. Cerrato, P., et al. Restricted dissociated sensory loss in a patient with a lateral medullary syndrome: A clinical-MRI study. *Stroke* 31, 3064–3066 (2000).
22. Kim, J. S. Pure lateral medullary infarction: clinical-radiological correlation of 130 acute, consecutive patients. *Brain* 126, 1864–1872 (2003).
23. Zhang, S. Q., Liu, M. Y., Wan, B. & Zheng, H. M. Contralateral body half hypalgesia in a patient with lateral medullary infarction: atypical Wallenberg syndrome. *Eur Neurol* 59, 211–215 (2008).
24. Kim, J. S., et al. Medial medullary infarction: abnormal ocular motor findings. *Neurology* 65, 1294–1298 (2005).
25. Nandhagopal, R., Krishnamoorthy, S. G. & Srinivas, D. Neurological picture. Medial medullary infarction. *J Neurol Neurosurg Psychiatry* 77, 215 (2006).
26. Nakajima, M., Inoue, M. & Sakai, Y. Contralateral pharyngeal paralysis caused by medial medullary infarction. *J Neurol Neurosurg Psychiatry* 76, 1292–1293 (2005).

11

Cranial and Spinal Nerve Overview and Skull Base

Spinal & Cranial Nerve Origins

Spinal & Cranial Nuclear Classification

Cranial Nerve Nuclei

Cranial Nerve Nuclei (Simplified)

Skull Base

Skull Foramina

Cavernous Sinus

Know-It Points

Spinal & Cranial Nerve Origins

- The trilaminar developing embryo contains ectoderm, mesoderm, and endoderm.
- The neural crests are neural tube derivatives that give rise to, amongst other things, the peripheral nervous system.
- Sclerotome differentiates into bone; dermatome derives the dermis; the myotomal masses derive skeletal muscle.
- An artery and nerve pair corresponds to each somite segment, and wherever the products of that somite go, the nerve and artery pair follows.
- The sulcus limitans separates the basal and alar plates.
- The basal plates, which produce the ventral roots, house motor cell columns.
- The alar plates, which receive the dorsal roots, house sensory cell columns.

Spinal & Cranial Nuclear Classification

- In the spinal cord:
  - The general somatic afferent column lies in the posterior horn.
  - The general somatic efferent column lies in the anterior horn.
  - The general visceral afferent column lies in the posterior intermediate horn.
  - The general visceral efferent column lies in the anterior intermediate horn.
- In the brainstem:
  - The general somatic efferent column lies medial to the general visceral efferent column.
  - The general visceral afferent column lies medial to the general somatic afferent column.
  - Within the upper medulla, the special somatic afferent column spans the width of the alar plate.
  - The special visceral cell columns hug the sulcus limitans.

Cranial Nerve Nuclei

- The somatomotor set is nearly exclusively general somatic efferent, but it also includes a single general visceral efferent nucleus.
- The solely special sensory set is exclusively special somatic afferent.
- The pharyngeal arch derivatives contain all of the cell column types except for the general somatic efferent and special somatic afferent cell columns.
- The somatomotor set lies in midline and comprises cranial nerves 3, 4, 6, 12, and 11.
- The solely special sensory set comprises cranial nerves 1, 2, and 8.
- The pharyngeal arch set comprises cranial nerves 5, 7, 9, and 10.

Skull Base

- The anterior cranial fossa comprises the frontal bone, ethmoid bone, jugum sphenoidale, and lesser wing of the sphenoid bone.
- The basal portions of the frontal lobes lie within anterior cranial fossae.
- The middle cranial fossa comprises the greater wing of the sphenoid bone, a portion of the squamous temporal bone, a portion of the petrous temporal bone, and the sella turcica of the sphenoid bone.

- The basal portions of the temporal lobes lie within the middle cranial fossae.
- The posterior cranial fossa comprises the posterior portion of the petrous bone, the occipital bone, and the clivus.
- The cerebellum and brainstem lie within the posterior cranial fossae.
- The occipital and parietal lobes lie superior to the plane of the skull base.

Skull Foramina

- The foramina of the cribriform plate of the ethmoid bone contain the olfactory nerve bundles (cranial nerve 1).
- The optic nerve (cranial nerve 2) traverses the optic canal.
- The oculomotor, trochlear, and abducens nerves (cranial nerves 3, 4, and 6, respectively) and the first division of the trigeminal nerve (the ophthalmic nerve [5(1)]) pass through the superior orbital fissure.
- The second division of the trigeminal nerve (the maxillary nerve [5(2)]) traverses foramen rotundum.

- The third division of the trigeminal nerve (the mandibular nerve [5(3)]) traverses foramen ovale.
- The facial nerve (cranial nerve 7) and vestibulocochlear nerve (cranial nerve 8) pass through the internal acoustic meatus.
- The glossopharyngeal nerve (cranial nerve 9), vagus nerve (cranial nerve 10), and spinal accessory nerve (cranial nerve 11) pass through the jugular foramen.
- The hypoglossal nerve (cranial nerve 12) passes through the hypoglossal canal.
- The spinal accessory nerve enters the cranium through the foramen magnum (and exits through the jugular foramen).

Cavernous Sinus

- The cavernous sinus is a major venous confluence with many venous communications.
- Along the lateral wall of the cavernous sinus, from superior to inferior, lie cranial nerves 3 and 4 and the first and second divisions of cranial nerve 5.
- Medial to the first division of cranial nerve 5 lies cranial nerve 6.

- Within the medial aspect of the cavernous sinus lies the internal carotid artery.
- The posterolateral cavernous sinus dura forms the medial upper third of Meckel's cave, which envelops the trigeminal ganglion.

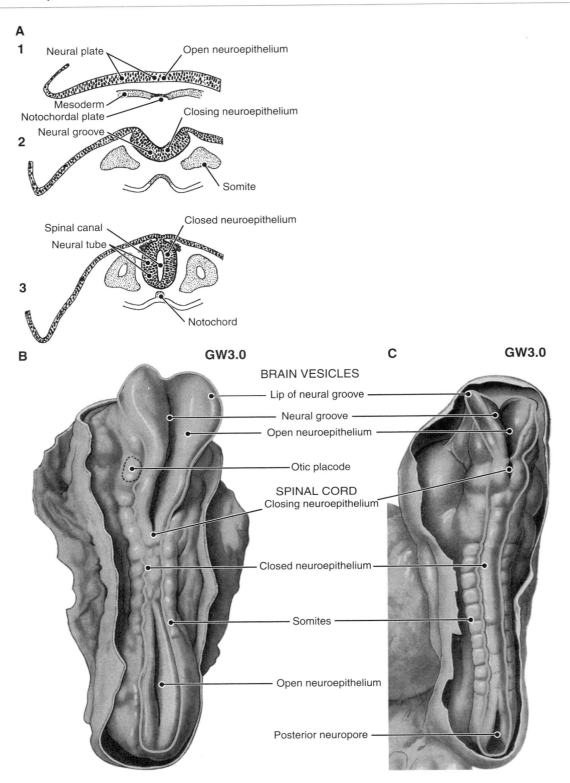

FIGURE 11-1 A. Axial section through the developing embryo and B. Neural tube model and axial section. Used with permission from Altman, Joseph, and Shirley A. Bayer. *Development of the Human Spinal Cord: An Interpretation Based on Experimental Studies in Animals.* Oxford; New York: Oxford University Press, 2001.

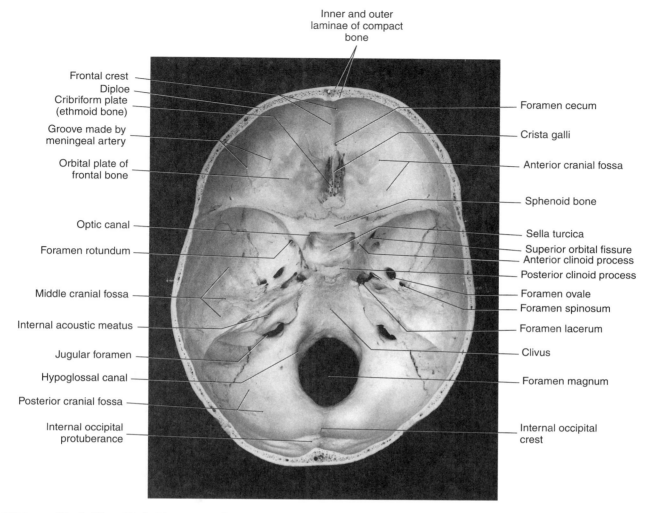

FIGURE 11-2 The skull base. Used with permission from Bruni, J. E. & Montemurro, D. G. *Human Neuroanatomy: A Text, Brain Atlas, and Laboratory Dissection Guide.* New York: Oxford University Press, 2009.

Spinal & Cranial Nerve Origins

To understand the origins of the spinal and cranial nerves, we will draw the developing embryo. First, draw a coronal section through the dorsal half of the embryo. Label the outer layer as the ectoderm; it derives the epidermis and neuroectoderm. Then, draw endoderm at the bottom of the diagram; it comprises most of the ventral half of the embryo and it forms the gut and respiratory contents of the developing embryo. Next, draw the notochord and indicate that it is mesoderm-derived. We have thus established the three main layers of the trilaminar developing embryo: the ectoderm, mesoderm, and endoderm.

The developing embryo forms around the notochord and the notochord eventually degenerates into the jelly-like substance of the intervertebral discs, called nucleus pulposus. If the notochord persists in its primitive state, it is considered chordoma—notochord tumor. The notochord induces the overlying ectoderm to develop into the neural plate. Its neural folds then invaginate to become the oval-shaped neural tube, which has a long, narrow cerebrospinal fluid space in its center, and, as mentioned, is ectoderm-derived. We will draw the details of the neural tube later.

Dorsolateral to the neural tube, draw the neural crests, which are neural tube derivatives that give rise to, amongst other things, the peripheral nervous system. Next, draw somite tissue masses lateral to the notochord; they, like the notochord, are mesoderm-derived. The neural crest cells and somite tissue masses develop early in embryogenesis and the somite masses derive sclerotomal, myotomal, and dermatomal cells. We will include the somites in our diagram along with their derivatives, albeit an anachronism, for simplicity.

Draw three arrows from one of the somite masses as follows. Direct one to the notochord and label it sclerotome: the sclerotome differentiates into bone. Indicate that the sclerotome around the notochord becomes vertebral bone. Next, draw another arrow dorsally to the surface of the embryo and label it dermatome, which derives the dermis: the skin layer underlying the epidermis. Then, direct the last arrow laterally to the myotomal masses, which derive skeletal muscle.

An artery and nerve pair corresponds to each somite segment, and wherever the products of that somite go, the nerve and artery pair follows. This is the anatomic basis of how we systematically assess dermatomal and myotomal levels during the neurologic exam. From the peripheral distribution of the deficit, we localize the rostral–caudal level of the lesion.

With that embryogenesis as a background, let's take a closer look at the origin of the cranial and spinal nerves. Separate the tissue within the neural tube into a ventral-lying basal plate and a dorsal-lying alar plate. Along the horizontal meridian, label the sulcus limitans: a small sulcus, which cuts into the lateral walls of the central-lying cerebrospinal fluid space and separates the basal and alar plates. Somite nerve pairs emanate from these neural plates as nerve roots: the ventral roots carry motor fibers and the dorsal roots carry sensory fibers (in accordance with the law of Bell and Magendie). This ventral–dorsal functional division applies to the neural tube, as well. The basal plates, which produce the ventral roots, house motor cell columns, and the alar plates, which receive sensory roots, house sensory cell columns. The ventral–motor/dorsal–sensory division that exists early in embryogenesis in the neural tube persists throughout development. This division provides the basis for the organization of the spinal and cranial nerves.[1-4]

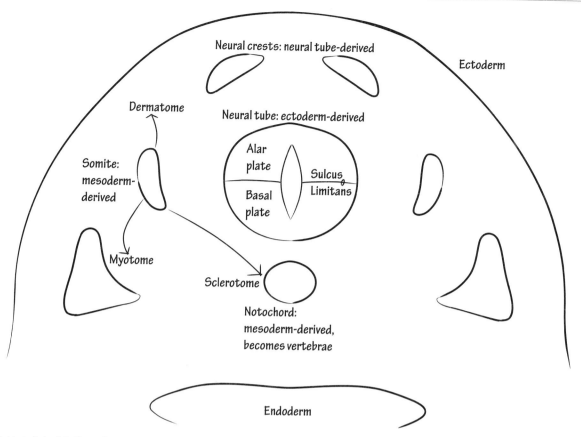

DRAWING 11-1 **Spinal & Cranial Nerve Origins**

Spinal & Cranial Nuclear Classification

Here, we will draw the spinal neurons and the brainstem cranial nerve nuclei in axial view. Draw an axial cross-section through the spinal cord. First, divide the spinal cord gray matter into alar (sensory) and basal (motor) plates. Then, divide the gray matter into three anatomic horns: posterior, intermediate, and anterior. Now, label the cell columns: general somatic afferent in the posterior horn, general somatic efferent in the anterior horn, general visceral afferent in the posterior intermediate horn, and general visceral efferent in the anterior intermediate horn.

Next, let's draw the cranial nerve nuclear cell columns. They share the same general layout as the spinal neurons but have two key anatomic differences. One difference is that in the brainstem, the posterior-lying alar plate shifts laterally to make room for the fourth ventricle; therefore, all of the cranial nerve nuclei end up oriented along the horizontal axis of the dorsal brainstem tegmentum. To understand this shift, imagine opening an orange—the dorsum of the orange swings out laterally. A second difference between the brainstem cell columns and the spinal cord is that the brainstem involves additional cell columns—the special visceral efferent and afferent cell columns and the special somatic afferent cell column. The special visceral cell columns are part of the pharyngeal arch (aka branchial arch) cranial nerve derivatives, which appear early in embryogenesis as bar-like ridges that contain the ectoderm, endoderm, and mesoderm that form the skeletal tissue, musculature, and linings of the head and neck. The pharyngeal arches produce cranial nerve, arterial, and musculoskeletal derivatives.[5]

Now, let's draw the cranial nuclear columns of the brainstem. Draw one side of an axial brainstem composite: a compression of all three brainstem levels. Divide it from posterior to anterior into tectum, tegmentum, and basis. The cranial nuclear cell columns lie within the dorsal tegmentum, just in front of the cerebrospinal fluid space. Next, label the sulcus limitans in the fourth ventricle; it separates the efferent from the afferent cell columns. Now, begin with the cranial homologues of the spinal nerves: in the basal plate, from medial to lateral, draw the general somatic efferent and general visceral efferent cell columns, and in the alar plate, from medial to lateral, draw the general visceral afferent and general somatic afferent cell columns. Next, include the special somatic afferent column; within the upper medulla, its constellation of subnuclei spans the width of the alar plate. Now, we need to address the special visceral cell columns, both of which hug the sulcus limitans. Draw the special visceral efferent cell column in the space between the general visceral efferent cell column and the sulcus limitans. Then, join the special visceral afferent cell column with the general visceral afferent column in the medial alar plate.

Note that some texts substitute the word "somatic" with the word "sensory" when referring to the general somatic afferent and special somatic afferent columns and refer to them, instead, as the general sensory and special sensory afferent columns.[6,7]

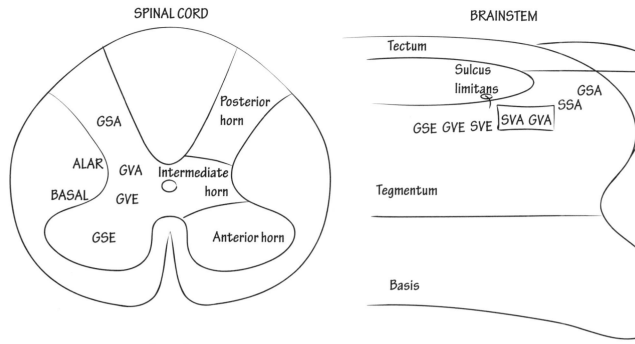

SPINAL CORD

BRAINSTEM

GSE - General Somatic Efferent
GVE - General Visceral Efferent
SVE - Special Visceral Efferent

GSA - General Somatic Afferent
GVA - General Visceral Afferent
SSA - Special Somatic Afferent
SVA - Special Visceral Afferent

DRAWING 11-2 **Spinal & Cranial Nuclear Classification**

Cranial Nerve Nuclei

Here, we will draw the organization of the cranial nerve nuclei in coronal view. Draw a coronal section through the brainstem and upper cervical spinal cord and mark the boundaries of the midbrain, pons, and medulla. Then, denote the sulcus limitans, which divides the brainstem into basal and alar plates. Along the top of the brainstem, list the positions of the cell columns. At the medial end of the basal plate (ie, at the midline of the brainstem), label the general somatic efferent column; lateral to it, label the general visceral efferent column; continuing laterally, label the special visceral efferent column; then, label the combined general visceral afferent and special visceral afferent columns; then, label the special somatic afferent column; and finally, label the general somatic afferent column.

We organize the cranial nerves into three groups of nerves: the somatomotor (aka somitic), solely special sensory, and pharyngeal arch derivatives. Each of the different cranial nerve sets involves various populations of cell columns. The somatomotor set is nearly exclusively general somatic efferent, but also includes a single general visceral efferent nucleus; the solely special sensory set is exclusively special somatic afferent; and the pharyngeal arch derivatives contain all of the cell column types except for the general somatic efferent and special somatic afferent cells.

Begin with the somatomotor set. It lies in midline and comprises cranial nerves 3, 4, 6, 12, and 11. The somatomotor set is considered the brainstem extension of the spinal neurons because it innervates somite tissue derivatives. However, whereas the spinal neurons contain general somatic efferent and afferent and general visceral efferent and afferent cells, the somatomotor cranial nerve set comprises only general somatic efferent cells and a single general visceral efferent nucleus—the Edinger–Westphal nucleus. To demonstrate the actions of the somatomotor cranial nerve set, move your eyes in all directions using cranial nerves 3, 4, and 6; protrude your tongue using cranial nerve 12; and shrug your shoulders using cranial nerve 11. Notice that these movements involve midline muscles, which helps us remember that the general somatic efferent cell column lies near to midline.

Now, in the general somatic efferent column, in descending order, draw the nuclei of the somatomotor set. Label the oculomotor nucleus of cranial nerve 3 (the oculomotor nerve): it extends from the upper to the lower midbrain, spanning the height of the superior colliculus and reaching the level of the inferior colliculus. Then, underneath the oculomotor nucleus, label the trochlear nucleus of cranial nerve 4 (the trochlear nerve): it is a small nucleus that lies in the caudal midbrain at the level of the inferior colliculus. Next, label the abducens nucleus of cranial nerve 6 (the abducens nerve): it spans from the mid to the lower pons. Now, show the hypoglossal nucleus of cranial nerve 12 (the hypoglossal nerve), which spans most of the height of the medulla. Then, label the accessory nucleus of cranial nerve 11 (the accessory nerve) in the upper cervical spinal cord: it spans the first five cervical spinal cord levels.

Next, in the general visceral efferent cell column, draw the Edinger–Westphal nucleus of cranial nerve 3 (the oculomotor nerve), which lies in the rostral midbrain. Note that although we distinguish this nucleus from the oculomotor nucleus, it is actually a rostral subnucleus of the oculomotor complex, which comprises all of the nuclei of cranial nerve 3.

Now, we will draw the solely special sensory set, which comprises cranial nerves 1, 2, and 8, all of which are purely sensory. Cranial nerve 1 is involved in olfaction, cranial nerve 2 in vision, and cranial nerve 8 in vestibular and auditory function. Only cranial nerve 8 resides within the brainstem. Cranial nerve 1 comprises tiny nerve filaments that traverse the cribriform plate, and cranial nerve 2 is the set of optic nerves that run underneath the base of the brain.

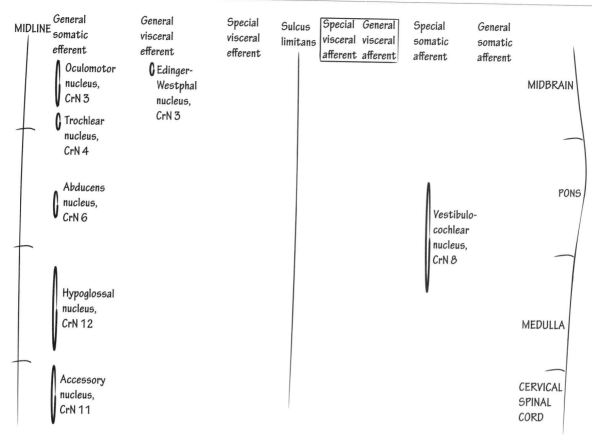

MIDLINE	General somatic efferent	General visceral efferent	Special visceral efferent	Sulcus limitans	Special visceral afferent	General visceral afferent	Special somatic afferent	General somatic afferent	
	Oculomotor nucleus, CrN 3	Edinger-Westphal nucleus, CrN 3							MIDBRAIN
	Trochlear nucleus, CrN 4								
	Abducens nucleus, CrN 6								PONS
							Vestibulo-cochlear nucleus, CrN 8		
	Hypoglossal nucleus, CrN 12								MEDULLA
	Accessory nucleus, CrN 11								CERVICAL SPINAL CORD

DRAWING 11-3 **Cranial Nerve Nuclei—Partial**

Cranial Nerve Nuclei (Cont.)

Next, in the special somatic afferent column, label the vestibulocochlear nucleus of cranial nerve 8 (the vestibulocochlear nerve), which spans from the upper pons to the mid-medulla. Although not shown as such, here, within the upper medulla, its constellation of subnuclei spans the width of the alar plate: from the sulcus limitans to the lateral edge of the brainstem.

Now, let's draw the pharyngeal arch set, which comprises the remaining cranial nerve nuclei: cranial nerves 5, 7, 9, and 10. According to the simplest, most common definition, the first pharyngeal arch derives cranial nerve 5, the second pharyngeal arch derives cranial nerve 7, the third pharyngeal arch derives cranial nerve 9, and the fourth and sixth pharyngeal arches derive cranial nerve 10. Charles Judson Herrick's early 1900s observations about the role of these cranial nerves in the gill arches of fish provides insight into their purpose in humans. Fish use these nerves to coordinate jaw movements that pump water across their gills for oxygen transfer. In humans, oxygen transfer occurs in the lungs, so we use the special visceral efferent component of these cranial nerves, instead, for other purposes, including chewing (cranial nerve 5), facial expression (cranial nerve 7), and speaking and swallowing (cranial nerves 9 and 10).

Taste is carried by special visceral afferents of cranial nerve 7 from the anterior two thirds of the tongue and by cranial nerves 9 and 10 from the posterior one third of the tongue and the epiglottis, respectively. Facial sensation is mostly carried by cranial nerve 5, but it is also carried by cranial nerves 7, 9, and 10, to a lesser extent. Finally, cranial nerves 7, 9, and 10 also provide parasympathetic innervation to the glands and viscera of the face and thoracoabdomen.

Now, let's draw the nuclei of the pharyngeal arch set. Start with the nuclei of the general visceral efferent cell column. Indicate that the superior salivatory nucleus of cranial nerve 7 (the facial nerve) is a small nucleus that sits at the inferior border of the pons. Then, underneath the superior salivatory nucleus, show that the inferior salivatory nucleus of cranial nerve 9 (the glossopharyngeal nerve) is a small nucleus in the upper medulla. Now, underneath the inferior salivatory nucleus, draw the dorsal motor nucleus of the vagus nerve, cranial nerve 10, as spanning from the inferior salivatory nucleus to the bottom of the medulla.

Next, let's draw the special visceral efferent cell column. Begin with the motor trigeminal nucleus of cranial nerve 5 (the trigeminal nerve) in the upper pons. Then, draw the facial nucleus of cranial nerve 7 (the facial nerve), which spans from the lower pons to the pontomedullary junction. Next, draw the nucleus ambiguus of cranial nerves 9 and 10, which spans the height of the medulla. Note that the nucleus ambiguus actually has both special visceral and general visceral efferent components.

Now, turn to the sensory cells in the alar plate. Begin with the combined special and general visceral afferent cell column; draw the solitary tract nucleus of cranial nerves 7, 9, and 10, which spans the height of the medulla. Then, move to the general somatic afferent cell column at the lateral end of the alar plate; draw the three subnuclei of the trigeminal nucleus: the mesencephalic trigeminal nucleus, which spans from the midbrain to the upper pons; the principal sensory trigeminal nucleus, which is restricted to the upper pons; and the spinal trigeminal nucleus, which spans from the upper pons to the upper cervical spinal cord. Cranial nerve 5 contributes to all three subdivisions of the trigeminal nucleus, and cranial nerves 7, 9, and 10 help supply the spinal trigeminal nucleus, only.[3,4,6–12]

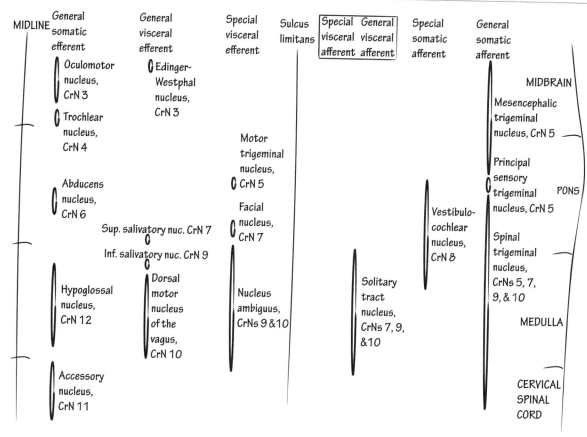

MIDLINE

General somatic efferent

Oculomotor nucleus, CrN 3

Trochlear nucleus, CrN 4

Abducens nucleus, CrN 6

Hypoglossal nucleus, CrN 12

Accessory nucleus, CrN 11

General visceral efferent

Edinger-Westphal nucleus, CrN 3

Sup. salivatory nuc. CrN 7

Inf. salivatory nuc. CrN 9

Dorsal motor nucleus of the vagus, CrN 10

Special visceral efferent

Motor trigeminal nucleus, CrN 5

Facial nucleus, CrN 7

Nucleus ambiguus, CrNs 9 & 10

Sulcus limitans

Special visceral afferent | General visceral afferent

Solitary tract nucleus, CrNs 7, 9, & 10

Special somatic afferent

Vestibulo-cochlear nucleus, CrN 8

General somatic afferent

Mesencephalic trigeminal nucleus, CrN 5

Principal sensory trigeminal nucleus, CrN 5

Spinal trigeminal nucleus, CrNs 5, 7, 9, & 10

MIDBRAIN

PONS

MEDULLA

CERVICAL SPINAL CORD

DRAWING 11-4 **Cranial Nerve Nuclei—Complete**

Cranial Nerve Nuclei *(Simplified)*

Here, we will consolidate the cranial nerve nuclei into a simple diagram we can recall at the bedside. Note that this compression is not a depiction of the complete cranial nerve nuclei but instead provides an easy way to remember the relative positions of the cranial nerves. Draw another coronal brainstem. Across the top, use the sulcus limitans to divide the brainstem into a medial, motor division and a lateral, sensory division. Then divide the rostral–caudal axis of the brainstem into the midbrain, pons, and medulla. Along the medial half of the motor division, draw the cranial nerve nucleus of cranial nerve 3 in the rostral midbrain, 4 in the caudal midbrain, 6 in the mid- to lower pons, 12 spanning the height of the medulla, and 11 in the cervical spinal cord. In the lateral motor area, draw the efferent cranial nerve nucleus of cranial nerve 5 in the rostral pons, 7 in the caudal pons, and 9 and 10 spanning the height of the medulla.

Next, in the medial sensory region, draw the afferent cranial nerve nuclei of cranial nerves 7, 9, and 10 spanning the height of the medulla. Then, draw the cranial nerve nucleus of cranial nerve 8 from the pons into the medulla. Next, at the lateral edge of the brainstem, show that the afferent nucleus of cranial nerve 5 spans from the midbrain to the upper cervical spinal cord, and also show that it receives additional afferent innervation from cranial nerves 7, 9, and 10.

The cranial nuclei are numbered by their rostral–caudal positions as they exit the base of the brain. Cranial nerve 1 lies rostral to 2, 2 to 3, 3 to 4, and so on. The only exception is cranial nerve 11, which originates from below cranial nerve 12. One way to recall this rostral–caudal organization is to imagine that you are a primordial fish swimming through the great sea. First, you smell food (cranial nerve 1, the olfactory nerve); then, you visualize it (cranial nerve 2, the optic nerve); next, you fix your eyes on it, for which you use your extraocular eye muscles—innervated by cranial nerve 3 (the oculomotor nerve), cranial nerve 4 (the trochlear nerve), and cranial nerve 6 (the abducens nerve); you chew the food using cranial nerve 5 (the trigeminal nerve) and then taste it and smile using cranial nerve 7 (the facial nerve). Then, you listen for predators with cranial nerve 8 (the vestibulocochlear nerve) while you swallow the meal with cranial nerves 9 (the glossopharyngeal nerve) and 10 (the vagus nerve); you lick your lips with cranial nerve 12 (the hypoglossal nerve); and toss your head from side to side with cranial nerve 11 (the accessory nerve).[3,4,6–12]

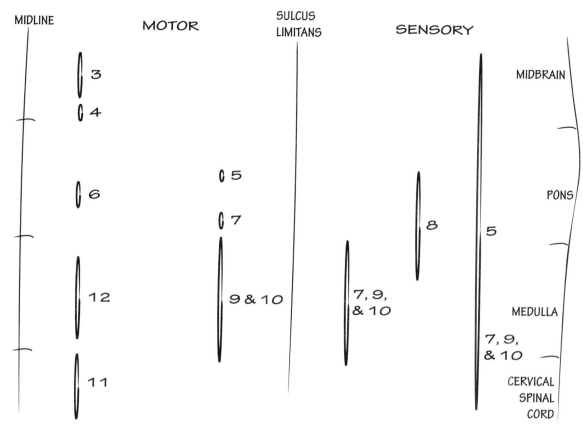

DRAWING 11-5 **Cranial Nerve Nuclei** (*Simplified*)

Skull Base

Here, we will draw the skull base in axial view. Draw an outline of one half of an axial view of the skull base and label its anterior one third as the frontal bone. Next, in midline, demarcate the ethmoid bone, which comprises the steeply peaked crista galli and the surrounding cribriform plate. Then, posterior to the frontal bone, draw the sphenoid bone, which subdivides into a body and lesser and greater wings. First, label the midline portion of the sphenoid bone as the sphenoid body. Show that it subdivides into the jugum sphenoidale, anteriorly, and the sella turcica, posteriorly. The posterior end of the midline sphenoid bone and the neighboring anterior occipital bone (drawn later), together, form the clivus. Now, draw the sphenoid wings. Label the lesser wing, anteriorly, and the greater wing, posteriorly. Topographically, the lesser sphenoid wing angles up over the greater sphenoid wing, which rolls downward. Label the protuberance along the posteromedial ridge of the lesser wing as the anterior clinoid process, an important anatomic landmark.

Next, draw the temporal bone posterior to the greater wing of the sphenoid bone. Label the squamous part, laterally, and the petrous part, medially. The squamous part makes up the bulk of the external surface of the temporal bone, whereas the petrous part makes up the bulk of the internal surface. Next, posteromedial to the temporal bone, draw the occipital bone; it extends back to the occiput. In the anterior one third of the occipital bone, draw the foramen magnum, which is the entry zone of the brainstem. Now, label the combined anterior occipital bone and posterior sphenoid bone as the clivus, which is steeply sloped. Next, along the lateral edge of the skull base, label the parietal bone. The parietal bones make up much of the lateral and superior surfaces of the skull.

Now, let's draw a sagittal section of the skull to illustrate how the peaks and valleys within the skull base form different fossae. Draw a downward-sloping line with two peaks. Label the anterior depression as the anterior cranial fossa, the middle depression as the middle cranial fossa, and the posterior depression as the posterior cranial fossa.[1]

Next, let's define the borders of these fossae in our axial diagram. First, let's include the major peaks within the skull base (the fossae comprise the valleys between these peaks). Dot a line along the lesser wing of the sphenoid bone. Anterior to it, label the anterior cranial fossa, which comprises the frontal bone, ethmoid bone, jugum sphenoidale, and lesser wing of the sphenoid bone—the basal portions of the frontal lobes lie within this fossa. Next, dot a diagonal line through the petrous temporal bone. Indicate that the middle cranial fossa lies between the lesser wing of the sphenoid bone and the petrous ridge of the temporal bone. The middle cranial fossa comprises the greater wing of the sphenoid bone, a portion of the squamous temporal bone, a portion of the petrous temporal bone, and the sella turcica of the sphenoid bone—the basal portions of the temporal lobes lie within this fossa. Lastly, posterior to the petrous ridge, label the posterior cranial fossa, which comprises the posterior portion of the petrous bone, the occipital bone, and the clivus—the cerebellum and brainstem lie within this fossa. Note that the occipital and parietal lobes lie superior to the plane of the skull base.[13]

Next, we will draw the foramina of the skull base. Skull base injuries and diseases present with unique patterns of neurologic deficit, so we need a good understanding of the skull foramina and their neurovascular contents to diagnose the various presentations of skull base injury.[3,4,6,13,14]

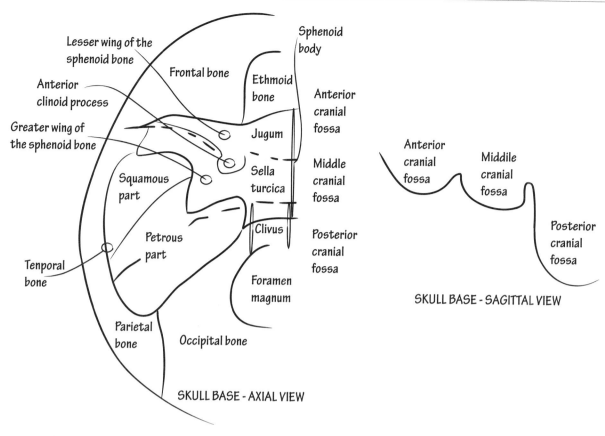

DRAWING 11-6 **Skull Base**

Skull Foramina

Here, we will draw the skull foramina. First, draw the anterior half of the skull base in axial view; include the following topographic landmarks: the frontal bone, ethmoid bone, lesser wing of the sphenoid bone (include its anterior clinoid process), and the ridge of the petrous portion of the temporal bone. Next, we will label the major neurovascular structures and cranial nerves that pass through the foramina; we will denote the cranial nerves in brackets. Show that the foramina of the cribriform plate of the ethmoid bone contain the olfactory nerve bundles (cranial nerve 1). Next, medial to the anterior clinoid process, label the optic canal and lateral to it label the superior orbital fissure. Show that the optic nerve (cranial nerve 2) traverses the optic canal and that the oculomotor, trochlear, and abducens nerves (cranial nerves 3, 4, and 6, respectively) and the first division of the trigeminal nerve (the ophthalmic nerve [5(1)]) pass through the superior orbital fissure. Next, show that the ophthalmic artery traverses the optic canal and that the superior ophthalmic vein passes through the superior orbital fissure. The ophthalmic artery is a direct branch of the internal carotid artery, which traverses the carotid canal; indicate that the carotid canal lies along the petrous ridge. Note that adjacent to the carotid canal is the foramen lacerum, which the internal carotid artery runs above in its lacerum segment (see Drawing 11-8).[15]

Next, posterior to the superior orbital fissure, within the greater wing of the sphenoid bone, from anterior to posterior, label foramen rotundum, foramen ovale, and foramen spinosum. Indicate that the second division of the trigeminal nerve (the maxillary nerve [5(2)]) traverses foramen rotundum and that the third division of the trigeminal nerve (the mandibular nerve [5(3)]) traverses foramen ovale. To remember that foramen *rotundum* houses the second division of the trigeminal nerve, think of the "Star Wars" character *R2D2*, whose round head and name (*R2D2*) should serve as a helpful mnemonic. Note that within the mandible is foramen mentum, which houses the distal mandibular nerve branch—the mental nerve, which provides sensory coverage to the mentum (the chin). Lastly, indicate that foramen spinosum contains the meningeal branch of the mandibular nerve (aka nervus spinosus) and also the middle meningeal artery—injury to this vessel can lead to intracranial epidural hematoma.[9,16]

Now, draw the posterior surface of the skull base in axial view; include the posterior extension of the petrous ridge and the foramen magnum as topographic landmarks.[17] First, along the petrous apex, draw the internal acoustic meatus. Indicate that both the facial nerve (cranial nerve 7) and vestibulocochlear nerve (cranial nerve 8) and the internal auditory artery (aka labyrinthine artery) pass through the internal acoustic meatus. Next, below the internal acoustic meatus, draw the jugular foramen, which lies at the border of the temporal and occipital bones. Show that the glossopharyngeal nerve (cranial nerve 9), vagus nerve (cranial nerve 10), and spinal accessory nerve (cranial nerve 11) pass through the jugular foramen; and also show that the internal jugular vein passes through the jugular foramen—it receives the sigmoid sinus and inferior petrosal sinus.[18] Now, along the foramen magnum, label the hypoglossal canal and show that both the hypoglossal nerve (cranial nerve 12) and also a venous plexus pass through the hypoglossal canal. Then, indicate that in addition to traversing the jugular foramen, the spinal accessory nerve also runs through foramen magnum; it originates in the cervical spinal cord, passes up through foramen magnum, and then passes out of the cranium through the jugular foramen. Finally, indicate that the vertebral arteries and spinal vessels traverse the foramen magnum as well.[3,4,6–11]

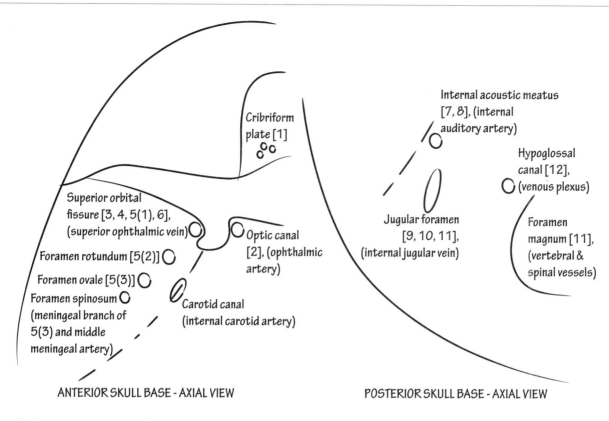

ANTERIOR SKULL BASE - AXIAL VIEW

Cribriform plate [1]

Superior orbital fissure [3, 4, 5(1), 6], (superior ophthalmic vein)

Foramen rotundum [5(2)]

Foramen ovale [5(3)]

Foramen spinosum (meningeal branch of 5(3) and middle meningeal artery)

Optic canal [2], (ophthalmic artery)

Carotid canal (internal carotid artery)

POSTERIOR SKULL BASE - AXIAL VIEW

Internal acoustic meatus [7, 8], (internal auditory artery)

Hypoglossal canal [12], (venous plexus)

Jugular foramen [9, 10, 11], (internal jugular vein)

Foramen magnum [11], (vertebral & spinal vessels)

[ ] - indicates cranial nerve #

DRAWING 11-7 **Skull Foramina**

Cavernous Sinus

Here, we will draw the cavernous sinus in coronal and oblique views. Begin with the coronal diagram; show its planes of orientation. Next, let's draw a few related anatomic landmarks: the sella turcica of the sphenoid bone and related pituitary body, the base of the brain and underlying optic nerves, and the medial edge of the temporal lobe. Then, draw one of the paired sphenoid sinuses within the sphenoid bone and indicate that it is air-filled.

Next, draw one of the bilateral cavernous sinuses between the sella turcica and the temporal lobe. Indicate that the cavernous sinuses are filled with venous trabeculations; the cavernous sinus is a major venous confluence with many venous communications. Next, let's draw the contents of one of the cavernous sinuses (we will label the cranial nerves in brackets). Along the lateral wall of the cavernous sinus, from superior to inferior, label cranial nerves 3 and 4 and then the first and second divisions of cranial nerve 5. Next, medial to the first division of cranial nerve 5, label cranial nerve 6. Then, within the medial aspect of the cavernous sinus, label the internal carotid artery. Finally, draw another portion of the internal carotid artery in between the roof of the cavernous sinus and the ipsilateral optic nerve—the carotid artery doubles back across the top of the cavernous sinus, as we will show in our oblique view, next. Within the cavernous sinus, the pupillosympathetic fibers run across cranial nerve 6 when they leave the internal carotid artery to join the first division of the fifth cranial nerve.

Now, we will draw an oblique view of the cavernous sinus. Begin with our planes of orientation and then let's draw the skull landmarks. Draw the anterior clinoid process, which is the posteromedial edge of the lesser wing of the sphenoid bone, and then draw the relevant foramina: medial to the anterior clinoid process, label the optic canal, and lateral to it, draw the superior orbital fissure; posterior to the superior orbital fissure, draw foramen rotundum, and posterior to it, draw foramen ovale.[19]

Next, indicate that cranial nerve 2 passes through the optic canal and then that cranial nerves 3, 4, and 6 pass through the superior orbital fissure. Then, show that cranial nerve 5(1) passes through the superior orbital fissure, 5(2) passes through foramen rotundum, and 5(3) (which does not pass through the cavernous sinus) passes through foramen ovale, and that all of these divisions of the trigeminal nerve join together as the trigeminal ganglion.

Now, let's draw the course of the internal carotid artery. Here, we follow Bouthillier's 1996 classification scheme. First, show that within the cervical segment, the artery ascends from the carotid bifurcation through the carotid space to the carotid canal; in the petrous segment, the carotid artery rises and passes forward within the carotid canal; in the lacerum segment, it exits the carotid canal and rises into the cavernous sinus; in the cavernous sinus segment, it rises within the cavernous sinus, then passes forward through it, and then rises out of the cavernous sinus, where it becomes the clinoid segment, which curves posteriorly; in the ophthalmic segment, the artery passes posteriorly and gives off the ophthalmic artery, which traverses anteriorly through the optic canal; lastly, within the communicating segment, the carotid artery rises into the suprasellar cistern and gives off the anterior choroidal and posterior communicating artery branches and bifurcates into the anterior and middle cerebral arteries.[20–22]

Finally, let's define the walls of the dura-enclosed cavernous sinus. Show that its roof underlies the level of the anterior clinoid process; that anteriorly, the cavernous sinus extends to the superior orbital fissure; that posteriorly, it reaches the apex of the petrous bone/upper clivus; that medially, it neighbors the lateral sella turcica; and that laterally, it neighbors the medial temporal lobe. Finally, show that the posterolateral cavernous sinus dura also forms the medial upper third of Meckel's cave, which envelops the trigeminal ganglion.[7,23]

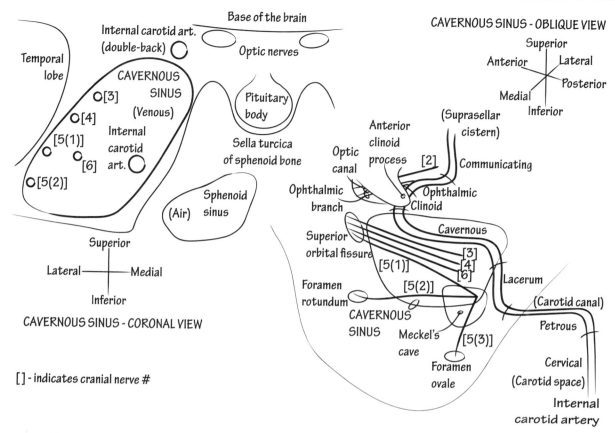

Base of the brain

Internal carotid art. (double-back)

Optic nerves

Temporal lobe

CAVERNOUS SINUS (Venous)

O[3]

O[4]

[5(1)]

O[6]

O[5(2)]

Internal carotid art.

Pituitary body

Sella turcica of sphenoid bone

(Air) Sphenoid sinus

Superior
Lateral — Medial
Inferior

CAVERNOUS SINUS - CORONAL VIEW

[ ] - indicates cranial nerve #

CAVERNOUS SINUS - OBLIQUE VIEW

Superior
Anterior   Lateral
Posterior
Medial   Inferior

(Suprasellar cistern)

Optic canal

Anterior clinoid process

[2]

Communicating

Ophthalmic branch

Ophthalmic

Clinoid

Cavernous

Superior orbital fissure

[5(1)]

[3]
[4]
[6]

[5(2)]

Lacerum

(Carotid canal)

Foramen rotundum

CAVERNOUS SINUS

Meckel's cave

[5(3)]

Petrous

Foramen ovale

Cervical (Carotid space)

Internal carotid artery

DRAWING 11-8 **Cavernous Sinus**

References

1. Jinkins, R. *Atlas of neuroradiologic embryology, anatomy, and variants* (Lippincott Williams & Wilkins, 2000).

2. Donkelaar, H. J. T., Lammens, M., Hori, A. & Cremers, C. W. R. J. *Clinical neuroembryology: development and developmental disorders of the human central nervous system* (Springer, 2006).

3. Haines, D. E. & Ard, M. D. *Fundamental neuroscience: for basic and clinical applications,* 3rd ed. (Churchill Livingstone Elsevier, 2006).

4. Standring, S. & Gray, H. *Gray's anatomy: the anatomical basis of clinical practice,* 40th ed. (Churchill Livingstone/Elsevier, 2008).

5. Rosen, C. J. & American Society for Bone and Mineral Research. *Primer on the metabolic bone diseases and disorders of mineral metabolism,* 7th ed., p. 953 (American Society for Bone and Mineral Research, 2008).

6. Wilson-Pauwels, L. *Cranial nerves: function and dysfunction,* 3rd ed. (People's Medical Pub. House, 2010).

7. Naidich, T. P. & Duvernoy, H. M. *Duvernoy's atlas of the human brain stem and cerebellum: high-field MRI: surface anatomy, internal structure, vascularization and 3D sectional anatomy* (Springer, 2009).

8. Sundin, L. & Nilsson, S. Branchial innervation. *J Exp Zool* 293, 232–248 (2002).

9. Binder, D. K., Sonne, D. C. & Fischbein, N. J. *Cranial nerves: anatomy, pathology, imaging* (Thieme, 2010).

10. Afifi, A. K. & Bergman, R. A. *Functional neuroanatomy: text and atlas,* 2nd ed. (Lange Medical Books/McGraw-Hill, 2005).

11. Nieuwenhuys, R., Voogd, J. & Huijzen, C. V. *The human central nervous system,* 4th ed. (Springer, 2008).

12. Buck, A. H. & Stedman, T. L. *A Reference handbook of the medical sciences: embracing the entire range of scientific and practical medicine and allied science,* 3rd ed. (W. Wood, 1913).

13. Netter, F. H. & Dalley, A. F. *Atlas of human anatom,* 2nd ed., Plates 4–7 (Novartis, 1997).

14. Swartz, J. D. & Loevner, L. A. *Imaging of the temporal bone.* 4th ed., p. 58 (Thieme, 2009).

15. Mafee, M. F., Valvassori, G. E. & Becker, M. *Imaging of the head and neck,* 2nd ed. (Thieme, 2005).

16. Vogl, T. J. *Differential diagnosis in head and neck imaging: a systematic approach to the radiologic evaluation of the head and neck region and the interpretation of difficult cases* (Thieme, 1999).

17. Fossett, D. T. & Caputy, A. J. *Operative neurosurgical anatomy* (Thieme, 2002).

18. Pensak, M. L. *Controversies in otolaryngology* (Thieme, 2001).

19. Cappabianca, P., Califano, L. & Iaconetta, G. *Cranial, craniofacial and skull base surgery* (Springer, 2010).

20. Sanna, M. *Atlas of microsurgery of the lateral skull base,* 2nd ed. (Thieme, 2008).

21. Macdonald, A. J. *Diagnostic and surgical imaging anatomy. Brain, head & neck, spine,* 1st ed., pp. 282–283 (Amirsys, 2006).

22. Osborn, A. G. & Jacobs, J. M. *Diagnostic cerebral angiography,* 2nd ed. (Lippincott Williams & Wilkins, 1999).

23. Bruni, J. E. & Montemurro, D. G. *Human neuroanatomy: a text, brain atlas, and laboratory dissection guide* (Oxford University Press, 2009).

12

Cranial Nerves 3, 4, 6, 12

Know-It Points

Cranial Nerves 3, 4, & 6: Anatomy

- Cranial nerve 3 emerges from the anterior, medial midbrain and enters the interpeduncular cistern; then, it passes through the prepontine cistern, the lateral dural wall of the cavernous sinus, and through the superior orbital fissure to enter the orbit.
- Cranial nerve 4 passes dorsally out of the posterior aspect of the midbrain and courses around the outside of the opposite cerebral peduncle through the ambient cistern; then, it passes through the lateral dural wall of the cavernous sinus and the superior orbital fissure to enter the orbit to innervate the superior oblique muscle on the side opposite its nucleus of origin.
- Cranial nerve 6 exits the brainstem at the pontomedullary sulcus, climbs the clivus, passes over the petrous apex, and then passes through the cavernous sinus and superior orbital fissure to enter the orbit.
- The posterior communicating artery, which connects the internal carotid artery and ipsilateral posterior cerebral artery, passes just above the oculomotor nerve.

Extraocular Movements

- Cranial nerve 3 innervates the majority of the extraocular muscles: the medial rectus, superior rectus, inferior rectus, and inferior oblique.
- Cranial nerve 6 innervates the lateral rectus.
- Cranial nerve 4 innervates the superior oblique.
- All of the extraocular muscles except for the inferior oblique attach at the orbital apex in a common tendinous ring: the annulus of Zinn.
- Cardinal positions of gaze: medial rectus—adduction, lateral rectus—abduction, superior rectus—elevation (with eye in abduction), inferior rectus—depression (with eye in abduction), superior oblique—depression (with eye in adduction), inferior oblique—elevation (with eye in adduction).
- Each muscle's chief action in primary position (ie, looking straight ahead) is its primary action.
- Each muscle's secondary and tertiary actions are its additional rotational effects on the eye.
- The mnemonic "SUPERIOR people do NOT extort" indicates that the superior muscles are both intorters.
- The mnemonic "OBLIQUE muscles rotate the eye OUT" indicates that the oblique muscles are abductors.

Oculomotor Nuclei (*Advanced*)

- The superior rectus subnuclei project contralaterally, the single levator palpebrae subnucleus projects bilaterally, and the remaining subnuclei project ipsilaterally.
- Superior rectus subnucleus lesions produce bilateral palsies because when the superior rectus fibers exit their subnucleus, they immediately pass through the contralateral subnucleus.
- The accommodation reflex (or near-response) is a three-part reflex that brings near objects into focus through lens thickening, pupillary constriction, and inward rotation of the eyes—eye convergence.
- The preganglionic perioculomotor cell group lies along the dorsal aspect of the oculomotor nucleus.
- The motoneuron division of the perioculomotor cell group lies along the medial aspect of the oculomotor nucleus.

Cranial Nerve 12

■ The hypoglossal nucleus spans most of the height of the medulla.

■ Cranial nerve 12 exits the medulla between the medullary pyramid and the inferior olive, passes through the premedullary cistern, and exits the skull base through the hypoglossal canal; then, it passes through the medial nasopharyngeal carotid space and terminates in the tongue musculature.

■ The hypoglossal nerve innervates the large intrinsic tongue muscle mass, and it innervates three of the four extrinsic tongue muscles: styloglossus, hyoglossus, and genioglossus.

■ Palatoglossus is the only extrinsic tongue muscle not innervated by cranial nerve 12; its innervation comes from cranial nerve 10, the vagus nerve.

■ When one side of the genioglossus is denervated, the tongue moves forward and toward the weakened side (away from the intact side).

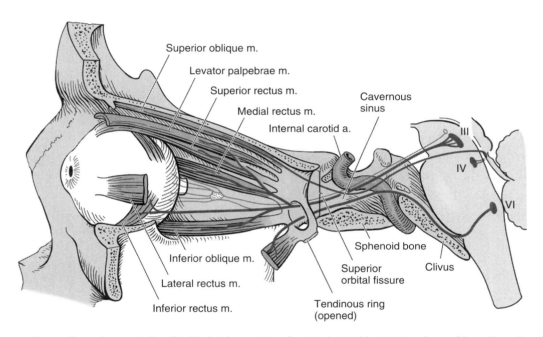

FIGURE 12-1 **Sagittal view of cranial nerves 3, 4, and 6. Used with permission from Baehr, Mathias, M. Frotscher, and Peter Duus.** *Duus' Topical Diagnosis in Neurology: Anatomy, Physiology, Signs, Symptoms,* **4th completely rev. ed. Stuttgart; New York: Thieme, 2005.**

Cranial Nerves 3, 4, & 6: Anatomy

Here, we will draw the course of cranial nerves 3, 4, and 6 in sagittal view. First, draw a midsagittal section through the brainstem from the midbrain to the pontomedullary sulcus; be sure to include a cerebral peduncle. Next, label the cavernous sinus, the superior orbital fissure, and the orbit. Note that cranial nerves 3 and 4 pass through the lateral dural wall of the cavernous sinus, whereas cranial nerve 6 passes through the cavernous sinus, itself. Also note that all of the extraocular muscles except for the inferior oblique share a common tendinous ring, called the annulus of Zinn; cranial nerves 3 and 6 pass through this ring to innervate their respective muscles, whereas cranial nerve 4 passes above it to innervate the superior oblique muscle.

Now, draw the oculomotor complex of cranial nerve 3 within the dorsal, center of the midbrain and indicate that it lies at the level of the superior colliculus. In axial view, show that the oculomotor fascicles emerge from the anterior, medial midbrain and enter the interpeduncular cistern. Then, in the sagittal diagram, show that the oculomotor nerve passes through the prepontine cistern, the lateral dural wall of the cavernous sinus, and the superior orbital fissure to enter the orbit.

Next, draw the trochlear nucleus of cranial nerve 4 at the level of the inferior colliculus. In axial view, indicate that the fourth nerve passes dorsally out of the posterior aspect of the midbrain and courses around the outside of the opposite cerebral peduncle through the ambient cistern. Then, in sagittal view, complete its course through the lateral dural wall of the cavernous sinus and through the superior orbital fissure to enter the orbit to innervate the superior oblique muscle on the side opposite its nucleus of origin. The trochlear nerve is the only cranial nerve to exit posteriorly from the brainstem and the only cranial nerve to send *all* of its fibers to the contralateral side. When the long, thin trochlear nerve is injured, the affected eye is elevated (aka hypertropic). Hold your fists with your index fingers straight out to demonstrate the direction of the eyes. To demonstrate a right fourth nerve palsy, elevate your right hand. Now, tilt your head both ways; tilting your head toward the elevated (affected) side worsens the disconjugate lines of vision whereas tilting it the opposite way (towards the normal side) brings the lines of vision into alignment: patients with a fourth nerve palsy tilt their head away from the affected eye.

Now, draw the clivus; it is a fusion of the sphenoid and occipital bones that sits directly across from the brainstem. Then, draw the abducens nucleus of cranial nerve 6 in the dorsal, inferior pons. Show that the sixth nerve exits the brainstem at the pontomedullary sulcus, climbs the clivus, passes over the petrous apex, and then passes through the cavernous sinus and superior orbital fissure to enter the orbit. Next, also indicate that as part of its path into the cavernous sinus (after crossing over the petrous apex), the sixth nerve passes through Dorello's canal: a dural channel within a basilar venous plexus. In this stretch, the abducens nerve is in close proximity to the first division of cranial nerve 5, and injury to both nerves, here, is called Gradenigo's syndrome. Note that cranial nerve 6 dysfunction is often a harbinger of increased intracranial pressure because the abducens nerve is fixed where it pierces the dura and can be stretched when there is downward herniation of the brainstem.

Next, let's show the arteries that can compress the aforementioned cranial nerves. First, show that the posterior cerebral artery (PCA) sits above both the third and fourth cranial nerves, and then that the superior cerebellar artery (SCA) sits below them. Next, show that the anterior inferior cerebellar artery (AICA) lies in close relation to the sixth cranial nerve as it exits the pontomedullary sulcus. Then, show that the internal carotid artery (ICA) lies within the cavernous sinus, and show that the posterior communicating artery (Pcomm) passes just above the oculomotor nerve to connect the ICA and PCA.[1–7]

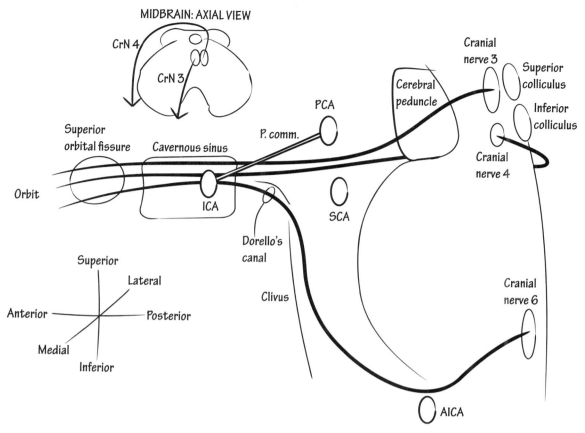

MIDBRAIN: AXIAL VIEW

CrN 4

CrN 3

Superior orbital fissure

Cavernous sinus

Orbit

ICA

PCA

P. comm.

Cerebral peduncle

Cranial nerve 3

Superior colliculus

Inferior colliculus

Cranial nerve 4

SCA

Dorello's canal

Clivus

Cranial nerve 6

Cranial nerve 12

Superior

Lateral

Anterior

Posterior

Medial

Inferior

AICA

DRAWING 12-1 **Cranial Nerves 3, 4, & 6: Anatomy**

Extraocular Movements

Here, we will draw the six cardinal positions of gaze and create a table for the complete extraocular muscle actions. Cranial nerve 3 innervates the majority of the extraocular muscles: the medial rectus, superior rectus, inferior rectus, and inferior oblique; cranial nerve 6 innervates the lateral rectus; and cranial nerve 4 innervates the superior oblique. We will draw the cardinal positions in coronal section, so first label the superior–inferior and lateral–medial axes and then identify our perspective as from the left eye. Show that the lateral rectus directs the eye laterally (called abduction) and that the medial rectus directs the eye medially (called adduction). Then, show that when the eye is abducted, the superior rectus directs the eye superiorly and the inferior rectus directs the eye inferiorly. Next, show that when the eye is adducted, the superior oblique directs the eye inferiorly and the inferior oblique directs the eye superiorly.

Now, in order to understand the complete movements, beyond just the six cardinal directions of gaze, let's first learn the relationship between the eye and the eye muscle plane. Draw an axial view of the eye within the orbit. Show the optical axis of the eye and then the eye muscle plane. The muscle plane originates from the orbital apex, which lies anterior to the orbital opening of the optic canal; all of the extraocular muscles except for the inferior oblique attach at the orbital apex in a common tendinous ring: the annulus of Zinn. The inferior oblique, instead, attaches to the medial orbital floor. Now, show that the primary position of the eye, the position of the eye when it is looking straight ahead, is 23 degrees nasal to the eye muscle plane. This angle results in the vertical eye muscles (superior and inferior rectus and superior and inferior oblique) all having three different actions on the eye in primary position: vertical, rotational, and horizontal.

Next, let's complete our eye muscle actions table. Across the top row, write cranial nerve (CrN), muscle, primary action, secondary action, and tertiary action. The muscle's chief action in primary position (ie, looking straight ahead) is its primary action, and the muscle's secondary and tertiary actions are its additional rotational effects on the eye. Begin with the medial rectus muscle, innervated by cranial nerve 3, and show that its primary action is adduction and that it does not have secondary or tertiary actions. Then, show that the cranial nerve 6-innervated lateral rectus muscle's primary action is abduction, and show that it also does not have either secondary or tertiary actions. In the next row, write that the cranial nerve 3-innervated superior rectus muscle's primary action is elevation, its secondary action is intorsion, and its tertiary action is adduction. Then, write that the cranial nerve 3-innervated inferior rectus muscle's primary action is depression, its secondary action is extorsion, and its tertiary action is adduction. Next, show that the cranial nerve 4-innervated superior oblique muscle's primary action is intorsion, its secondary action is depression, and its tertiary action is abduction. Finally, show that the cranial nerve 3-innervated inferior oblique muscle's primary action is extorsion, its secondary action is elevation, and its tertiary action is abduction.

Now, include the following two mnemonics: "SUPERIOR people do NOT extort," which means that the superior muscles are both intorters, and "OBLIQUE muscles rotate the eye OUT," which means that the oblique muscles are abductors.[8,9]

SIX CARDINAL POSITIONS OF GAZE

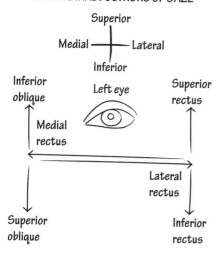

TABLE OF EXTRAOCULAR MOVEMENTS

CRN	MUSCLE	PRIMARY ACTION	SECONDARY ACTION	TERTIARY ACTION
3	Medial rectus	Adduction	X	X
6	Lateral rectus	Abduction	X	X
3	Superior rectus	Elevation	Intorsion	Adduction
3	Inferior rectus	Depression	Extorsion	Adduction
4	Superior oblique	Intorsion	Depression	Abduction
3	Inferior oblique	Extorsion	Elevation	Abduction

"SUPERIOR people do NOT EXTORT"

"OBLIQUE muscles move the eye OUT"

EYE IN THE ORBIT: AXIAL VIEW

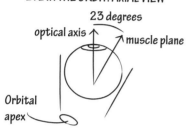

DRAWING 12-2 **Extraocular Movements**

Extraocular Muscles: Recti Muscles

Here, we will draw the actions of the recti muscles: horizontal (ie, medial and lateral) and vertical (ie, superior and inferior). First, establish the anterior–posterior and medial–lateral axes. Then, draw two eyeballs in primary position in axial section. On one, attach a medial rectus muscle; on the other, attach a lateral rectus muscle. Indicate that the medial rectus, which is innervated by cranial nerve 3, rotates the eye medially and that the lateral rectus, which is innervated by cranial nerve 6, rotates it laterally. Next, draw axial sections with the eyes rotated medially (adducted) and also laterally (abducted), and show that in both of these positions, the medial rectus still adducts the eye and the lateral rectus still abducts it. The horizontal recti only move the eye within the horizontal plane. As a clinical corollary, when the lateral rectus fails, the eye has trouble turning outward and the patient has difficulty with far vision, whereas when the medial rectus fails, the patient has difficulty with eye convergence and near vision.

Now, we will use our hands to feel the horizontal recti rotational pull on the eye. The medial and lateral recti muscles are the simplest. Make a fist with your right hand to represent your right eyeball. Your thumb is your right medial rectus. Grip your thumb with your left hand and pull on it (not so hard that you pull the eye out of its orbit!). Notice that whether your fist is directed straight ahead, adducted, or abducted, the force from your left hand always rotates your wrist medially along the horizontal plane. To demonstrate the lateral rectus rotational pull, flip your fist over and pull your thumb backward. Again, whether your fist is directed straight ahead, adducted, or abducted, the lateral rectus rotates it laterally.

Next, let's learn the vertical recti muscles: superior and inferior. For this drawing, add the superior–inferior axis. At the extremes of horizontal gaze, the vertical recti produce pure actions, but in primary position, the actions are mixed. Start with the eyes in abduction: superior rectus inserts on the top of the eyeball and inferior rectus inserts on the bottom. Show that in this position, superior rectus rotates the eye up and inferior rectus rotates it down. Next, show that in adduction, superior rectus rotates the eye internally around the anterior–posterior axis: it intorts it, meaning the medial aspect of the eye lowers and the lateral aspect of the eye elevates. Then, show that in adduction, inferior rectus externally rotates the eye: it extorts it, meaning the medial aspect of the eye raises and the lateral aspect of the eye lowers. Finally, in primary position, show that superior rectus produces elevation, intorsion, and adduction, and that inferior rectus produces depression, extorsion, and adduction.

Now, let's use our hands again to feel the vertical recti rotations. Use your right fist as your right eye and hook your left index finger (the right superior rectus) over the top of it at an angle. First, with your hand fully abducted pull on your wrist: the fist rotates superiorly. Then position your fist straight ahead and pull: you can feel your fist adduct (note, however, that superior rectus has multiple actions in this position). Finally, position your fist in full adduction and continue to pull. The fist is unable to rotate medially any farther, and instead it intorts. Note that the eye muscle always overpowers the eye (ie, your left finger should overpower your right fist). Next, let's do the same for the inferior rectus. Flip your right hand over (knuckles down) and hook your left index finger underneath your fist. Fully abduct your fist and pull; the downward/backward force of the inferior rectus depresses the eye. Then, direct your fist straight ahead and pull to feel your fist adduct (note, however, that inferior rectus has multiple actions in this position). Finally, in full adduction, continue to pull down and back: the fist is unable to rotate medially any farther, and instead it extorts.[6,8,9]

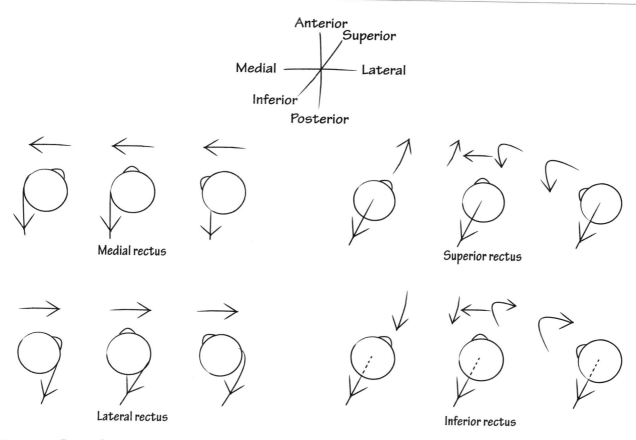

DRAWING 12-3 **Extraocular Muscles: Recti Muscles**

Extraocular Muscles: Oblique Muscles

Here, we will draw the oblique muscles. Once again, establish the anterior–posterior, medial–lateral, and superior–inferior axes. First, draw an axial view of the superior oblique muscle in adduction. Show that the superior oblique muscle runs across the superior surface of the eyeball, hooks around the trochlea, which is Latin for "pulley," and runs along the medial wall of the orbit. Next, show that in this position, the superior oblique rotates the eye down. Then, show that when the eye is fully abducted, superior oblique force causes the eye to intort. With the eye looking straight ahead, show that the superior oblique causes intorsion, depression, and also abduction.

For the inferior oblique, let's use a coronal plane because the inferior oblique attaches to the medial nasal floor (unlike the other extraocular muscles, which attach at the orbital apex at the annulus of Zinn). Draw the inferior oblique first in adduction. Show that in this position, the inferior oblique causes elevation; then, show that in abduction, it causes extortion; and lastly, show that in primary position, it causes extorsion, elevation, and abduction.

Now, let's use our fist to demonstrate the rotational pull of these eye muscles; we'll start with the superior oblique. Your right fist is again the eyeball. Hook your left thumb around your right index finger. The left thumb is the trochlea and the right index finger is the superior oblique. Pay attention to the spread between your index and middle fingers. When the eye is fully adducted, force along the trochlea depresses the eye; when the eye is abducted, force along the trochlea intorts the eye; use primary position to feel the superior oblique cause eye abduction (although the superior oblique has multiple actions in this position). For the inferior oblique, we have to reverse our anterior–posterior plane: here, the knuckles are posterior and the wrist is anterior; thus, when the wrist is facing toward the body, it is in adduction, and when it is facing away from the body, it is in abduction. With your wrist adducted, grip your right index finger and pull; the eye elevates; then, in full abduction, feel the inferior oblique cause the eye to extort; use primary position to feel the inferior oblique cause eye abduction (although the inferior oblique has multiple actions in this position).[6,8,9]

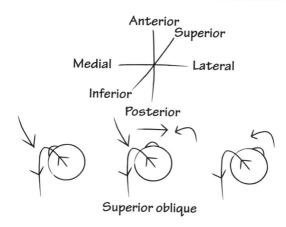

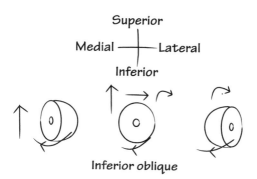

DRAWING 12-4 **Extraocular Muscles: Oblique Muscles**

Oculomotor Nuclei (*Advanced*)

Here, we will draw the Warwick model of the oculomotor complex and the perioculomotor cell group model. Let's begin with the oculomotor complex. In the 1950s, R. Warwick created a classic model for the oculomotor complex, and although details of this model have been updated over time, its basic construct remains unchanged. The model shows that the superior rectus subnuclei project contralaterally, the single levator palpebrae subnucleus projects bilaterally, and the remaining subnuclei project ipsilaterally. As an important clinical corollary, levator palpebrae subnucleus lesions naturally cause bilateral eye muscle palsies and superior rectus subnucleus lesions also produce bilateral palsies because when the superior rectus fibers exit their subnucleus, they immediately pass through the contralateral subnucleus.

Now, let's draw Warwick's model of the oculomotor complex in sagittal view. Label the rostral–caudal and dorsal–ventral planes of orientation. First, let's draw the lateral subnuclei from ventral to dorsal. Draw the long, narrow ventral subnucleus; designate it as innervating the medial rectus (although in actuality, three separate oculomotor regions supply the medial rectus muscle). Above the ventral subnucleus, draw the intermediate subnucleus, which innervates the inferior oblique; and above it, draw the dorsal subnucleus, which innervates the inferior rectus. Medial to these subnuclei, draw the medial subnucleus, which innervates the contralateral superior rectus (note: this subnucleus is commonly unnamed). Then, on the dorsocaudal surface, draw the small central caudal subnucleus, which innervates the bilateral levator palpebrae. On the rostral surface, draw the visceral nuclei, which include the Edinger–Westphal nucleus, anteromedian nucleus, and the nucleus of Perlia.[10]

Next, let's draw the perioculomotor cell group, which places the Edinger–Westphal nucleus, anteromedian nucleus, and nucleus of Perlia into a larger context of neural substrate responsible for the accommodation reflex. The accommodation reflex (or near-response) is a three-part reflex that brings near objects into focus

through lens thickening, pupillary constriction, and inward rotation of the eyes—eye convergence. First, indicate that our diagram is in coronal view. Then, draw a large, long nucleus to represent a consolidation of the oculomotor complex; note that this representation excludes the visceral nuclei, which will be drawn as part of the perioculomotor cell group. Next, along the dorsal aspect of the oculomotor nucleus, draw the preganglionic perioculomotor cell group; show that the Edinger–Westphal nucleus lies within this part of the perioculomotor cell group. The preganglionic cell group is responsible for producing the lens thickening and pupillary constriction responses of the accommodation reflex. Next, along the rostral–caudal length of the medial aspect of the oculomotor nucleus, draw the motoneuron division of the perioculomotor cell group; it innervates the multiply innervated muscle fibers of the accommodation reflex, which produce the eye convergence response. Show that the motoneuron division of the perioculomotor cell group encompasses the anteromedian nucleus, anteriorly, and the nucleus of Perlia in mid-anteroposterior position. Note that due to the actual complexity of this nuclear complex, we should not attempt to draw discrete functional meaning from the positions of the Edinger–Westphal nucleus, anteromedian nucleus, and nucleus of Perlia from this diagram—these nuclei are included, here, only to provide historical/anatomic context to our perioculomotor cell group model, and we should still simply consider them to broadly enact the visceral actions of the oculomotor nerve.

Finally, in regards to the accommodation reflex, itself, consider that supranuclear control of the perioculomotor cell group comes from widely distributed areas, which include the supraoculomotor area (which lies within the mesencephalic reticular formation just dorsal to the oculomotor complex) and numerous cerebral and cerebellar smooth pursuit centers described in Chapter 23.[2,6–9,11,12]

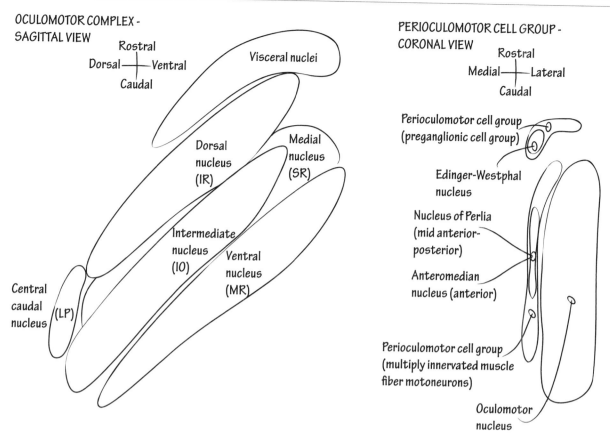

OCULOMOTOR COMPLEX -
SAGITTAL VIEW

Rostral
Dorsal——Ventral
Caudal

Visceral nuclei

Dorsal
nucleus
(IR)

Medial
nucleus
(SR)

Intermediate
nucleus
(IO)

Ventral
nucleus
(MR)

Central
caudal
nucleus

(LP)

PERIOCULOMOTOR CELL GROUP -
CORONAL VIEW

Rostral
Medial——Lateral
Caudal

Perioculomotor cell group
(preganglionic cell group)

Edinger-Westphal
nucleus

Nucleus of Perlia
(mid anterior-
posterior)

Anteromedian
nucleus (anterior)

Perioculomotor cell group
(multiply innervated muscle
fiber motoneurons)

Oculomotor
nucleus

DRAWING 12-5 **Oculomotor Nuclei**

Cranial Nerve 12

Here we will draw the hypoglossal nerve (cranial nerve 12) course in sagittal view and then we will create a diagram to understand the actions of the extrinsic tongue muscles that it innervates. We begin with the hypoglossal nerve path from the medulla to the tongue. First, draw an axial view of the medulla and label the hypoglossal nucleus within the posterior medulla; it spans from the upper to the lower regions of the medulla. Next, label a few key structures along the hypoglossal nerve course: the inferior olive, the vertebral artery, and the hypoglossal canal. Now, show that the hypoglossal nerve passes anteriorly through the medulla and exits between the medullary pyramid and the inferior olive at the ventrolateral (aka preolivary) sulcus. Then, show that the hypoglossal nerve passes through the premedullary cistern, lateral to the vertebral artery, to exit the skull base through the hypoglossal canal.

Now, show that after the hypoglossal nerve exits the hypoglossal canal, it passes through the medial nasopharyngeal carotid space, where it descends in close proximity to the carotid and internal jugular vasculature before approaching the hyoid bone and terminating in the tongue musculature. The proximity of cranial nerve 12 to the internal carotid artery makes it susceptible to injury from carotid dissection, because clot formed from dissection can expand the carotid wall enough to compress the adjacent nerves. Cranial nerves 9, 10, and 11 also run within this space, so a combined cranial nerve 9, 10, 11, and 12 injury suggests a possible carotid dissection.

Next, let's show the termination of the hypoglossal nerve under the tongue, or "glossus" (hence the name "hypoglossal nerve"). The hypoglossal nerve innervates the large intrinsic tongue muscle mass, which comprises the superior and inferior longitudinal muscles and the transverse and vertical muscles, and it innervates three of the four extrinsic tongue muscles: styloglossus, hyoglossus, and genioglossus. Palatoglossus is the only extrinsic tongue muscle not innervated by cranial nerve 12; its innervation comes from cranial nerve 10, the vagus nerve. Genioglossus is the most clinically important of these three extrinsic tongue muscles because whereas the other tongue muscles receive bilateral cortical innervation, genioglossus receives predominately contralateral cortical innervation; therefore, it is the most helpful for clinical localization, as we discuss at the end.[13]

To understand the action of all of these muscles, we will draw a sagittal schematic of their innervation. Show that styloglossus attaches the tongue to the styloid process; indicate that it pulls the tongue up and back. Then, show that hyoglossus attaches the tongue to the hyoid bone; indicate that it depresses the tongue. Finally, show that genioglossus attaches the tongue to the anterior mandible; indicate that it provides tongue protrusion.

Now, in axial section, show that both genioglossi point towards the center of the anterior mandible. Their opposing horizontal angles cancel, and so the tongue is directed forward when it is activated (you can also feel the tongue curl when you protrude it because the genioglossi pull the center of the tongue downward, as well). Thus, when one side of the genioglossus is impaired (either from genioglossus atrophy or from hypoglossal nerve or nucleus injury), the tongue moves forward and toward the side of the lesion (away from the intact side). Demonstrate this with your index fingers. Hold your fists in front of you and point your index fingers toward midline. Now drop one of your fists: the tongue protrudes toward the side of the lesion (away from the intact side). Corticonuclear innervation to the portion of each hypoglossal nucleus that innervates the genioglossus is predominantly contralateral, however. Therefore, with lesions proximal to the hypoglossal nucleus, tongue protrusion is either normal or it points away from the side of the lesion: for instance, in a right-side hemispheric lesion, the left genioglossus will be weak, so the tongue will deviate toward the left (away from the injured side of the brain).[1–4,6,7]

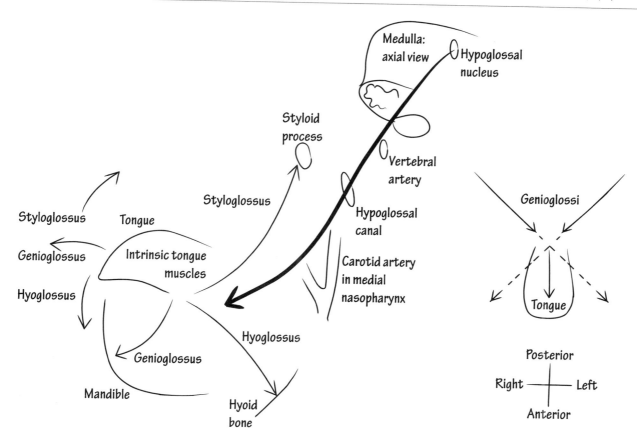

DRAWING 12-6 **Cranial Nerve 12**

References

1. Binder, D. K., Sonne, D. C. & Fischbein, N. J. *Cranial nerves: anatomy, pathology, imaging* (Thieme, 2010).

2. Brazis, P. W., Masdeu, J. C. & Biller, J. *Localization in clinical neurology,* 5th ed. (Lippincott Williams & Wilkins, 2007).

3. Haines, D. E. & Ard, M. D. *Fundamental neuroscience: for basic and clinical applications,* 3rd ed. (Churchill Livingstone Elsevier, 2006).

4. Macdonald, A. J. *Diagnostic and surgical imaging anatomy. Brain, head & neck, spine,* 1st ed., pp. 282–283 (Amirsys, 2006).

5. Takahashi, S. O. *Neurovascular imaging: MRI & microangiography* (Springer, 2010).

6. Wilson-Pauwels, L. *Cranial nerves: function and dysfunction,* 3rd ed. (People's Medical Pub. House, 2010).

7. Naidich, T. P. & Duvernoy, H. M. *Duvernoy's atlas of the human brain stem and cerebellum: high-field MRI: surface anatomy, internal structure, vascularization and 3D sectional anatomy* (Springer, 2009).

8. Leigh, R. J. & Zee, D. S. *The neurology of eye movements* (Oxford University Press, 2006).

9. Wong, A. M. F. *Eye movement disorders* (Oxford University Press, 2008).

10. Warwick, R. A study of retrograde degeneration in the oculomotor nucleus of the rhesus monkey, with a note on a method of recording its distribution. *Brain* 73, 532–543 (1950).

11. Horn, A. K., et al. Perioculomotor cell groups in monkey and man defined by their histochemical and functional properties: reappraisal of the Edinger-Westphal nucleus. *J Comp Neurol* 507, 1317–1335 (2008).

12. Miller, N. R., Walsh, F. B. & Hoyt, W. F. *Walsh and Hoyt's clinical neuro-ophthalmology,* 6th ed. (Lippincott Williams & Wilkins, 2005).

13. Conn, P. M. *Neuroscience in medicine,* 3rd ed. (Humana Press, 2008).

13

Cranial Nerves 5, 7, 9, 10

Know-It Points

Cranial Nerve 5: Peripheral Innervation

- The peripheral divisions of the trigeminal nerve are division 1—the ophthalmic division, which covers the eyes; division 2—the maxillary division, which covers the cheeks; and division 3—the mandibular division, which covers the jaw.
- The main function of the trigeminal motor system is mastication (ie, chewing), which requires the trigeminally innervated medial and lateral pterygoids, masseter, and temporalis muscles.
- In a lower trigeminal motor neuron lesion (eg, when a trigeminal motor nucleus or nerve is injured or when a lateral pterygoid is damaged), the jaw deviates toward the injured side.

Cranial Nerve 5: Nuclei

- The trigeminal ganglion lies in Meckel's cave: a dural-based, cerebrospinal fluid-filled cavern that lies along the posterolateral aspect of the cavernous sinus.
- The ophthalmic division traverses the superior orbital fissure; the maxillary division traverses foramen rotundum; and the mandibular division traverses foramen ovale.
- The ophthalmic and maxillary divisions (divisions 1 and 2, respectively) pass through the lateral wall of the cavernous sinus and then merge together along with the mandibular division to form the trigeminal ganglion within Meckel's cave.
- The trigeminal motor nucleus and the principal sensory nucleus lie in parallel just above the abducens nucleus in the upper pons.
- The mesencephalic nucleus spans from the upper pons to the level of the superior colliculus (in the midbrain).
- The spinal trigeminal nucleus and tract span from the upper pons to the upper cervical spinal cord.
- The motor division of the trigeminal nerve passes through the cerebellopontine angle cistern and joins the mandibular division as it exits the middle cranial fossa through foramen ovale.

Cranial Nerve 5: Tracts (*Advanced*)

- The central sensory afferents of the trigeminal nerve relay to the cortex through two different trigeminothalamic pathways: anterior and posterior.
- Small fiber sensory modality trigeminal nerve fibers project to the spinal trigeminal tract and nucleus and large fiber sensory modality trigeminal nerve fibers project to the principal sensory nucleus.
- The spinal trigeminal nucleus divides from superior to inferior into pars oralis, pars interpolaris, and pars caudalis.

Cranial Nerve 7: Innervation

- The upper division of the facial nucleus receives bilateral corticonuclear projections and the lower division receives contralateral projections, only.
- Fibers from the upper division innervate the upper face and fibers from the lower division innervate the lower face.
- In a right cerebral cortical stroke, the left upper face is strong and the left lower face is weak.
- In a left Bell's palsy, both the left upper face and left lower face are weak.

Cranial Nerve 7: Anatomy

- The facial nucleus houses special visceral efferent (SVE) cells and innervates the muscles of facial expression.
- The superior salivatory nucleus houses general visceral efferent cells (GVE) and provides parasympathetic innervation to the pterygopalatine and submandibular ganglia.
- The solitary tract nucleus receives the special visceral afferent (SVA) fibers of cranial nerve 7, which carry taste sensation from the anterior two thirds of the tongue.

- The pars caudalis portion of the spinal trigeminal nucleus receives the general sensory afferent (GSA) fibers of cranial nerve 7, which carry sensory information from select portions of the external ear.
- The facial nerve divides into four segments: an extracranial segment—where the nerve emerges from the petrous portion of the temporal bone; an intratemporal segment—where it passes through the petrous bone; a cisternal segment—where it passes through the cerebellopontine angle cistern; and an intra-axial segment—its brainstem course.

Cranial Nerves 9 & 10

- The inferior salivatory nucleus innervates the otic ganglion, which provides parasympathetic innervation to the parotid gland.
- The dorsal motor nucleus of the vagus provides parasympathetic innervation to smooth muscle of the oropharynx and parasympathetic innervation to viscera within the thoracoabdomen.
- Nucleus ambiguus innervates the throat muscles and provides parasympathetic innervation to select cardiovascular structures.
- The spinal trigeminal nucleus, pars caudalis receives a small portion of its cutaneous sensory

reception from the glossopharyngeal and vagus nerves.
- The solitary tract nucleus receives sensory afferents for taste, sensory afferents from the epiglottis, and parasympathetic afferents from widespread thoracoabdominal regions.
- The glossopharyngeal and vagus nerves exit the medulla through the post-olivary sulcus to enter the cerebellomedullary cistern, and they traverse the skull base through the jugular foramen.

The Gag Reflex

- The gag reflex relies on the glossopharyngeal nerve for its afferent loop and the vagus nerve for its efferent loop.

- In a lower motor neuron injury (such as a direct lesion to the nucleus ambiguus itself or its exiting fibers), there is unilateral palatal paralysis on the side of the lower motor neuron lesion.

Cranial Nerve 5: Peripheral Innervation

Here, we will draw the peripheral sensory coverage of the trigeminal nerve and the trigeminal motor innervation of the muscles of mastication. The peripheral divisions of the trigeminal nerve are division 1—the ophthalmic division, which covers the eyes; division 2—the maxillary division, which covers the cheeks; and division 3—the mandibular division, which covers the jaw. First, draw a head. Next, mark a dot on the superior-posterior curvature of the head, then mark one at the corner of the eye, and then the tip of the nose. Now, connect these dots and label the region supero-anterior to this line as division 1—the ophthalmic division. Next, midway along that line make another dot, then make a dot at the maxilla, and then the corner of the mouth. Join these dots and label the region between this line and division 1 as division 2—the maxillary division. Finally, mark a dot at the original superior-posterior point, then at the tragus, and then at the mentum. Connect these dots and label the region between this line and division 2 as division 3—the mandibular division. Now tap these points on your own face for sense-memory.

Two key details of facial sensory coverage are that division 3 of the trigeminal nerve covers neither the outer ear nor the angle of the mandible. The coverage of the outer ear is complex: it involves the great auricular nerve (supplied by C2, C3) and cranial nerves 7, 9, and 10; the angle of the mandible is covered by the great auricular nerve. Thus, sensory examination of the outer ear and angle of the mandible should be normal in isolated peripheral trigeminal nerve injury. Lastly, note that the coverage of the trigeminal nerve extends posteriorly past the superior pole of the head, and thus the sensory loss in peripheral trigeminal nerve injury should continue posterior to the superior pole of the head.

The main function of the trigeminal motor system is mastication (chewing). Mastication requires the trigeminally innervated medial and lateral pterygoids, masseter, and temporalis muscles. Feel just above and in front of the angle of your mandible and clench and relax your jaw. The contracting muscles under your fingertips are the masseters. Next, look at your temples and cheeks; the temporalis muscles fill out your facial contour. Atrophy to these muscles is an important potential clue of trigeminal neuronal degeneration. The medial pterygoids, temporalis, and masseter muscles elevate the mandible to close the jaw, whereas the lateral pterygoids help to open it (although much of the work in jaw opening actually relies on the digastric muscle, which is partially innervated by the trigeminal nerve, and the geniohyoid muscle). Open your jaw and extend your mandible forward to activate your lateral pterygoids.

Next, draw the lateral pterygoids at an angle to one another; show that they push the mandible forward. Then, point your index fingers towards one another to represent the lateral pterygoids. Drop one of your fingers to represent a weakened lateral pterygoid; the intact finger points toward the weak side. In a lower motor neuron lesion (eg, when a trigeminal motor nucleus or nerve is injured or when a lateral pterygoid is damaged), the jaw deviates toward the injured side. Cortical innervation of the trigeminal motor nuclei is bilateral with contralateral predominance; thus, in cortical injury, if jaw deviation occurs, it is directed away from the injured side. For instance, in a right hemispheric stroke, the left trigeminal nucleus is unable to activate the left lateral pterygoid and so the jaw may deviate to the left (away from the right cerebral hemispheric injury).[1–8]

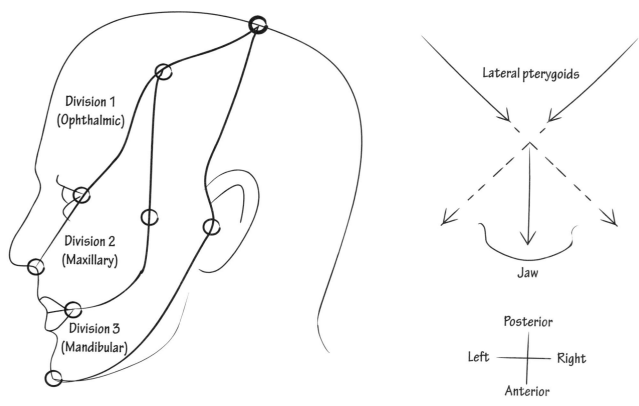

DRAWING 13-1 **Cranial Nerve 5: Peripheral Innervation**

Cranial Nerve 5: Nuclei

Here, we will draw the trigeminal nuclei in sagittal view. First, draw the trifurcated sensory ganglion of the trigeminal nerve, called the trigeminal ganglion, which means the "three twins." It lies in a low depression known as the trigeminal impression at the apex of the petrous temporal bone. The trigeminal ganglion is enveloped in Meckel's cave: a dural-based, cerebrospinal fluid-filled cavern that lies adjacent to the posterolateral aspect of the cavernous sinus. Now show that from rostral to caudal, the divisions of the trigeminal ganglion are the ophthalmic, maxillary, and mandibular divisions—their central projections terminate in the various trigeminal nuclei. Next, show that the ophthalmic division traverses the superior orbital fissure; the maxillary division traverses foramen rotundum; and the mandibular division traverses foramen ovale. As they proceed centrally, the ophthalmic and maxillary divisions (divisions 1 and 2, respectively) pass through the lateral wall of the cavernous sinus; they then merge together along with the mandibular division to form the trigeminal ganglion within Meckel's cave.[9]

Now, let's draw a sagittal section through the brainstem in order to show the four different trigeminal nuclei: one motor, three sensory. We will use the upper pons as the central point of the trigeminal nuclei, so also draw an axial cross-section through the upper pons for reference. Next, establish the position of the trigeminal motor nucleus and the principal sensory nucleus in the upper pons. They lie in parallel just above the abducens nucleus. Show that the trigeminal motor nucleus lies medial to the principal sensory nucleus—their positions follow the general organization of the cranial nerves (see Drawings 11-2 and 11-4). Whereas the principal sensory and motor trigeminal nuclei are restricted to this upper pontine level, the two other trigeminal sensory nuclei combined span the height of the brainstem and upper cervical spinal cord. Return, now, to the sagittal diagram and show that the mesencephalic nucleus spans from the upper pons to the level of the superior colliculus (in the midbrain), and then show that the spinal trigeminal nucleus and tract span from the upper pons to the upper cervical spinal cord (their termination is variably listed as anywhere from C2 to C4). Trigeminal sensory afferents descend the spinal trigeminal tract and then synapse in the adjacent spinal trigeminal nucleus in a specific somatotopic pattern (see Drawing 13-3). The caudal end of the spinal trigeminal nucleus is continuous with the substantia gelatinosa, which lies within the dorsal horn of the spinal cord, and the spinal trigeminal tract is continuous with the posterolateral fasciculus (aka Lissauer's tract), which lies along the dorsal edge of the dorsal horn of the spinal cord (see Drawings 7-1 and 7-2).

Next, show that the motor division of the trigeminal nerve passes ventrolaterally through the cerebellopontine angle cistern to exit the brainstem (all of the pharyngeal arch derivatives leave the brainstem along a ventrolateral path) and joins the mandibular division as it exits the middle cranial fossa through foramen ovale to innervate the muscles of mastication.

The mesencephalic nucleus contains the primary sensory neurons for proprioceptive afferents from the muscles of mastication, which ascend through the mandibular division of the trigeminal nerve. Thus, the mesencephalic nucleus is the only central nervous system nucleus to house primary sensory neurons (the primary sensory neurons of the mesencephalic sensory afferents do *not* lie within a peripheral ganglion). The mesencephalic nucleus projects to other sensory nuclei and also to the trigeminal motor nucleus to produce the masseter reflex (ie, the jaw jerk). When the muscles of mastication are stretched, they activate the mesencephalic nucleus, which triggers the jaw jerk. A brisk jaw jerk can suggest pathologic disinhibition of suppressive corticopontine fibers to cranial nerve 5.

We discuss the principal sensory and spinal trigeminal nuclei next.[1–6,10]

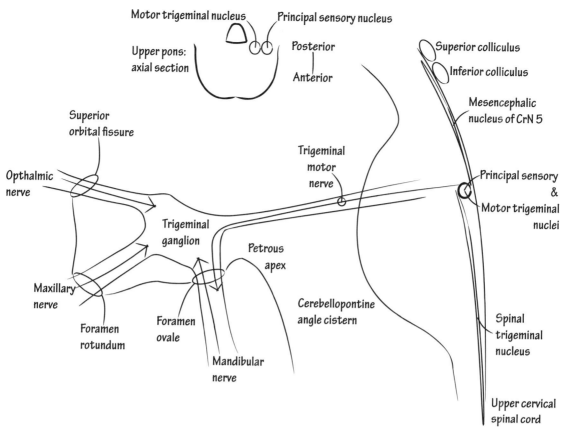

DRAWING 13-2 **Cranial Nerve 5: Nuclei**

Cranial Nerve 5: Tracts (*Advanced*)

Here, we will draw the trigeminothalamic tracts and the somatotopic organization of the spinal trigeminal nucleus. The central sensory afferents of the trigeminal nerve relay to the cortex through two different trigeminothalamic pathways: anterior and posterior. Draw a coronal view of the brainstem. Then, draw the trigeminal ganglion and show that the small fiber sensory modality trigeminal nerve fibers project to the spinal trigeminal tract and nucleus and that the large fiber sensory modality trigeminal nerve fibers project to the principal sensory nucleus. Note that although the principal sensory nucleus is often considered the trigeminal functional equivalent of the gracile and cuneate nuclei and the spinal trigeminal nucleus is often considered the trigeminal functional equivalent of the anterolateral system (ie, spinothalamic tract), postsynaptic interconnections within the trigeminal system make this an imperfect relationship and we are unable to use it, clinically.[3]

Now, let's draw the trigeminothalamic projections. First, show that the anterolateral portion of the principal sensory nucleus projects via the anterior trigeminothalamic tract to the contralateral ventroposterior medial nucleus of the thalamus, and then show that the posteromedial portion of the principal sensory nucleus projects via the posterior trigeminothalamic tract to the ipsilateral ventroposterior medial nucleus of the thalamus. Then, indicate that the spinal trigeminal nucleus projects via the anterior trigeminothalamic tract to the contralateral ventroposterior medial nucleus of the thalamus. Note that in regards to the somatotopy of the principal sensory nucleus, the mandibular division of the trigeminal nerve synapses posteriorly within the principal sensory nucleus and the ophthalmic division synapses anteriorly; the maxillary division synapses intermediately between the mandibular and ophthalmic divisions.[3]

Next, let's draw the spinal trigeminal nucleus. It runs medial to the spinal trigeminal tract, has an onionskin somatotopy, and divides into three different cytoarchitectural regions. In sagittal view, show that the spinal trigeminal nucleus spans from the pons to the upper cervical spinal cord. Indicate that within the spinal trigeminal nucleus, pars oralis is the superior-most subnucleus: it spans from the pons to the mid-medulla; show that pars interpolaris is the middle subnucleus: it lies in the mid-medulla; and, finally, indicate that pars caudalis is the inferior-most subnucleus: it spans from the lower medulla to the upper cervical spinal cord. Its inferior extent is variably listed as anywhere from C2 to C4. Next, show that the somatotopic features of the face in the spinal trigeminal somatotopic map are stretched and distorted to fit into the proportions of the long, columnar spinal trigeminal nucleus (imagine pulling a rubber mask off of your face to visualize the distortion). The superior features of the face (eg, the eyes) lie anterior and the inferior features (eg, the jaw) lie posterior; the most superior portion of the pars caudalis subnucleus receives the lips and perioral area and the most inferior component receives the outer ears. Note that our somatotopic discussion of the spinal trigeminal nucleus refers to the pars caudalis subnucleus, only; therefore, the most superior area is the inferior medulla and the most inferior area is the upper cervical spinal cord. Clinically, when we discuss the spinal trigeminal nucleus, we generally are referring to the pars caudalis subnucleus of the spinal trigeminal nucleus, only.

Now, let's draw the onion-skin layers of the spinal trigeminal somatotopic map: the central sensory processing map for pain/temperature information in the face. Draw an undistorted face. Show that the lips and perioral area constitute the outermost layer of the onion—they lie within the most superior area of the pars caudalis subnucleus of the spinal trigeminal nucleus; the next innermost layer, moving inferiorly within pars caudalis, comprises the nose, eyes, and outer oral areas; then, continuing downward, lies the cheeks and forehead; then the vertical band just in front of the ears; and finally lies the partial spinal trigeminal sensory coverage of the external ear (from cranial nerves 7, 9, and 10).[1–6,8,10]

TRIGEMINAL THALAMIC PROJECTIONS

SPINAL TRIGEMINAL SOMATOTOPY

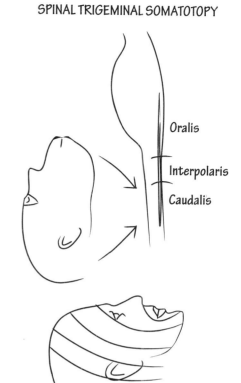

Ipsilateral thalamus

Contralateral thalamus

Posterior trigemino-thalamic tract

Anterior trigemino-thalamic tract

Anterolateral projection

Posteromedial projection

Principal sensory nucleus

Trigeminal ganglion

Spinal trigeminal tract & nucleus

Oralis

Interpolaris

Caudalis

DRAWING 13-3 **Cranial Nerve 5: Tracts**

Cranial Nerve 7: Innervation

Here, we will address the corticonuclear innervation of cranial nerve 7, the facial nerve. We focus on this subject in particular because testing facial weakness can help us differentiate an upper motor neuron injury (eg, cortical stroke) from a lower motor neuron injury (eg, Bell's palsy). First, draw the left half of a face; label its upper and lower divisions. At the bedside, we test the upper face with forehead wrinkle and the lower face with forced smile. Note that an involuntary smile (aka mimetic or emotional smile) has a different innervation pattern than what we will draw, here, so be careful not to make your patients laugh at this point in the exam.

Next, draw the bilateral cerebral hemispheres. Then, draw the left facial nucleus and divide it into its upper and lower divisions. First, show that the upper division receives bilateral corticonuclear projections and then show that the lower division receives contralateral projections, only. Now, draw fibers from the upper division to the upper face and then show fibers from the lower division to the lower face. The fact that the upper face receives bilateral corticonuclear innervation and the lower face receives contralateral corticonuclear innervation allows us to distinguish upper motor neuron from lower motor neuron lesions, as we will see when we walk through the two clinical vignettes, next.[2]

Vignette one involves a right cerebral cortical stroke that affects the facial fibers. Redraw the hemispheres, facial nucleus, and face. Then encircle the cortex of the right hemisphere to indicate damage from the stroke. In this situation, contralateral facial nuclear innervation is lost. However, show that ipsilateral upper division facial nuclear innervation is preserved. As a result, show that the left upper face is strong and the left lower face is weak. Thus, in cerebral cortical injury, there is contralateral lower facial weakness with preserved upper facial strength. As a small clinical pearl, when there is facial weakness due to upper motor neuron injury, the palpebral fissure on the paretic side of the face will often be wider than on the normal side of the face because the facial droop will pull down the lower eyelid.

Vignette two involves a left Bell's palsy. Again, redraw the hemispheres, facial nucleus, and face. Here, encircle the facial nucleus, itself, to indicate damage from the Bell's palsy. Show that in this clinical circumstance, innervation to the facial nucleus is preserved bilaterally, but peripheral innervation to the face is lost. As a result, show that both the left upper face and left lower face are weak. In Bell's palsy, there is paralysis of the complete ipsilateral side of the face. Note that Bell's palsy can occur anywhere along the seventh cranial nerve; therefore, the full clinical presentation of a Bell's palsy depends on where along its course the facial nerve is affected. The next diagram will help us to understand why there are such a wide variety of presentations for Bell's palsy and what those potential presentations can be.[1–6,8,10]

NORMAL INNERVATION PATTERN

UPPER MOTOR NEURON LESION

LOWER MOTOR NEURON LESION

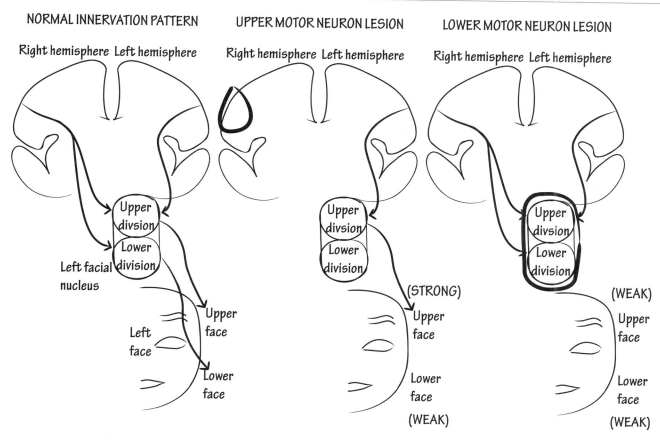

DRAWING 13-4 **Cranial Nerve 7: Innervation**

Cranial Nerve 7: Anatomy

Here, we will draw the four components of cranial nerve 7, the facial nerve. To begin, divide the nerve into four segments: an extracranial segment—where the nerve emerges from the petrous portion of the temporal bone (the petrous bone); an intratemporal segment—where it passes through the petrous bone; a cisternal segment—where it passes through the cerebellopontine angle cistern; and an intra-axial segment—its brainstem course. Now, let's establish the relevant cranial nerve 7 nuclei and their end targets, and then we'll illustrate their paths.

First, for reasons that will become clear later, draw the abducens nucleus of cranial nerve 6, which spans from the mid to lower pons. Then, draw the facial nucleus, which spans from the lower pons to the pontomedullary junction and houses special visceral efferent (SVE) cells. Indicate that this component innervates the muscles of facial expression. Next, draw the superior salivatory nucleus, which lies just above the pontomedullary junction and houses general visceral efferent cells (GVE). Indicate that this component provides preganglionic parasympathetic innervation to the pterygopalatine and submandibular ganglia. Now, draw the solitary tract nucleus, which spans the height of the medulla and receives the special visceral afferent (SVA) fibers of cranial nerve 7. Indicate that these fibers carry taste sensation from the anterior two thirds of the tongue. Next, draw the pars caudalis portion of the spinal trigeminal nucleus, which spans from the inferior medulla to the upper cervical spinal cord and receives the general sensory afferent (GSA) fibers of cranial nerve 7. Indicate that these fibers carry sensory information from select portions of the external ear.

Now, let's establish several key anatomic features of the facial nerve course. First, label the internal genu; this is the sweeping path the facial nerve takes over the top of the abducens nucleus—it generates a small bump in the

floor of the fourth ventricle, called the facial colliculus. Next, in the cisternal segment, at the level of the pontomedullary junction, label the motor root, which consists of special visceral efferent (SVE) fibers, only, and then label the nervus intermedius (of Wrisberg), which consists of the remaining three fiber types. Now, label the internal acoustic meatus (aka internal auditory canal), which is where the facial nerve enters the petrous bone. The motor root and nervus intermedius merge together within the internal acoustic meatus. Next, label the geniculate ganglion, which houses the cell bodies for the pseudo-unipolar facial sensory afferents. Then, label the nerve to the stapedius muscle (an SVE branch). This small muscle contracts the neck of the stapes to prevent the transmission of high-energy sounds through the middle ear ossicles; note that it may also serve to extract meaningful sound from background noise. Now, label the greater petrosal nerve, which carries the GVE (upper division) fibers. Next, label the chorda tympani, which is the nerve bundle of the combined GVE (lower division) and the SVA fibers. And finally, draw the stylomastoid foramen, which is the opening through which the SVE and GSA fibers exit the petrous bone.

Before we draw the nerve paths, themselves, let's subdivide the intratemporal segment of the facial nerve into four descriptive segments. First, label the meatal segment, which is the segment wherein the facial nerve passes through the internal acoustic meatus. Next, label the labyrinthine segment, which is the segment wherein the facial nerve exits the meatal segment and enters the facial canal. This segment terminates at the geniculate ganglion, which is identified by its abrupt bend, the external genu. Next, label the horizontal (aka tympanic) segment, wherein the facial nerve runs posteriorly (horizontally). Lastly, label the mastoid segment. In this segment, the facial nerve drops straight down and exits the skull through the stylomastoid foramen.

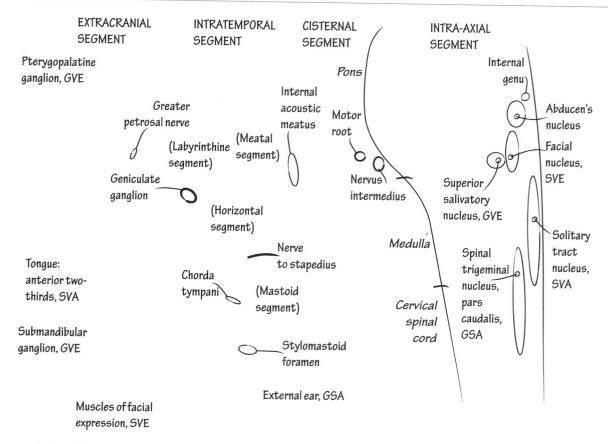

EXTRACRANIAL
SEGMENT

INTRATEMPORAL
SEGMENT

CISTERNAL
SEGMENT

INTRA-AXIAL
SEGMENT

Pterygopalatine
ganglion, GVE

Greater
petrosal nerve

(Labyrinthine
segment)

Geniculate
ganglion

(Horizontal
segment)

(Meatal
segment)

Internal
acoustic
meatus

Nerve
to stapedius

Chorda
tympani

(Mastoid
segment)

Stylomastoid
foramen

Tongue:
anterior two-
thirds, SVA

Submandibular
ganglion, GVE

Muscles of facial
expression, SVE

External ear, GSA

Pons

Motor
root

Nervus
intermedius

Medulla

Cervical
spinal
cord

Internal
genu

Abducen's
nucleus

Facial
nucleus,
SVE

Superior
salivatory
nucleus, GVE

Spinal
trigeminal
nucleus,
pars
caudalis,
GSA

Solitary
tract
nucleus,
SVA

DRAWING 13-5 Cranial Nerve 7: Anatomy—Partial

Cranial Nerve 7: Anatomy (Cont.)

Now, we will show the nerve path for each facial nerve fiber type. Begin with the SVE fiber component; show that it originates from the facial nucleus, sweeps over the abducens nucleus in the internal genu, exits the brainstem at the pontomedullary junction as the motor root, passes through the cerebellopontine angle cistern, enters the petrous bone through the internal acoustic meatus, and then passes through the meatal, labyrinthine, and horizontal segments. Show that it gives off the stapedius nerve branch at the beginning of the mastoid segment and then drops straight down and exits the skull through the stylomastoid foramen and divides into several nerve branches, which innervate the muscles of facial expression.

Next, let's draw the GSA fibers; they originate from small portions of the external ear, which comprises the auricle (aka pinna) and external acoustic meatus (aka external ear canal). The peripheral process of the GSA component enters the skull through the stylomastoid foramen, ascends the mastoid segment, and traverses the horizontal segment, and its cell bodies reside in the geniculate ganglion. The central process of the GSA component emerges from the geniculate ganglion; passes through the labyrinthine segment, through the internal acoustic meatus, and through the cerebellopontine angle cistern within the nervus intermedius; enters the brainstem at the pontomedullary junction; and descends the spinal trigeminal tract to synapse in the inferior portion of the pars caudalis portion of the spinal trigeminal nucleus.

Now, let's illustrate the SVA fibers, which originate from the anterior two thirds of the tongue. Indicate that the peripheral process of the SVA component joins the chorda tympani, ascends the mastoid segment, and traverses the horizontal segment, and its cell bodies lie within the geniculate ganglion. From the geniculate ganglion, show that its central process traverses the labyrinthine

and meatal segments, crosses the cerebellopontine angle cistern within the nervus intermedius, enters the brainstem at the pontomedullary junction, and synapses in the superior portion of the solitary tract nucleus.

Next, let's draw the GVE fibers, which carry preganglionic parasympathetic fibers. The GVE component originates from the superior salivatory nucleus; it exits the brainstem at the pontomedullary junction, traverses the cerebellopontine angle cistern within the nervus intermedius, passes through the meatal segment, and divides at the end of the labyrinthine segment (ie, at the geniculate ganglion). The upper division exits the petrous bone through a hiatus along the anterior petrous surface as the greater petrosal nerve; it passes through foramen lacerum and then the pterygoid canal to innervate the pterygopalatine ganglion, which provides parasympathetic postganglionic innervation to the nasal, palatine, and lacrimal glands. The lower division continues with the rest of the facial nerve through the horizontal segment and then through the superior portion of the mastoid segment, where it joins the chorda tympani to innervate the submandibular ganglion, which provides postganglionic parasympathetic innervation to the submandibular and sublingual glands.

Finally, let's include some associated nerve structures that either join or run alongside the facial nerve. First, show that the vestibulocochlear nerve also passes through the internal acoustic meatus along with the facial nerve. Then, show that the chorda tympani merges with the lingual nerve, a branch of the mandibular division of the trigeminal nerve, which carries sensory afferent information from the floor of the mouth. Lastly, show that the sympathetic deep petrosal nerve joins the greater petrosal nerve in the pterygoid canal; together they form the nerve of the pterygoid canal (aka the vidian nerve).[1–8,10–12]

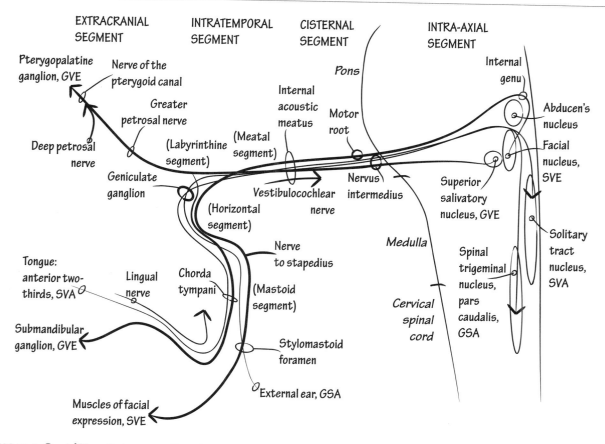

EXTRACRANIAL SEGMENT

INTRATEMPORAL SEGMENT

CISTERNAL SEGMENT

INTRA-AXIAL SEGMENT

Pterygopalatine ganglion, GVE

Nerve of the pterygoid canal

Greater petrosal nerve

Deep petrosal nerve

(Labyrinthine segment)

Geniculate ganglion

(Horizontal segment)

Internal acoustic meatus

(Meatal segment)

Vestibulocochlear nerve

Pons

Motor root

Nervus intermedius

Internal genu

Abducen's nucleus

Facial nucleus, SVE

Superior salivatory nucleus, GVE

Solitary tract nucleus, SVA

Medulla

Spinal trigeminal nucleus, pars caudalis, GSA

Cervical spinal cord

Tongue: anterior two-thirds, SVA

Lingual nerve

Chorda tympani

Nerve to stapedius

(Mastoid segment)

Submandibular ganglion, GVE

Stylomastoid foramen

External ear, GSA

Muscles of facial expression, SVE

DRAWING 13-6 Cranial Nerve 7: Anatomy—Complete

Cranial Nerves 9 & 10

Here, we will draw the glossopharyngeal nerve (cranial nerve 9) and the vagus nerve (cranial nerve 10), together. First, draw a sagittal view of the brainstem. Begin with the inferior salivatory nucleus, which is a small nucleus in the upper medulla. Indicate that it innervates the otic ganglion with GVE fibers of the glossopharyngeal nerve. The otic ganglion provides parasympathetic innervation to the parotid gland. Next, directly underneath the inferior salivatory nucleus, draw the dorsal motor nucleus of the vagus, which spans the remainder of the medulla. Indicate that it provides parasympathetic innervation to smooth muscle of the oropharynx and parasympathetic innervation to viscera within the thoracoabdomen through GVE fibers of the vagus nerve. Its actions include pulmonary bronchiole constriction, heart rate reduction, and augmentation of gut peristalsis. Now, draw nucleus ambiguus, which spans the height of the medulla. Indicate that it innervates the throat muscles with SVE fibers of the glossopharyngeal and vagus nerves. Its glossopharyngeal innervation is to stylopharyngeus, which elevates the pharynx during speech and swallowing, and its vagal innervation is to the pharynx, larynx, select palatine muscles, and one tongue muscle: palatoglossus. Next, show that nucleus ambiguus also provides parasympathetic GVE innervation to the carotid body and carotid sinus through the glossopharyngeal nerve, and to the heart and aortic bodies through the vagus nerve.

Now, draw the spinal trigeminal nucleus, pars caudalis, which spans from the inferior medulla to the upper cervical spinal cord. Indicate that inferiorly it receives cutaneous sensory reception from GSA fibers of the glossopharyngeal and vagus nerves (and the facial nerve). Its sensory afferents originate from many sites of the head and neck, including the oropharynx, external ear, and the tympanic membrane; also, the GSA component of the vagus nerve carries posterior cranial fossa dura mater sensory input.

Finally, draw the solitary tract nucleus, which spans the height of the medulla. Show that within its upper (gustatory) region, it receives taste afferents from the posterior third of the tongue via SVA fibers of the glossopharyngeal nerve and from the epiglottis via SVA fibers of the vagus nerve. Then, indicate that within its lower (cardiorespiratory) region, it receives GVA fibers of the glossopharyngeal nerve from the carotid body chemoreceptors and the carotid sinus (aka carotid bulb) baroreceptors. Lastly, indicate that the solitary tract nucleus receives GVA fibers of the vagus nerve from the thoracoabdomen: specifically, from the heart, baroreceptors in the aortic arch, chemoreceptors in the aortic bodies, pharynx, larynx, lungs, and proximal gut.[13]

Next, note that both the glossopharyngeal and vagus nerves each have superior and inferior sensory ganglia that are protected by the skull base; they lie within or near to the jugular foramen. Cell bodies of the GSA fibers lie in the superior ganglia and those of the GVA and SVA fibers lie in the inferior ganglia.[10]

Now, draw an axial view of the medulla. Show that the glossopharyngeal and vagus fibers exit the medulla laterally through the post-olivary sulcus to enter the cerebellomedullary cistern (aka inferior cerebellopontine cistern). Then, return to our sagittal diagram and show that these nerve fibers traverse the skull base through the jugular foramen along with the accessory nerve (cranial nerve 11) and the internal jugular vein. Next, show that within the periphery, within the carotid space, cranial nerves 9, 10, and 11 and also cranial nerve 12 (the hypoglossal nerve) and the internal jugular vein and internal carotid artery run together.[1–8,10–12]

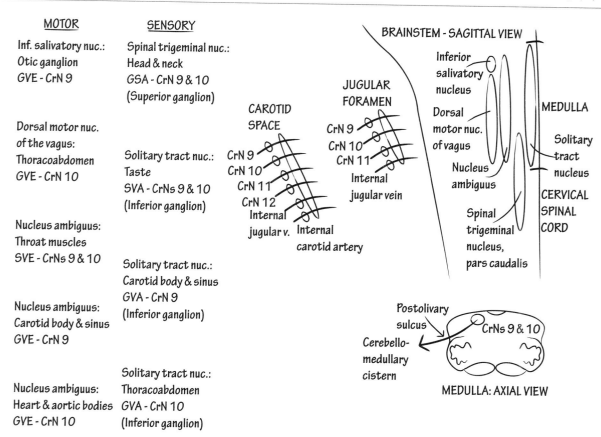

MOTOR

Inf. salivatory nuc.:
Otic ganglion
GVE - CrN 9

Dorsal motor nuc.
of the vagus:
Thoracoabdomen
GVE - CrN 10

Nucleus ambiguus:
Throat muscles
SVE - CrNs 9 & 10

Nucleus ambiguus:
Carotid body & sinus
GVE - CrN 9

Nucleus ambiguus:
Heart & aortic bodies
GVE - CrN 10

SENSORY

Spinal trigeminal nuc.:
Head & neck
GSA - CrN 9 & 10
(Superior ganglion)

Solitary tract nuc.:
Taste
SVA - CrNs 9 & 10
(Inferior ganglion)

Solitary tract nuc.:
Carotid body & sinus
GVA - CrN 9
(Inferior ganglion)

Solitary tract nuc.:
Thoracoabdomen
GVA - CrN 10
(Inferior ganglion)

CAROTID
SPACE
CrN 9
CrN 10
CrN 11
CrN 12
Internal
jugular v.   Internal
carotid artery

JUGULAR
FORAMEN
CrN 9
CrN 10
CrN 11
Internal
jugular vein

BRAINSTEM - SAGITTAL VIEW
Inferior
salivatory
nucleus
Dorsal
motor nuc.
of vagus
Nucleus
ambiguus
Spinal
trigeminal
nucleus,
pars caudalis

MEDULLA
Solitary
tract
nucleus
CERVICAL
SPINAL
CORD

Postolivary
sulcus
Cerebello-
medullary
cistern

CrNs 9 & 10

MEDULLA: AXIAL VIEW

DRAWING 13-7   Cranial Nerves 9 & 10

The Gag Reflex

In neurology, the gag reflex is often tested to assess the integrity of the brainstem and cranial nerves. We brush the patient's soft palate and observe for the characteristic gag response. The gag reflex relies on the glossopharyngeal nerve for its afferent loop and the vagus nerve for its efferent loop, and it also involves the motor division of the trigeminal nerve and the hypoglossal nerve for additional motor effects. Although certain details of the gag reflex remain poorly understood, enough of its neuroanatomy has been elucidated that we are able create a reliable diagram for it.

First, show that soft palate stimulation sends a volley of afferent impulse along the glossopharyngeal nerve; it is unclear whether this afferent impulse is somatic or visceral. Next, draw the glossopharyngeal sensory nuclei; include both the spinal trigeminal nucleus for the GSA fibers and the solitary tract nucleus for the GVA fibers (as either may be involved). Then, show that these nuclei excite motor neurons in nucleus ambiguus and indicate that nucleus ambiguus sends efferent impulse via the vagus nerve for pharyngeal constriction. Thus, the glossopharyngeal nerve provides the afferent limb of the gag reflex and the vagus nerve provides the efferent limb. However, the gag reflex additionally involves jaw opening and tongue thrust, so also show that nucleus ambiguus stimulates the trigeminal motor nucleus in the pons, which is largely responsible for jaw opening via cranial nerve 5, and the hypoglossal nucleus in the medulla, which provides tongue thrust via cranial nerve 12.

Next, let's illustrate the supranuclear innervation of the palate in order to demonstrate the cortical innervation to the special visceral efferent component of the glossopharyngeal and vagus nerves. First, draw the bilateral nucleus ambiguus nuclei. Then, show that each nucleus ambiguus innervates the ipsilateral side of the palate. Next, show that each cerebral hemisphere projects corticonuclear fibers to each nucleus ambiguus, but show that the predominance of fibers go to the contralateral nucleus.

Now, we will use prototypical injury patterns to show what happens in both upper motor neuron and lower motor neuron lesions to solidify our understanding of this arrangement. Redraw the hemispheres and bilateral nucleus ambiguus nuclei. Show that in an upper motor neuron lesion (such as a cortical stroke), the side of the palate contralateral to the stroke is weak and the side contralateral to the intact hemisphere is strong: the majority of fibers from the intact hemisphere go to the contralateral nucleus ambiguus and the minority go to the ipsilateral nucleus ambiguus. Note, however, that many texts deny that there is any difference in the innervation to the ipsilateral and the contralateral nucleus ambiguus nuclei and simply state that cortical innervation to the nucleus ambiguus nuclei is bilateral without ipsilateral or contralateral predominance. When that is the case, a unilateral upper motor neuron lesion (eg, a cortical stroke) has no effect on the gag reflex.

Next, again draw the hemispheres and bilateral nucleus ambiguus nuclei. Show that in a lower motor neuron injury (such as a direct lesion to the nucleus ambiguus, itself, or its exiting fibers), the corticonuclear innervation is preserved but there is complete peripheral fiber loss on the side of the lesion and, therefore, there is unilateral palatal paralysis on the side of the lower motor neuron lesion.[11]

When we evaluate for palatal weakness, the side of the palate that hangs lower is the side that is weak; dismiss trying to determine the directionality of the uvula—this only adds an unnecessary layer of complexity to our assessment. Paralysis of the muscles of the soft palate results in failure of closure of the nasopharyngeal aperture; as a consequence, air escapes through the nose during speech and liquids are regurgitated into the nasal cavity during swallowing. In amyotrophic lateral sclerosis (ALS), there is often loss of corticonuclear innervation to the nucleus ambiguus, with resultant characteristic nasal pattern speech.

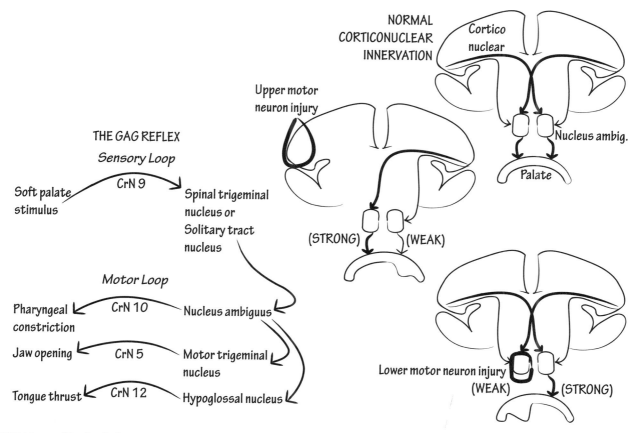

NORMAL
CORTICONUCLEAR
INNERVATION

Cortico
nuclear

Nucleus ambig.

Palate

Upper motor
neuron injury

(STRONG)   (WEAK)

THE GAG REFLEX

Sensory Loop

CrN 9

Soft palate
stimulus

Spinal trigeminal
nucleus or
Solitary tract
nucleus

Motor Loop

Pharyngeal
constriction   CrN 10   Nucleus ambiguus

Jaw opening   CrN 5   Motor trigeminal
nucleus

Tongue thrust   CrN 12   Hypoglossal nucleus

Lower motor neuron injury
(WEAK)   (STRONG)

DRAWING 13-8 **The Gag Reflex**

References

1. Binder, D. K., Sonne, D. C. & Fischbein, N. J. *Cranial nerves: anatomy, pathology, imaging* (Thieme, 2010).

2. Brazis, P. W., Masdeu, J. C. & Biller, J. *Localization in clinical neurology,* 5th ed. (Lippincott Williams & Wilkins, 2007).

3. Haines, D. E. & Ard, M. D. *Fundamental neuroscience: for basic and clinical applications,* 3rd ed. (Churchill Livingstone Elsevier, 2006).

4. Naidich, T. P. & Duvernoy, H. M. *Duvernoy's atlas of the human brain stem and cerebellum: high-field MRI: surface anatomy, internal structure, vascularization and 3D sectional anatomy* (Springer, 2009).

5. Netter, F. H. & Dalley, A. F. *Atlas of human anatomy*, 2nd ed. (Novartis, 1997).

6. Wilson-Pauwels, L. *Cranial nerves: function and dysfunction,* 3rd ed. (People's Medical Pub. House, 2010).

7. Willoughby, E. W. & Anderson, N. E. Lower cranial nerve motor function in unilateral vascular lesions of the cerebral hemisphere. *Br Med J (Clin Res Ed)* 289, 791–794 (1984).

8. Standring, S. & Gray, H. *Gray's anatomy: the anatomical basis of clinical practice,* 40th ed. (Churchill Livingstone/Elsevier, 2008).

9. Mafee, M. F., Valvassori, G. E. & Becker, M. *Imaging of the head and neck,* 2nd ed. (Thieme, 2005).

10. Macdonald, A. J. *Diagnostic and surgical imaging anatomy. Brain, head & neck, spine,* 1st ed. (Amirsys, 2006).

11. Conn, P. M. *Neuroscience in medicine,* 3rd ed. (Humana Press, 2008).

12. Sundin, L. & Nilsson, S. Branchial innervation. *J Exp Zool* 293, 232–248, doi:10.1002/jez.10130 (2002).

13. Fritsch, H. & Kühnel, W. *Color atlas of human anatomy. Volume 2, Internal organs,* 5th ed., Chapter 11 (Thieme, 2007).

14

Vestibular and Auditory Systems

The Ear

The Vestibular System

Central Auditory Pathways

Auditory Physiology (Advanced)

Know-It Points

The Ear

- The external and middle ear canals lie within the tympanic portion of the temporal bone.
- The middle ear canal contains three ossicles—from lateral to medial: the malleus, incus, and stapes.
- The stapes abuts the oval window; when sound is transmitted through the ossicles, the stapes pushes the oval window into the inner ear.
- The inner ear canal lies within the petrous portion of the temporal bone.
- The inner ear canal divides into three different parts: the semicircular canals, which serve vestibular function; the cochlea, which serves auditory function; and the vestibule, which is involved in both auditory and vestibular functions.
- Three ducts form within the cochlea: the cochlear duct (scala media), the vestibular duct (scala vestibuli), and the tympanic duct (scala tympani).

- Reissner's membrane separates the vestibular duct from the cochlear duct, and the basilar membrane separates the cochlear duct from the tympanic duct.
- The vestibular and tympanic ducts are filled with perilymphatic fluid, and the cochlear duct is filled with endolymphatic fluid.
- The three semicircular canals (anterior, horizontal, and posterior) lie perpendicular to one another and detect rotational acceleration.
- From the observer's perspective, the anterior canals produce upward eye movement; the posterior canals produce downward eye movement; the right-side canals produce clockwise torsional eye movement; and the left-side canals produce counterclockwise torsional eye movement.

The Vestibular System

- The vestibular nuclear complex excites the contralateral abducens nucleus and the abducens nucleus excites the contralateral oculomotor nucleus, which is ipsilateral to the vestibular nuclear complex where the impulse originated.
- The vestibular nuclear complex spans from the upper pons to the inferior floor of the fourth ventricle (in the medulla).

- The medial division of the vestibular nuclear complex comprises the superior nucleus and medial nucleus.
- The lateral division of the vestibular nuclear complex comprises the lateral nucleus and inferior nucleus.

Central Auditory Pathways

- The ventral cochlear nucleus lies at the pontomedullary junction.
- The dorsal cochlear nucleus lies in the upper medulla.
- The superior olivary complex lies in the mid-pons.
- The inferior colliculi lie in the inferior midbrain.
- The lateral lemniscus tracts project to the inferior colliculi.

- Each inferior colliculus projects to the ipsilateral medial geniculate nucleus via the brachium of the inferior colliculus.
- Each medial geniculate nucleus projects to the ipsilateral transverse temporal gyri (Heschl's gyri)—the primary auditory cortex.

Auditory Physiology (*Advanced*)

- Preservation of tone localization throughout the central auditory system is called tonotopy.
- The base of the cochlea encodes high-frequency sounds and the apex encodes low-frequency sounds.
- Low-frequency sounds lie anterior within the ventral and dorsal cochlear nuclei.
- High-frequency sounds lie posterior within the ventral and dorsal cochlear nuclei.

- Within the transverse temporal gyri (Heschl's gyri), low-frequency sounds localize laterally whereas high-frequency sounds localize medially.
- When there is a unilateral lesion to the central auditory pathway, hearing is preserved from the duplication of auditory information in the contralateral cerebral hemisphere.

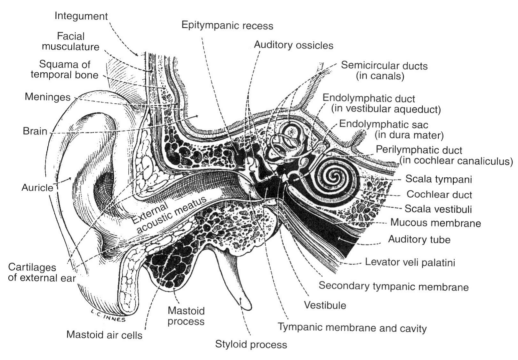

FIGURE 14-1 **Outer, middle, and inner ear.** Used with permission from Baloh, Robert W., and Vicente Honrubia. *Clinical Neurophysiology of the Vestibular System,* 3rd ed. Contemporary Neurology Series 63. Oxford; New York: Oxford University Press, 2001.

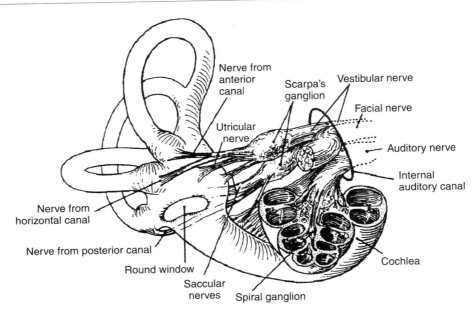

FIGURE 14-2 **Inner ear.** Used with permission from Baloh, Robert W., and Vicente Honrubia. *Clinical Neurophysiology of the Vestibular System,* 3rd ed. Contemporary Neurology Series 63. Oxford; New York: Oxford University Press, 2001.

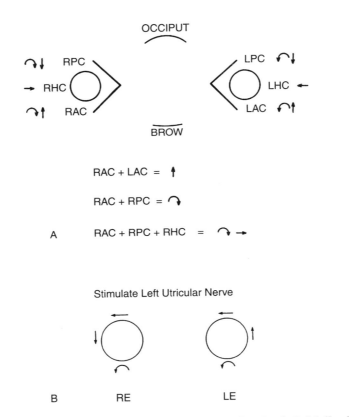

FIGURE 14-3 **Oculomotor effects of semicircular canal stimulation.** Used with permission from Leigh, R. J. & Zee, D. S. *The Neurology of Eye Movements.* Oxford; New York: Oxford University Press, 2006.

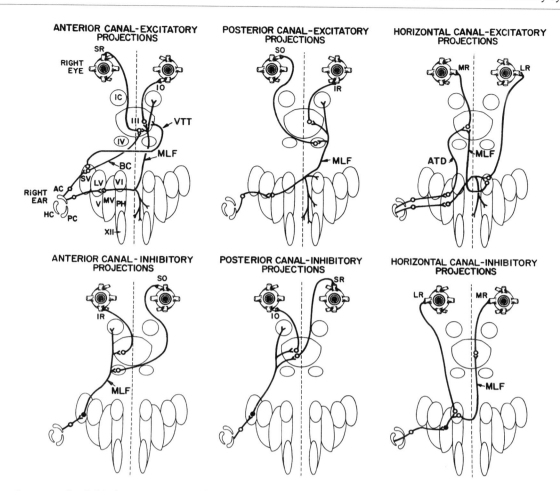

FIGURE 14-4 Summary of probable direct connections of vestibulo-ocular reflex, based upon findings from a number of species. Excitatory neurons are indicated by open circles, inhibitory neurons by filled circles. III: oculomotor nuclear complex; IV: trochlear nucleus; VI: abducens nucleus; XII: hypoglossal nucleus; AC: anterior semicircular canal; ATD: ascending tract of Deiters; BC: brachium conjunctivum; HC: "horizontal" or lateral semicircular canal; IC: interstitial nucleus of Cajal; IO: inferior oblique muscle; IR: inferior rectus muscle; LR: lateral rectus muscle; LV: lateral vestibular nucleus; MLF: medial longitudinal fasciculus; MR: medial rectus muscle; MV: medial vestibular nucleus; PC: posterior semicircular canal; PH: prepositus nucleus; SV: superior vestibular nucleus; SO; superior oblique muscle; SR: superior rectus muscle; V: inferior vestibular nucleus; VTP: ventral tegmental pathway. Used with permission from Leigh, R. J. & Zee, D. S. *The Neurology of Eye Movements.* Oxford; New York: Oxford University Press, 2006.

The Ear

Here, we will draw a coronal view of the ear with the subject facing towards us. Begin with our planes of orientation. First, draw the medial–lateral plane; then, the anterior–posterior plane; and finally, the superior–inferior plane. Now, draw the outer ear. Then, draw the external ear canal, which extends through the tympanic portion of the temporal bone, just in front of the mastoid process. Next, draw the tympanic membrane. Indicate that sound waves pass through the external ear canal to vibrate the tympanic membrane.

Now, draw the middle ear canal, which also lies mostly within the tympanic portion of the temporal bone. Indicate that it contains three ossicles—from lateral to medial, the malleus, incus, and stapes, which are the Latin terms for their shapes: "hammer," "anvil," and "stirrup," respectively. Next, indicate that the stapes abuts the oval window. When sound is transmitted through the ossicles, the stapes pushes the oval window into the inner ear (drawn soon). Now, show that the eustachian tube extends from the middle ear into the nasopharynx; it causes your middle ears to equilibrate with the atmospheric pressure in your nasopharynx when you swallow. Two important muscles exist within the middle ear canal: the tensor tympani, which is innervated by the trigeminal nerve and which acts on the tympanic membrane, and the stapedius muscle, which is innervated by the facial nerve and which acts on the stapes.

Next, we will draw the inner ear canal, which lies within the petrous portion of the temporal bone. Divide the inner ear into three different parts. First, draw the semicircular canals, which lie in superior-lateral position and serve vestibular function; then, draw the cochlea, which is shaped like a snail's shell, and which lies in anterior-inferior position and serves auditory function; and finally, draw the vestibule, which lies in between them and is involved in both auditory and vestibular functions—it transmits sound waves from the oval window to the cochlea and contains the otolith organs, which provide vestibular cues.[1]

Now, let's draw the three ducts that form within the cochlea. First, draw the cochlear duct (scala media); then, label the vestibular duct (scala vestibuli), which is continuous with the vestibule; and finally, label the tympanic duct (scala tympani), which ends in the round window (aka the secondary tympanic membrane). Show that the vestibular and tympanic ducts connect at the apex of the cochlea (aka the helicotrema). Reissner's membrane separates the vestibular duct from the cochlear duct and the basilar membrane separates the cochlear duct from the tympanic duct. The vestibular and tympanic ducts are filled with perilymphatic fluid, whereas the cochlear duct is filled with endolymphatic fluid. Perilymphatic fluid is like extracellular fluid in that it is high in sodium and low in potassium, whereas endolymphatic fluid is like intracellular fluid in that it is high in potassium and low in sodium. Patients with Ménière's syndrome, which causes bouts of vertigo, low-frequency hearing loss, and ear fullness, are commonly treated with salt-wasting diuretic medications because the syndrome is thought to be due to pathologically elevated endolymphatic sodium concentration. In more severe cases of Ménière's syndrome, vestibular ablation is performed and, also, aminoglycosides (specifically gentamicin and streptomycin) are used to destroy the vestibular end-organ with relative preservation of the auditory cells.

Now, indicate that when the oval window vibrates, a fluid wave passes through the vestibule, which then passes through the vestibular duct, across the apex of the cochlea into the tympanic duct, and then through the tympanic duct to push the round window into the air-filled middle ear canal. In this process, the auditory sensory organ, the organ of Corti, which lies along the basilar membrane, is activated for sound detection. High-frequency sounds activate hair cells at the base of the cochlea (near the oval and round windows) whereas low-frequency sounds activate hair cells at the apex of the cochlea. The basilar membrane is thinnest at its base and widest at its apex.

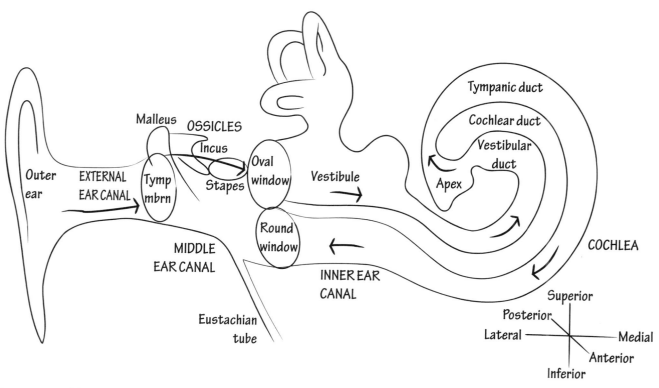

DRAWING 14-1 **The Ear—Partial**

The Ear (Cont.)

Next, return to the vestibule so we can show the otolith organs. First, draw the saccule, which detects vertical movement (ie, gravity), and then draw the utricle, which perceives horizontal (forward/backward) movement. The macula (the neuroepithelial sensory detection region) of the saccule is principally vertically oriented and its attached hair cells are horizontally oriented to detect vertical movement, whereas the macula of the utricle is principally horizontally oriented and its attached hair cells are vertically oriented to detect horizontal movement.

Now, let's label the semicircular canals: the anterior semicircular canal, horizontal semicircular canal, and posterior semicircular canal. These three semicircular canals lie perpendicular to one another and detect rotational acceleration. To understand their directionality, include within our figure an axial view of them. Draw an oval-shaped cranium and label its anterior and posterior aspects. Then, draw the left anterior semicircular canal facing anterolaterally and the left posterior semicircular canal perpendicular to it. The posterior canal lies along the axis of the petrous ridge. Next, include the laterally facing left horizontal canal. In normal, upright head position, the horizontal canal is tilted upward about 30 degrees to the horizontal plane and the anterior and posterior canals are roughly within the vertical plane. When sitting upright, if the head is tilted down 30 degrees, the horizontal canals are brought into the earth-horizontal plane. Now, draw the right-side semicircular canals as mirror images of the left.

At the utricular end of each canal is a membranous enlargement, called the ampulla, which contains the sensory cell system of the semicircular canal. Attached to the ampulla is the cupula, which is a gelatinous mass that deflects during angular acceleration. When the cupula bows, the hair cells are activated and, as a result, the semicircular canals generate eye movements in their plane of orientation. Show that the left anterior canal and the right posterior canal drive the eyes along the same diagonal, from left anterior to right posterior; then, show that the right anterior and left posterior canals drive the eyes along the same diagonal, from right anterior to left posterior; and finally, indicate that the horizontal canals drive the eyes laterally.[1]

Next, we will divide the directionality of the eye movements generated by the anterior and posterior semicircular canals (the vertical canals) based on whether the canal is anterior or posterior, right or left. Label across the top of the page that we will show the eye movement directionality from the observer's perspective in coronal view. Also, to avoid confusion, since eye movements are commonly addressed in regards to the nystagmus they produce, indicate that we are showing the slow phase of the nystagmus. Now, indicate that the anterior canals produce upward movements and that the posterior canals produce downward movements, and, again, from the observer's perspective, indicate that the right-side canals produce torsional movements in a clockwise direction whereas the left-side canals produce torsional movements in a counterclockwise direction.[2]

In benign paroxysmal positional vertigo, calcium carbonate crystals from the utricle fall into one of the semicircular canals—most often the posterior canal—and stimulate positional vertigo. If the right posterior canal is activated, then from the observer's perspective, the slow phase of the nystagmus is downward with clockwise rotation. The fast phase, which is how the nystagmus is actually named, is in the opposite direction: upward and counterclockwise.[2]

To conclude our diagram, let's draw the vestibulocochlear nerve, which transmits the vestibular and auditory impulses from the inner ear to the vestibulocochlear nuclei in the brainstem. First, draw the vestibular segment of the vestibulocochlear nerve and then the cochlear segment. Indicate that the vestibulocochlear nerve passes through the internal acoustic meatus (along with the facial nerve) and crosses the pontocerebellar cistern to enter the brainstem at the pontomedullary junction.

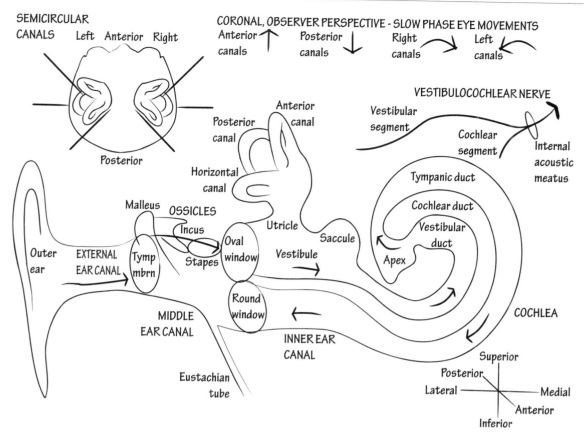

DRAWING 14-2 **The Ear—Complete**

The Vestibular System

Here, we will draw the vestibulo-ocular reflex, vestibulospinal pathways, and a few additional central vestibular projections. We will begin with the vestibulo-ocular reflex. Each of the semicircular canals has its own projection pattern (see Figure 14-4); here, we will draw the horizontal canal's excitation of the ocular nuclei because it is the most clinically helpful pathway to learn. Draw a coronal view of the brainstem and include an axial section through a pair of eyes. Next, draw the left vestibular nuclear complex, which spans much of the height of the pons and the medulla. Now, label the left oculomotor nucleus and also the right abducens nucleus. Show that the vestibular nuclear complex excites the contralateral abducens nucleus, which causes the right lateral rectus muscle to produce eye *ab*duction: it drives the right eye to the right. Then, indicate that the abducens nucleus also projects fibers across midline that ascend the medial longitudinal fasciculus and excite the contralateral oculomotor nucleus, which causes the left medial rectus muscle to produce eye *ad*duction: it drives the left eye to the right. Lastly, show that the vestibular nuclear complex also sends direct projections to the ipsilateral oculomotor nucleus via the ascending tract of Deiters. Note that the vestibular nuclear complex simultaneously inhibits the ipsilateral abducens nucleus and contralateral oculomotor nucleus, and also note that of the four vestibular nuclei (drawn later), the medial and lateral nuclei have the most robust ocular projections.[2]

For a simple way to remember this circuitry at the bedside, hold your fists in front of you and show that the left vestibular nuclear complex drives the eyes to the right and the right vestibular nuclear complex drive the eyes to the left. Next, drop one fist to demonstrate that when one vestibular nuclear complex is damaged, the eyes deviate toward the damaged side, away from the intact side.

Next, we will draw the vestibulospinal pathways. Redraw a brainstem. Include an outline of the vestibular nuclear complex, which spans from the upper pons to the inferior floor of the fourth ventricle (in the medulla). To draw the individual nuclei of the vestibular nuclear complex, divide the complex into medial and lateral divisions. Label the top of the medial division as the superior nucleus and the rest as the medial nucleus; then, label the top half of the lateral division as the lateral nucleus and the bottom half as the inferior nucleus. The lateral nucleus is also called Deiters' nucleus and the inferior nucleus is also called the descending nucleus. Note that although not shown as such in our diagram, the lateral and inferior nuclei actually overlap in the low pons and the medial and superior nuclei overlap in the mid-pons.

Now, to continue our vestibulospinal pathway diagram, include upper and lower levels of the spinal cord. Indicate that the lateral vestibular nucleus projects uncrossed descending fibers, which descend the ventral spinal cord and innervate extensor motor neurons throughout the spinal cord, and label this projection as the lateral vestibulospinal tract. Then, indicate that the medial vestibular nucleus projects crossed and uncrossed fibers that descend the medial spinal cord to innervate extensor motor neurons in the upper spinal cord, only, and label this as the medial vestibulospinal tract. Note that the medial vestibulospinal tract also receives minor inputs from the lateral and inferior vestibular nuclei, as well. These vestibulospinal pathways provide antigravity movements for the maintenance of posture, as do the reticulospinal tracts (see Drawing 7-3).

Next, let's list a few additional central vestibular functions. Indicate that the vestibular nuclei project to the thalamus for somatosensory detection of vestibular movement and to the reticular formation, which induces nausea and vomiting. Lastly, indicate that the vestibulocolic reflex maintains the head at a level position during movement.[2–4]

HORIZONTAL CANAL PROJECTIONS - EXCITATORY

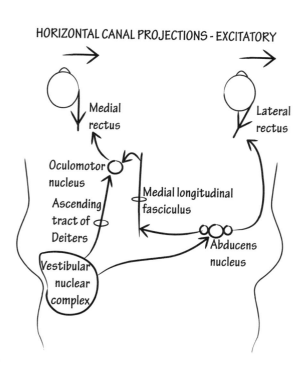

Medial rectus

Lateral rectus

Oculomotor nucleus

Ascending tract of Deiters

Medial longitudinal fasciculus

Vestibular nuclear complex

Abducens nucleus

VESTIBULOSPINAL TRACTS

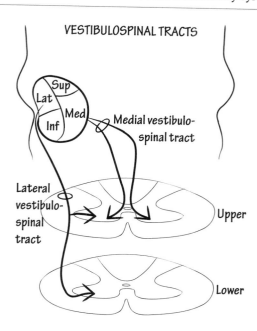

Sup
Lat
Med
Inf

Medial vestibulo-spinal tract

Lateral vestibulo-spinal tract

Upper

Lower

ADDITIONAL CENTRAL VESTIBULAR PROJECTIONS

Thalamic projections - somatosensory detection

Reticular projections - nausea/vomiting

Vestibulocolic reflex - level head

DRAWING 14-3 **The Vestibular System**

Central Auditory Pathways

Here, we will create a simplified diagram of the central auditory pathways. First, draw a coronal view of the brainstem. On the left side, label the ventral cochlear nucleus at the pontomedullary junction and then, just below it, in the upper medulla, label the dorsal cochlear nucleus. Note that the ventral cochlear nucleus is often further subdivided into its anterior and posterior subnuclei. Next draw an axial view of the posterolateral wedge of the upper medulla/pontomedullary junction to illustrate the anterior–posterior relationship of the ventral and dorsal cochlear nuclei. Draw the restiform body of the inferior cerebellar peduncle and then show that the ventral cochlear nucleus lies along its ventrolateral surface and that the dorsal cochlear nucleus lies along its dorsolateral surface.[5]

Now, in the coronal diagram, label the bilateral superior olivary complexes in the mid-pons. Each superior olivary complex comprises three separate nuclei: a nucleus of the trapezoid body, medial superior olivary nucleus, and lateral superior olivary nucleus. Surrounding the superior olivary complexes are peri-olivary cells. Next, in the inferior midbrain, label the bilateral inferior colliculi. Then, show projection fibers from the bilateral superior olivary complexes to their respective inferior colliculi and label these projections as the lateral lemniscus tracts. Next, label the left medial geniculate nucleus, which is part of the metathalamus, and then, label the left transverse temporal gyri (aka Heschl's gyri) continuous with the superior temporal gyrus in the Sylvian fissure. Now, draw a representative projection from the left inferior colliculus to the left medial geniculate nucleus via the brachium of the inferior colliculus. And finally, draw a projection from the left medial geniculate nucleus to the ipsilateral transverse temporal gyri (Heschl's gyri)—the primary auditory cortex. Note that the same projections exist on the right side, as well.

Next, let's show the projection fibers from the ventral and dorsal cochlear nuclei. Three acoustic striae exist: ventral, dorsal, and intermediate. First, let's draw the ventral stria. To begin, show projection fibers from the left ventral cochlear nucleus to the bilateral superior olivary complexes. Then, add another pathway that projects from the ventral cochlear nucleus to the contralateral inferior colliculus via the lateral lemniscus without synapsing in the superior olivary complex. Label the ventral cochlear to bilateral superior olivary complex and ventral cochlear to contralateral inferior colliculus projection fibers as the ventral acoustic stria, and indicate that they are also referred to as the trapezoid body. Next, in our axial diagram show that the ventral acoustic stria passes ventral to the restiform body.

Now, return to the coronal diagram and show that the dorsal cochlear nucleus projects to the contralateral inferior colliculus via the lateral lemniscus without forming a synapse in the superior olivary complex, and label this projection as the dorsal acoustic stria. In the axial diagram, show that the dorsal acoustic stria emerges from the dorsal cochlear nucleus and passes dorsally around the restiform body.

Next, back in the coronal diagram, show that the ventral cochlear nucleus sends additional projection fibers to the contralateral inferior colliculus, which ascend via the lateral lemniscus tract without synapsing in the superior olivary complex. Label these fibers as the intermediate acoustic stria. In our axial diagram, show that the intermediate acoustic stria emerges from the dorsal portion of the ventral cochlear nucleus and passes dorsally around the restiform body.

A simple acronym for the central auditory pathways is "S-L-I-M," which denotes a few of the key steps in the pathway: superior olivary complex to lateral lemniscus to inferior colliculus to medial geniculate body. A common electrophysiologic test of the auditory system is the brainstem auditory evoked response, which helps localize central auditory pathway lesions and helps detect asymptomatic central nervous system lesions in the diagnostic evaluation of multiple sclerosis.[3,6]

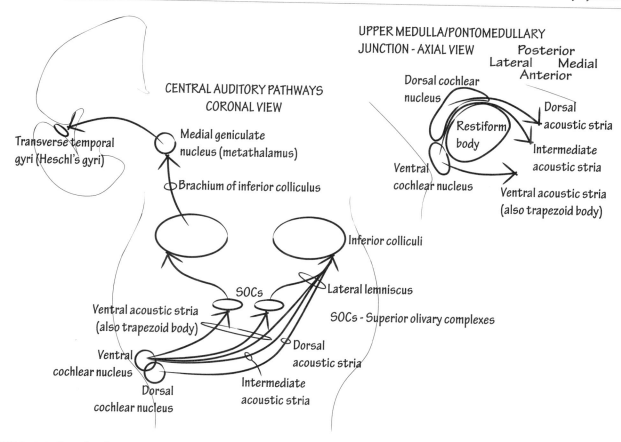

CENTRAL AUDITORY PATHWAYS CORONAL VIEW

Transverse temporal gyri (Heschl's gyri)

Medial geniculate nucleus (metathalamus)

Brachium of inferior colliculus

Inferior colliculi

SOCs

Lateral lemniscus

SOCs - Superior olivary complexes

Ventral acoustic stria (also trapezoid body)

Ventral cochlear nucleus

Dorsal cochlear nucleus

Dorsal acoustic stria

Intermediate acoustic stria

UPPER MEDULLA/PONTOMEDULLARY JUNCTION - AXIAL VIEW

Posterior
Lateral   Medial
Anterior

Dorsal cochlear nucleus

Restiform body

Dorsal acoustic stria

Intermediate acoustic stria

Ventral cochlear nucleus

Ventral acoustic stria (also trapezoid body)

DRAWING 14-4 Central Auditory Pathways

Auditory Physiology (*Advanced*)

Here, we will learn the physiology of tonotopy (the topographic organization of sound) and also the physiology of binaural and monaural sound localization. First, we will show the tonotopy of select regions of the auditory pathway. Indicate that the base of the cochlea encodes high-frequency sounds and that the apex encodes low-frequency sounds. Then, within the ventral and dorsal cochlear nuclei, show that low-frequency sounds lie anterior whereas high-frequency sounds lie posterior. Finally, indicate that within the transverse temporal gyri (Heschl's gyri) (the primary auditory cortex), low-frequency sounds localize laterally whereas high-frequency sounds localize medially. Thus, there is preservation of tonotopy throughout the central auditory system.[7,8]

Each cerebral hemisphere receives similar input from each set of cochlear nuclei, so when there is a unilateral lesion to any of the steps in the central auditory pathway, hearing is preserved from the duplication of auditory information in the contralateral cerebral hemisphere. The auditory system has this central duplication of sensory information whereas other sensory systems, such as the visual and somatosensory systems, do not because the peripheral receptors of the visual and somatosensory systems are topographically arranged to encode for stimulus localization, whereas the cochlea is tonotopically arranged, instead.

Tonotopy informs the brain about sound frequency but not location; therefore, sound localization must occur through other means. Sound reaches each ear (the near ear and far ear) at slightly different times and intensities. These are the two main interaural (between ear) differences: the interaural time difference and the interaural level difference (where "time" refers to the time the sound reaches each ear and "level" refers to the sound intensity level at each ear). Sound reaches the near ear before it reaches the far ear to create the interaural time difference, and the head, itself, attenuates the sound before it reaches the far ear to create the interaural level difference. In accordance with the duplex theory of sound localization, time differences are best detected for low-frequency sounds whereas level differences are best detected for high-frequency sounds.

Now, let's incorporate these interaural differences into the core pathways for binaural sound localization. First, in coronal view, on both sides of the brainstem, draw the following superior olivary complex nuclei: the medial nucleus of the trapezoid body, medial superior olivary nucleus, and lateral superior olivary nucleus. Low-frequency sounds are encoded within the spherical bushy cells of the ventral cochlear nucleus. Indicate that they project bilaterally to the medial superior olivary nuclei, which are sensitive to interaural *time* differences.

High-frequency sounds are encoded within the ventral cochlear nucleus in both the spherical bushy cells and globular bushy cells. Both cell types project to the lateral superior olivary nucleus, which is sensitive to interaural *level* differences. Show that the spherical bushy cells send exclusively ipsilateral, excitatory projections to the lateral superior olivary nucleus. On the contrary, using the ventral cochlear nucleus on the opposite side, show that the globular bushy cells send excitatory projections to the contralateral medial nucleus of the trapezoid body, which in turn sends inhibitory projections to the ipsilateral lateral superior olivary nucleus (thus the globular bushy cells inhibit the contralateral lateral superior olivary nucleus via the medial nucleus of the trapezoid body).[9–16]

These pathways establish the physiology of binaural sound localization, but plug one of your ears, close your eyes, and snap your fingers at different points in space. Even with only one ear, you can still localize sound stimuli fairly well because of your monaural sound localization skills. Monaural localization of sound relies on the head-related transfer function, which shapes sound waves as they propagate toward the eardrum. Through monaural sound localization mechanisms, the head, torso, and pinna distort sound waves into spectral patterns that the central auditory system uses in the localization of sound.[15]

TONOTOPY

BINAURAL SOUND LOCALIZATION

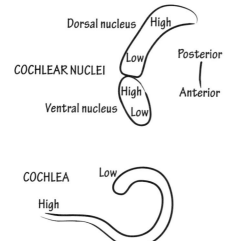

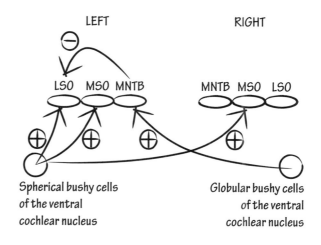

MEDIAL superior olivary nucleus sensitive to interaural TIME difference
LATERAL superior olivary nucleus sensitive to interaural LEVEL difference

MNTB - medial nucleus of the trapezoid body
MSO - medial superior olivary nucleus
LSO - lateral superior olivary nucleus

DRAWING 14-5 **Auditory Physiology**

References

1. Swartz, J. D. & Loevner, L. A. *Imaging of the temporal bone,* 4th ed. (Thieme, 2009).

2. Leigh, R. J. & Zee, D. S. *The neurology of eye movements* (Oxford University Press, 2006).

3. Wilson-Pauwels, L. *Cranial nerves: function and dysfunction,* pp. 143–165 (People's Medical Publishing House, 2010).

4. Waxman, S. G. *Clinical neuroanatomy,* 25th ed., p. 53 (Lange Medical Books/McGraw-Hill, Medical Pub. Division, 2003).

5. Rajimehr, R. & Tootell, R. Organization of human visual cortex. In *The senses: a comprehensive reference* (ed. A. I. Basbaum) (Elsevier Inc., 2008).

6. Covey, E. Inputs to the inferior colliculus. In *The senses: a comprehensive reference* (ed A. I. Basbaum) (Elsevier Science, 2008).

7. Winer, J. A. & Schreiner, C. *The auditory cortex,* p. 659 (Springer, 2011).

8. Ehret, G. & Romand, R. *The central auditory system,* pp. 161–163 (Oxford University Press, 1997).

9. Burkard, R. F., Eggermont, J. J. & Don, M. *Auditory evoked potentials: basic principles and clinical application,* pp. 217–218 (Lippincott Williams & Wilkins, 2007).

10. Benarroch, E. E. *Basic neurosciences with clinical applications,* p. 503 (Butterworth Heinemann Elsevier, 2006).

11. Woodin, M. A. & Maffei, A. *Inhibitory synaptic plasticity,* pp. 40–42 (Springer Verlag, 2010).

12. Bronzino, J. D. *The biomedical engineering handbook,* 3rd ed., pp. 5–11, 5–12 (CRC/Taylor & Francis, 2006).

13. Tollin, D. J. Encoding of interaural level differences for sound localization. In *The senses: a comprehensive reference* (ed A. I. Basbaum) (Elsevier Science, 2008).

14. Burger, R. M. & Rubel, E. W. Encoding of interaural timing for binaural hearing. In *The senses: a comprehensive reference* (ed A. I. Basbaum) (Elsevier Science, 2008).

15. Middlebrooks, J. Sound localization and the auditory cortex. In *The senses: a comprehensive reference* (ed A. I. Basbaum) (Elsevier Science, 2008).

16. Kaas, J. H. & Hackett, T. A. The functional neuroanatomy of the auditory cortex. In *The senses: a comprehensive reference* (ed A. I. Basbaum) (Elsevier Inc., 2008).

Cerebellum

Know-It Points

Lobes, Zones, & Modules

- The primary fissure divides the corpus cerebelli into anterior and posterior lobes.
- The posterolateral fissure separates the corpus cerebelli from the flocculonodular lobe.
- The vestibulocerebellum is important for equilibrium and eye movements.

- The spinocerebellum plays a major role in postural stability.
- The pontocerebellum is geared towards goal-directed, fine motor movements.

Somatotopy & Lobules

- Unilateral cerebellar lesions affect the ipsilateral side of the body.
- The midline cerebellum plays a role in posture whereas the lateral cerebellum assists in fine motor, goal-oriented skills.

- The midline, vermian cerebellum divides into ten different lobules.
- The cerebellar hemispheres divide into nine different lobules.

Peduncles, Midline Structures, Arteries

- The middle and inferior cerebellar peduncles are afferent pathways into the cerebellum.
- The superior cerebellar peduncle is an efferent pathway out of the cerebellum.
- Notable exceptions to the aforementioned rules are:
  - The anterior spinocerebellar tract enters the cerebellum through the superior cerebellar peduncle

  - Select midline cerebellar tracts exit the cerebellum through the inferior cerebellar peduncle
- The flocculonodular lobe lies in anterior, mid-cerebellar position.

Nuclei & Circuitry (*Advanced*)

- The two main classes of cerebellar nuclei are the cerebellar cortical neurons and the deep cerebellar nuclei.
- The cerebellar cortical cell layers, from outside to inside, are the molecular layer, Purkinje layer, and granule layer.
- From lateral to medial, the deep cerebellar nuclei are the dentate, emboliform, globose, and fastigial nuclei.

- The fastigial nucleus plays a role in both the vestibulocerebellum and spinocerebellum.
- The interposed nuclei (the combined globose and emboliform nuclei) are part of the spinocerebellum.
- The dentate nucleus is part of the pontocerebellum.
- Climbing fibers are excitatory fibers that originate solely from the inferior olive and project to the cerebellum via the contralateral inferior cerebellar peduncle.

Corticopontocerebellar Pathway

- The corticopontocerebellar fibers descend to the pontine nuclei.
- The pontine nuclei project across midline through the middle cerebellar peduncle into the contralateral cerebellar cortex.
- The cerebellar cortex projects to the dentate nucleus.

- The dentate nucleus projects through the superior cerebellar peduncle across midline within the midbrain, inferior to the red nucleus, to synapse in the ventrolateral nucleus of the thalamus and also in the red nucleus.
- The thalamus projects back to the primary motor strip to complete the corticopontocerebellar pathway.

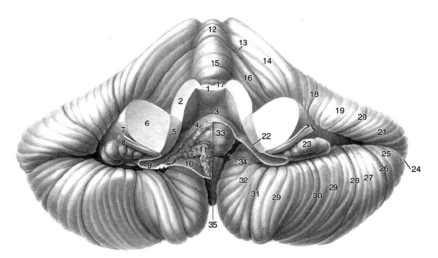

1	Superior medullary velum	12	Culmen
2	Superior cerebellar peduncle (brachium conjunctivum)	13	Preculminate fissure
		14	Anterior quadrangular lobule
3	Fastigium	15	Central lobule
4	Inferior medullary velum	16	Ala (wing) of the central lobule
5	Inferior cerebellar peduncle (restiform body)	17	Lingula
		18	Primary fissure
6	Middle cerebellar peduncle (brachium pontis)	19	Posterior quadrangular lobule (lobulus simplex)
7	Intermediate nerve	20	Superior posterior fissure
8	Vestibulocochlear nerve	21	Superior semilunar lobule
9	Lateral recess of the fourth ventricle	22	Floccular peduncle
10	Roofplate of the fourth ventricle	23	Flocculus
11	Choroid plexus of the fourth ventricle	24	Horizontal fissure

25	Inferior semilunar lobule
26	Ansoparamedian fissure
27	Gracile lobule
28	Prebiventral fissure
29	Biventral lobule
30	Intrabiventral fissure
31	Secondary fissure
32	Tonsil
33	Nodulus
34	Posterolateral fissure
35	Uvula

FIGURE 15-1 **Anterior cerebellum.** Used with permission from Nieuwenhuys, Rudolf, Christiaan Huijzen, Jan Voogd, and SpringerLink (Online service). "The Human Central Nervous System." Berlin, Heidelberg: Springer Berlin Heidelberg, 2008.

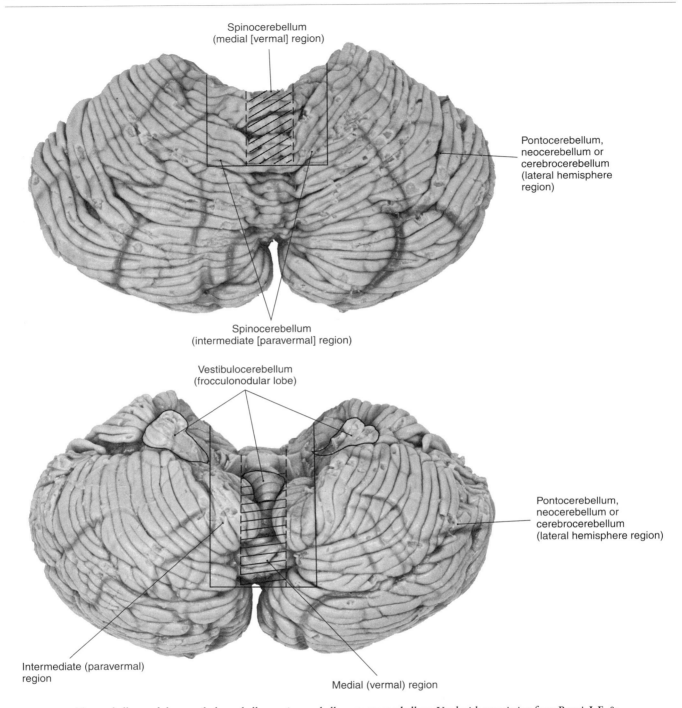

Spinocerebellum
(medial [vermal] region)

Pontocerebellum,
neocerebellum or
cerebrocerebellum
(lateral hemisphere
region)

Spinocerebellum
(intermediate [paravermal] region)

Vestibulocerebellum
(frocculonodular lobe)

Pontocerebellum,
neocerebellum or
cerebrocerebellum
(lateral hemisphere region)

Intermediate (paravermal)
region

Medial (vermal) region

FIGURE 15-2 The cerebellar modules: vestibulocerebellum, spinocerebellum, pontocerebellum. Used with permission from Bruni, J. E. & Montemurro, D. G. *Human Neuroanatomy: A Text, Brain Atlas, and Laboratory Dissection Guide.* New York: Oxford University Press, 2009.

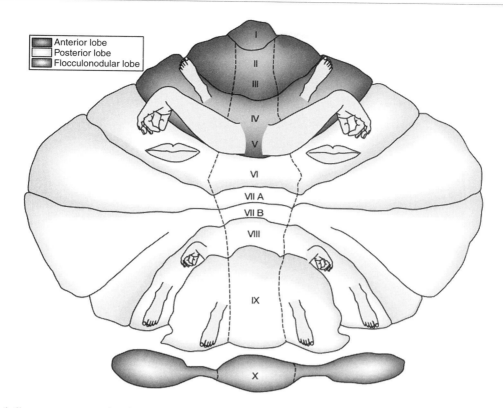

FIGURE 15-3 **Cerebellar somatotopy. Used with permission from Manni, E., and L. Petrosini. A Century of Cerebellar Somatotopy: A Debated Representation.** *Nat Rev Neurosci* **5, no. 3 (2004): 241-9.**

Lobes, Zones, & Modules

Here, we will use a flattened perspective of the cerebellum to learn the cerebellar anatomic lobes, zones, and functional modules. To understand how unfolding the cerebellum affects our perspective of it, draw a sagittal section of the folded cerebellum and then show that we peel back the anterior cerebellum so that the anterior lobe ends up at the top of the diagram and the flocculonodular lobe ends up at the bottom.

Now, draw the corpus cerebelli, which comprises the anterior and posterior cerebellar lobes and constitutes the bulk of the cerebellum. On the right, we will draw the cerebellar lobes, and on the left, we will draw the cerebellar zones.

Begin with the lobes: show that the primary fissure separates the corpus cerebelli such that the anterior one-third of the corpus cerebelli forms the anterior lobe and the posterior two-thirds forms the posterior lobe. Next, below the corpus cerebelli, draw the propeller-shaped flocculonodular lobe: label its nodule in midline and flocculus out laterally. Show that the posterolateral fissure separates the corpus cerebelli from the flocculonodular lobe.

Now, let's draw the cerebellar zones. Indicate that the midline cerebellum is the vermis (which means worm-like); then, lateral to it, denote the paravermis (aka the intermediate zone); and lateral to it, label the hemisphere (aka the lateral zone).

Next, let's address the functional modules; show that we will specifically address the module name, its anatomy and function, and the exam deficit observed when the module is injured.

Indicate that the flocculonodular lobe combines with the anterior tip of the vermis (the lingula) to form the vestibulocerebellum. The vestibulocerebellum receives its name because of its midline vestibulo- and olivocerebellar fibers, which project to the deep, medial-lying cerebellar fastigial nuclei. Show that this functional module is important for equilibrium and eye movements.

Next, show that the anterior lobe combines with the majority of the vermian and paravermian posterior lobe to form the spinocerebellum. The spinocerebellum receives its name from its major input fibers: the spinocerebellar tracts. Show that this functional module plays a major role in postural stability.

Now, indicate that the remainder of the posterior lobe forms the pontocerebellum, which receives its name because it acts through the corticopontocerebellar pathway. Show that this functional module is geared towards goal-directed, fine motor movements.

In acute alcohol intoxication, the entire cerebellum is affected: show that in this setting, nystagmus occurs from toxicity to the vestibulocerebellum, truncal ataxia occurs from toxicity to the spinocerebellum, and incoordination occurs from toxicity to the pontocerebellum. In contrast, in alcoholic cerebellar degeneration, the pathology is predominantly restricted to the anterior superior cerebellar vermis; therefore, truncal ataxia is sometimes the sole deficit. We may miss this exam finding, if we fail to ask our patients to stand during the exam.

As a final note on nomenclature, indicate that each functional module is synonymously named based on its stage of phylogenic development. The vestibulocerebellum is phylogenetically the oldest portion of the cerebellum and is referred to as the archicerebellum; the spinocerebellum is phylogenetically the next oldest and is referred to as the paleocerebellum; and the pontocerebellum is phylogenetically the newest portion of the cerebellum and is referred to as the neocerebellum.[1-11]

Module	Anatomy	Function	Exam deficit
Vestibulocerebellum or archicerebellum	Flocculonodular lobe (& lingula: ant. tip of vermis)	Equilibrium & eye movements	Nystagmus
Spinocerebellum or paleocerebellum	Anterior lobe & vermian & paravermian posterior lobe	Postural stability	Truncal ataxia
Pontocerebellum or neocerebellum	Lateral posterior lobe	Fine motor movement	Incoordination

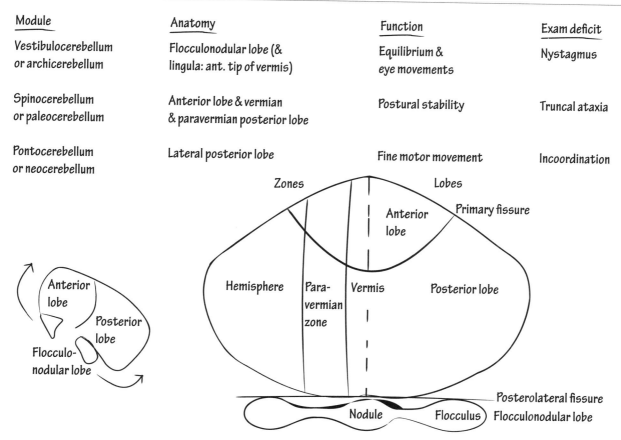

DRAWING 15-1 **Lobes, Zones, & Modules**

Somatotopy & Lobules

Here, we will use a flattened perspective of the cerebellum to learn the cerebellar somatotopic map and the classification of the cerebellar lobules. Once again, to understand how unfolding the cerebellum affects our perspective of it, draw a sagittal section of the folded cerebellum and then show that we peel back the anterior cerebellum so that the anterior lobe ends up at the top of the diagram and the flocculonodular lobe ends up at the bottom.

To begin our diagram, draw the corpus cerebelli and show that the primary fissure separates the anterior lobe from the posterior lobe. Next, draw the flocculonodular lobe and indicate that the posterolateral fissure separates it from the corpus cerebelli.

First, let's address the somatotopic map of the cerebellum. In clinical practice, remember the following: (1) unilateral cerebellar lesions affect the ipsilateral side of the body and (2) the midline cerebellum plays a role in posture whereas the lateral cerebellum assists in fine motor, goal-oriented skills. For instance, to stand upright, you need the midline cerebellum, and to play the piano, you need the lateral cerebellar hemispheres.

Now, show that the somatotopic map in the anterior lobe looks like someone lying in a bathtub—arms and legs coming out of the water. Next, show that the hands extend into the posterior lobe. Then, draw the mouth beneath the fingers. Now, show that there is duplication of the arms and legs in the posterior lobe.

As mentioned, the somatotopic map of the cerebellum is in concert with its functional layout: the role of the spinocerebellar anterior lobe is to provide postural stability, which requires the limbs and trunk, and the role of the neocerebellar posterior lobe is to provide goal-oriented, fine motor movements, such as those of the fingers and mouth.

Now, we will draw the classification of the cerebellar lobules—its numbering system and nomenclature is quite confusing, so keep track. The midline, vermian cerebellum divides into ten different lobules and the hemispheres divide into nine lobules. We'll draw the vermian lobules, first, and then the hemispheric lobules.

Indicate that vermian lobule 1 sits above the superior lip of the fourth ventricle and is named the lingula. Next, show that lobules 2 and 3, together, form the central lobule and then that lobules 4 and 5 form the culmen. Posterior to the primary fissure, label lobule 6, which is the declive. Show that lobule 7A is the folium and that lobule 7B is the tuber; then, indicate that lobule 8 is the pyramis and that lobule 9 is the uvula. Lobule 10 is the nodule of the flocculonodular lobe.

Now, let's label the classification of the cerebellar hemispheric lobules. Show that except for lobule 1, each vermian lobule has a hemispheric counterpart. Hemispheric lobules 2 and 3 form the wing (or ala) of the central lobule; lobules 4 and 5 form the anterior quadrangular lobule; posterior to the primary fissure is lobule 6, the simple lobule (aka the posterior quadrangular lobule); lobule 7A is quite large and forms the superior and inferior semilunar lobules (aka the ansiform lobule); lobule 7B is the gracile lobule; lobule 8 is the biventral lobule; lobule 9 is the tonsil. Finally, show that lobule 10 is the flocculus of the flocculonodular lobe.[1-11]

Hemispheric lobules

H 2 & 3	Wing of central lobule
H 4 & 5	Anterior quadrangular lobule
H 6	Simple lobule
H 7A	Superior semilunar lobule
	Inferior semilunar lobule
H 7B	Gracile lobule
H 8	Biventral lobule
H 9	Tonsil
H 10	Flocculus

Vermian lobules

1	Lingula
2 & 3	Central lobule
4 & 5	Culmen
6	Declive
7A	Folium
7B	Tuber
8	Pyramis
9	Uvula
10	Nodule

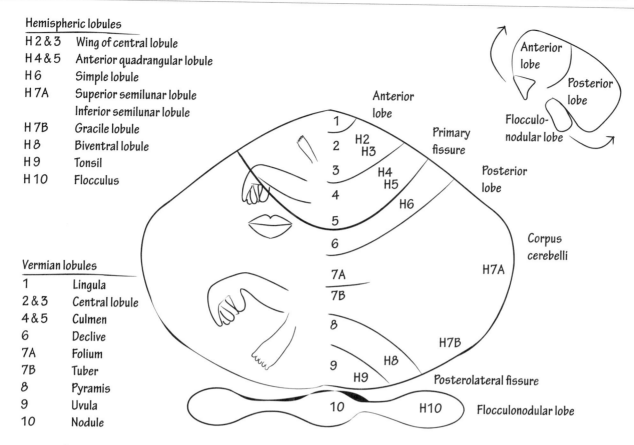

DRAWING 15-2 **Somatotopy & Lobules**

Peduncles, Midline Structures, Arteries

Here, we will draw the cerebellar peduncles, the flocculonodular lobe and paired tonsils, and the cerebellar arterial supply.

I. Cerebellar Peduncles

Begin with one of the saddle-shaped cerebellar hemispheres. Next, add the cerebellar peduncles: superior, middle, and inferior. To illustrate the flow through these pathways, redraw the cerebellar peduncles adjacent to the rest of our diagram.

First, show that the middle cerebellar peduncle is an afferent pathway into the cerebellum; it is reserved for fibers that originate in pontine nuclei. Next, indicate that the inferior cerebellar peduncle is also an afferent pathway into the cerebellum; it receives fibers from throughout the brainstem and spinal cord. Now, show that the cerebellum sends efferent fibers out through the superior cerebellar peduncle. Thus, the main inflow pathways into the cerebellum are the middle and inferior cerebellar peduncles and the main outflow peduncle from the cerebellum is the superior cerebellar peduncle.

Next, let's list the main exceptions to this rule. Indicate that the anterior spinocerebellar tract enters the cerebellum through the superior cerebellar peduncle, which defies this peduncle's role as an outflow pathway. Then, indicate that select midline cerebellar tracts exit the cerebellum through the inferior cerebellar peduncle, which defies this peduncle's role as an inflow pathway. Specifically, these midline pathways are the fastigiobulbar fibers, the fibers from the flocculonodular lobe to the brainstem vestibular nucleus, and certain monosynaptic cerebello-spinal connections.

Now, let's expound upon the major pathways that do follow the general inflow/outflow rule. Show that the middle cerebellar peduncle comprises corticopontocerebellar fibers (see Drawing 15-7), which are critical for the modulation of movement. Then, indicate that three of the four spinocerebellar pathways enter the cerebellum through the inferior cerebellar peduncle: the posterior spinocerebellar tract, cuneocerebellar tract, and rostral spinocerebellar tract. As mentioned, the fourth spinocerebellar tract, the anterior spinocerebellar tract, defies the general organization of cerebellar inflow and enters the cerebellum through the superior cerebellar peduncle. Next, show that the brainstem pathways that enter the cerebellum through the inferior cerebellar peduncle are the reticulo- and trigeminocerebellar fibers, the olivocerebellar fibers (known as climbing fibers), and fibers from the vestibular nucleus and nerve, itself.

Now, indicate that the pathways that exit the cerebellum through superior cerebellar peduncle are the dentatorubal and dentatothalamic tracts, which project rostrally; the dentatoreticular tract, which projects caudally; and fibers from the globose and emboliform nuclei, which reach the region of the red nucleus responsible for the rubrospinal tract.

MCP pathway
Corticopontocerebellar

ICP pathways
Spinal cord: PST, CST, & RST
Brainstem: Reticulo-, trigemino-
olivo-, & vestibulocerebellar
pathways, & direct vestibular
nerve fibers

SCP pathways
Pathways from the dentate &
interposed nuclei

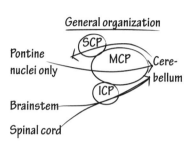

General organization

Pontine
nuclei only
SCP
MCP
ICP
Cere-
bellum

Brainstem

Spinal cord

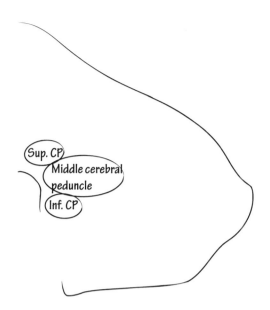

Sup. CP
Middle cerebral
peduncle
Inf. CP

Exceptions:
1. AST uses SCP for inflow
2. Select midline cerebellar
pathways use ICP for outflow

DRAWING 15-3 **Peduncles, Midline Structures, Arteries—Partial**

Peduncles, Midline Structures, Arteries (Cont.)

II. Midline Structures

Now, in order to draw the flocculonodular lobe and cerebellar tonsils, first label the fourth ventricle and indicate that the midline portion of the cerebellum is the vermis, and also show that the outer aspect of the cerebellum is the hemisphere. Next, include in our diagram the two components of the flocculonodular lobe: in the hemisphere, show the flocculus, and in the vermis, show the nodule. We show these structures, here, because the unfolded schematic of the cerebellum, which is so commonly used to represent the cerebellum, places the flocculonodular lobe at the bottom of the diagram, and we need to appreciate that the flocculonodular lobe actually lies in anterior, mid-cerebellar position. Also, above the fourth ventricle, include the lingula: the slender vermian tip of the anterior cerebellar lobe. The lingula combines with the flocculonodular lobe to form the vestibulocerebellum (or archicerebellum), which influences equilibrium and eye movements.

Next, include one of the paired cerebellar tonsils; we include the cerebellar tonsils because this paired, midline structure is an important aspect of a common neurologic condition, Chiari malformation. Chiari malformation is a wide-ranging syndrome divided into three different subtypes: types I, II, and III. Type I is the most mild and type III is the most severe. Chiari malformation always involves downward displacement of the cerebellar tonsils through the foramen magnum, but what determines its morbidity is the degree of cerebellar displacement and the degree of displacement of additional brainstem structures. Also, what determines its morbidity is the associated pathologic involvement of other areas of the central nervous system. Notably, type I Chiari malformation is found in roughly two thirds of cases of syringomyelia (a central cavitation of the spinal cord), and type II Chiari malformation (aka Arnold-Chiari malformation) is almost universally associated with myelomeningocele (a protrusion of the spinal cord and meninges through a defect in the posterior vertebral column). Patients with Chiari malformation range from being entirely asymptomatic (when the malformation is only incidentally found on radiographic imaging) to being severely affected with considerable developmental delay and substantial motor–sensory deficits.[12–15]

III. Arterial Supply

Lastly, let's show the basic arterial supply of the cerebellum. First, let's draw the vertebrobasilar arterial arrangement and then show its cerebellar perfusion pattern. Show that paired vertebral arteries derive the basilar artery, which branches into the paired posterior cerebral arteries. Then, indicate that the posterior inferior cerebellar arteries emerge from the vertebral arteries. Next, at the base of the basilar artery, show that paired anterior inferior cerebellar arteries emerge and, finally, at the upper portion of the basilar artery, show that the paired superior cerebellar arteries emerge. Now, show that on the anterior surface of the cerebellum, the posterior inferior cerebellar arteries perfuse the inferior cerebellum; the anterior inferior cerebellar arteries perfuse the mid-lateral cerebellum; and the superior cerebellar arteries perfuse the superior cerebellum. We show the discrete vascular cerebellar territories in Drawing 19-6.[1–11,16,17]

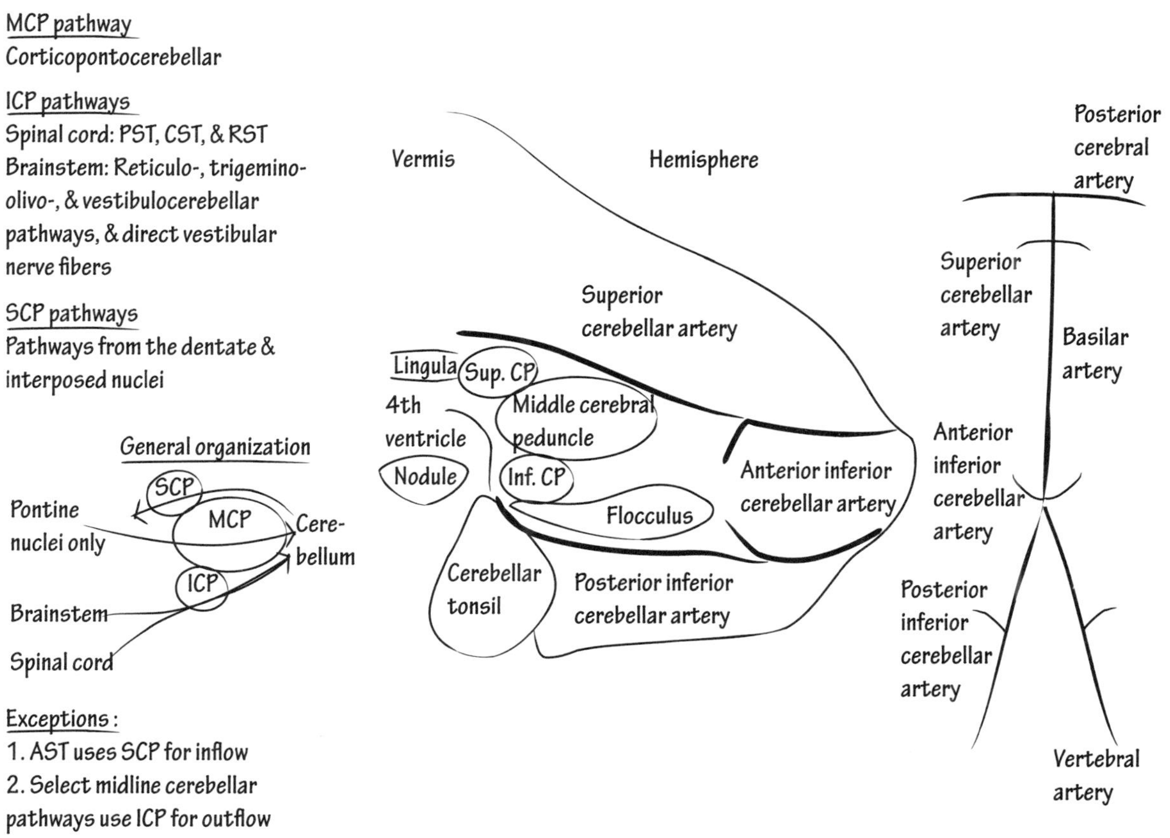

MCP pathway
Corticopontocerebellar

ICP pathways
Spinal cord: PST, CST, & RST
Brainstem: Reticulo-, trigemino-
olivo-, & vestibulocerebellar
pathways, & direct vestibular
nerve fibers

SCP pathways
Pathways from the dentate &
interposed nuclei

General organization

Pontine
nuclei only

SCP

MCP

Cere-
bellum

ICP

Brainstem

Spinal cord

Exceptions:
1. AST uses SCP for inflow
2. Select midline cerebellar
pathways use ICP for outflow

Vermis   Hemisphere

Superior
cerebellar artery

Lingula Sup. CP
4th
ventricle
Nodule
Middle cerebral
peduncle
Inf. CP
Flocculus

Cerebellar
tonsil
Posterior inferior
cerebellar artery

Anterior inferior
cerebellar artery

Posterior
cerebral
artery

Superior
cerebellar
artery

Basilar
artery

Anterior
inferior
cerebellar
artery

Posterior
inferior
cerebellar
artery

Vertebral
artery

DRAWING 15-4 Peduncles, Midline Structures, Arteries—Complete

Nuclei & Circuitry (*Advanced*)

Here, we will draw the cerebellar nuclei and circuitry. Label the left side of the page as the cerebellar nuclei. Begin this diagram with a saddle-shaped cerebellar hemisphere. Include along the surface a single fold, called a folium. The folding of the cerebellum into lobes, lobules, and folia allows it to assume a tightly packed, inconspicuous appearance in the posterior fossa. The cerebellum has a vast surface area, however, and when stretched, it has a rostrocaudal expanse of roughly 120 centimeters, which allows it to hold an estimated one hundred billion granule cells—more cells than exist within the entire cerebral cortex. Note that this is in part due to the small size of the granule cells, themselves. It is presumed that the cerebellum's extraordinary cell count plays an important role in the remarkable rehabilitation commonly observed in cerebellar stroke.[8,9,18]

Now, indicate that the two main classes of cerebellar nuclei are the cerebellar cortical neurons and the deep cerebellar nuclei. Draw a magnified view of the folium in order to show the different cerebellar cortical cell layers. Indicate that on the outside is the molecular layer, underneath it is the interposed Purkinje layer, and on the inside is the granule layer with the subcortical white matter underneath it. Show that the molecular layer primarily comprises cell processes but also contains stellate and basket cells; the Purkinje layer contains a single layer of large Purkinje cell bodies; and the granule layer is highly cellular: it contains granule cells, Golgi cells, and unipolar brush cells.

Next, let's address the centrally located deep cerebellar nuclei. At the bottom of the page, list their names. From medial to lateral, they are the fastigial, globose, emboliform, and dentate nuclei. Show that together the globose and emboliform nuclei are also known as the interposed nuclei. An acronym for the lateral to medial organization of the deep nuclei is "Don't Eat Greasy Food," for dentate, emboliform, globose, and fastigial.

The deep cerebellar nuclei parse into specific functional modules. The fastigial nucleus plays a role in both the vestibulocerebellum and spinocerebellum; the interposed nuclei are part of the spinocerebellum; and the dentate nucleus is part of the pontocerebellum.

Now, let's show the flow of information through the cerebellum. Label the right-hand side of the page as cerebellar circuitry. First, indicate that there are three main types of cerebellar afferent fibers: climbing fibers, mossy fibers, and multilayered fibers, which are also known as monoaminergic fibers.

Show that climbing fibers are excitatory fibers that originate solely from the inferior olive and pass via the contralateral inferior cerebellar peduncle to the cerebellum. Debate exists as to whether climbing fibers use the excitatory neurotransmitter aspartate or glutamate, but it seems most probable that they use glutamate. These olivocerebellar fibers are distinct in that each Purkinje cell is innervated by a single olivocerebellar climbing fiber. Note that this pathway represents the inferior arm of the triangle of Guillain-Mollaret, discussed in Chapter 9.

Now, show that the mossy fibers are excitatory fibers derived from diffuse cell populations within the brainstem and spinal cord. They, like the climbing fibers, mostly use the excitatory neurotransmitter glutamate.

Lastly, show that the multilayered fibers are derived from neurobehavioral centers in the brainstem and diencephalon, such as the locus coeruleus, raphe nucleus, and the tuberomammillary nucleus of the hypothalamus. Whereas the climbing and mossy fibers are unquestionably excitatory, the role of the multilayered fibers is less uniform. They are considered monoaminergic because their cells of origin are generally associated with a single neurotransmitter type: the locus coeruleus is noradrenergic, the raphe nucleus is serotinergic, and the tuberomammillary nucleus is histaminergic.

Now, show that all three fibers innervate both the deep cerebellar nuclei and cerebellar cortex.

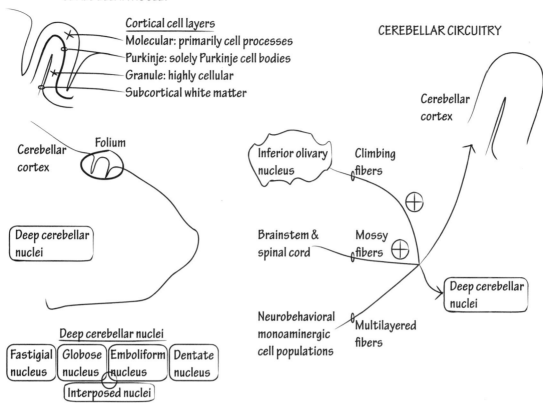

CEREBELLAR NUCLEI

Cortical cell layers
Molecular: primarily cell processes
Purkinje: solely Purkinje cell bodies
Granule: highly cellular
Subcortical white matter

CEREBELLAR CIRCUITRY

Cerebellar cortex

Cerebellar cortex

Folium

Deep cerebellar nuclei

Inferior olivary nucleus

Climbing fibers

Brainstem & spinal cord

Mossy fibers

Deep cerebellar nuclei

Neurobehavioral monoaminergic cell populations

Multilayered fibers

Deep cerebellar nuclei

| Fastigial nucleus | Globose nucleus | Emboliform nucleus | Dentate nucleus |

Interposed nuclei

DRAWING 15-5 **Nuclei & Circuitry—Partial**

Nuclei & Circuitry (*Advanced*) (Cont.)

Next, show that the deep cerebellar nuclei send excitatory fibers to structures throughout the central nervous system. The majority of efferent information that leaves the cerebellum does so from the deep cerebellar nuclei, which act through the excitatory neurotransmitter glutamate, most notably.

Now, indicate that the molecular and granule cell layers filter and temporally pattern information as it is transmitted to the Purkinje layer. Indicate that the Purkinje layer, which is the sole recipient of this post-processed information, sends inhibitory fibers to the deep cerebellar nuclei. Thus the cerebellar cortex, acting through the Purkinje layer, is an important modulating force on the deep cerebellar nuclei. The Purkinje cells act through the inhibitory neurotransmitter gamma-aminobutyric acid (GABA).[1–11,19–23]

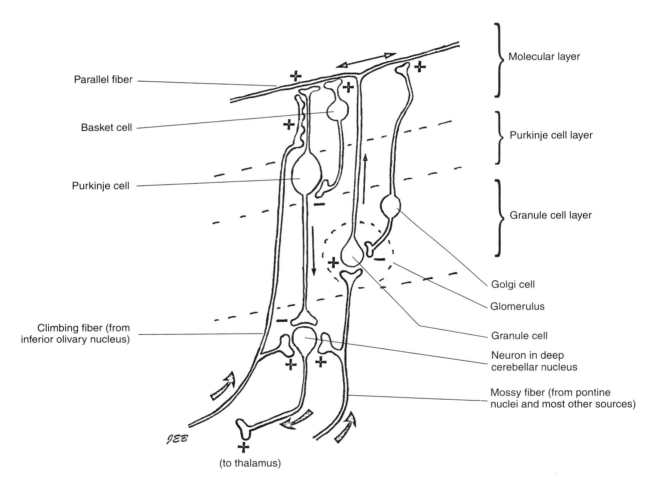

FIGURE 15-4 **Cerebellar histological architecture. Used with permission from Bruni, J. E. & Montemurro, D. G.** *Human Neuroanatomy: A Text, Brain Atlas, and Laboratory Dissection Guide.* **New York: Oxford University Press, 2009.**

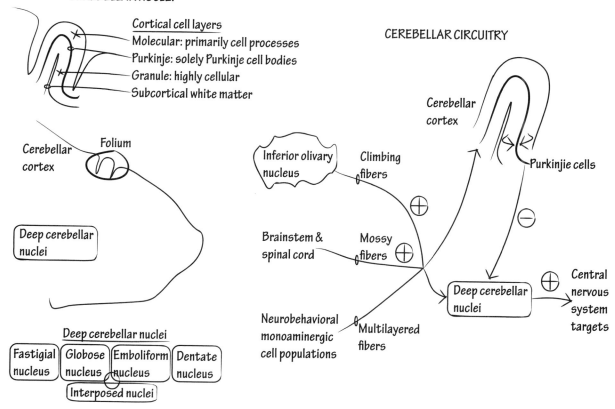

CEREBELLAR NUCLEI

Cortical cell layers
Molecular: primarily cell processes
Purkinje: solely Purkinje cell bodies
Granule: highly cellular
Subcortical white matter

Cerebellar cortex

Folium

Deep cerebellar nuclei

Deep cerebellar nuclei

| Fastigial nucleus | Globose nucleus | Emboliform nucleus | Dentate nucleus |

Interposed nuclei

CEREBELLAR CIRCUITRY

Cerebellar cortex

Purkinjie cells

Inferior olivary nucleus

Climbing fibers

Brainstem & spinal cord

Mossy fibers

Neurobehavioral monoaminergic cell populations

Multilayered fibers

Deep cerebellar nuclei

Central nervous system targets

DRAWING 15-6 **Nuclei & Circuitry—Complete**

Corticopontocerebellar Pathway

Here, we will draw the corticopontocerebellar pathway. For this diagram, we need to draw one side of the brain, the brainstem, and then the opposite side of the cerebellum, and we need to establish the midline of the diagram. Indicate that the bulk of the pathway originates in the primary motor and sensory cortices; we exclude the lesser contributions from more wide-reaching brain regions. To get a sense of the corticopontocerebellar pathway's importance in movement, consider that nearly 20 million fibers are dedicated to the corticopontocerebellar pathway, whereas only 1 million fibers are dedicated to the corticospinal tract.[24]

Now, show that the corticopontocerebellar fibers first descend to the pontine nuclei, where they make their primary synapse. Next, show that the pontine nuclei project across midline through the middle cerebellar peduncle into the contralateral cerebellar cortex. As a reminder, the inferior and middle cerebellar peduncles are the main inflow pathways into the cerebellum, and the superior cerebellar peduncle is the main outflow pathway from the cerebellum.

Then, show that the cerebellar cortex projects to the dentate nucleus, which lies deep within the cerebellum. Now, draw the superior cerebellar peduncle, red nucleus, and ventrolateral nucleus of the thalamus. Indicate that the dentate projects fibers out of the cerebellum through the superior cerebellar peduncle, which cross midline within the midbrain, inferior to the red nucleus, to synapse in the ventrolateral nucleus of the thalamus. Then, show that select fibers synapse directly in the red nucleus, instead. Note that the red nucleus projections typically originate from the globose and emboliform nuclei, which lie medial to the dentate nucleus, whereas the thalamic projections typically originate from the dentate nucleus. Now, show that the thalamus projects back to the primary motor strip to complete the corticopontocerebellar pathway.

The clinical application of this pathway comes in the analysis of cerebellar deficits. Cerebellar injuries cause ipsilateral deficits. If a person has a cerebellar deficit (for instance, incoordination), then either the ipsilateral cerebellum or a portion of this pathway (somewhere along its course) is affected. If the area of injury localizes contralateral to the side of the body that is affected, think of a corticopontocerebellar pathway lesion. Consider a stroke in which there is a left third nerve palsy and right-side hemiataxia. Where could the injury lie? On a separate sheet of paper, draw the midbrain. Define right and left. Draw the left third nerve and its exiting fascicles and then draw the right cerebellum. How can we connect these disparate regions? Show that fibers exit the right cerebellum through the superior cerebellar peduncle and pass adjacent to the third nerve fibers on the left. Indicate that injury here produces the aforementioned deficits (see Drawing 10-3, Claude's syndrome, for details).[1,3,7–11]

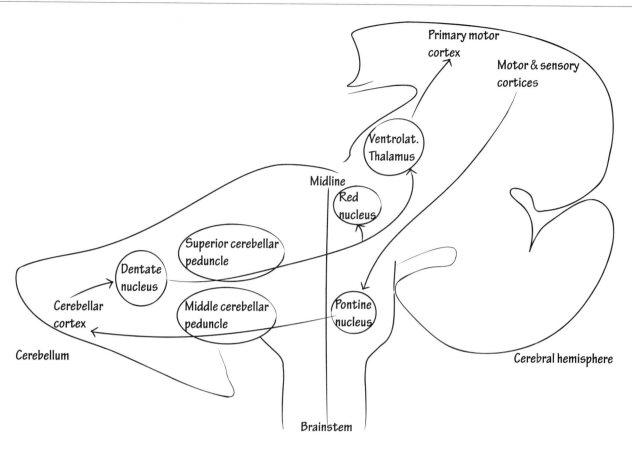

DRAWING 15-7 **Corticopontocerebellar Pathway**

References

1. Afifi, A. K. & Bergman, R. A. *Functional neuroanatomy: text and atlas,* 2nd ed. (Lange Medical Books/McGraw-Hill, 2005).

2. Duvernoy, H. M. & Bourgouin, P. *The human brain: surface, three-dimensional sectional anatomy with MRI, and blood supply,* 2nd completely rev. and enl. ed. (Springer, 1999).

3. Haines, D. E. & Ard, M. D. *Fundamental neuroscience: for basic and clinical applications,* 3rd ed. (Churchill Livingstone Elsevier, 2006).

4. Mai, J. K., Voss, T. & Paxinos, G. *Atlas of the human brain,* 3rd ed. (Elsevier/Academic Press, 2008).

5. Manni, E. & Petrosini, L. A century of cerebellar somatotopy: a debated representation. *Nat Rev Neurosci* 5, 241–249 (2004).

6. Manto, M.-U. & Pandolfo, M. *The cerebellum and its disorders* (Cambridge University Press, 2002).

7. Naidich, T. P. & Duvernoy, H. M. *Duvernoy's atlas of the human brain stem and cerebellum: high-field MRI: surface anatomy, internal structure, vascularization and 3D sectional anatomy* (Springer, 2009).

8. Nieuwenhuys, R., Voogd, J. & Huijzen, C. V. *The human central nervous system,* 4th ed. (Springer, 2008).

9. Noback, C. R. *The human nervous system: structure and function,* 6th ed. (Humana Press, 2005).

10. Paxinos, G. & Mai, J. K. *The human nervous system,* 2nd ed., Chapter 11 (Elsevier Academic Press, 2004).

11. Voogd, J. & Glickstein, M. The anatomy of the cerebellum. *Trends Neurosci* 21, 370–375 (1998).

12. Bailey, B. J., Johnson, J. T. & Newlands, S. D. *Head & neck surgery—otolaryngology,* 4th ed., p. 2311 (Lippincott Williams & Wilkins, 2006).

13. Chen, H. *Atlas of genetic diagnosis and counseling,* pp. 157–159 (Humana Press, 2006).

14. Rowland, L. P., Pedley, T. A. & Kneass, W. *Merritt's neurology,* 12th ed., p. 551 (Wolters Kluwer Lippincott Williams & Wilkins, 2010).

15. Sarnat, H. B. & Curatolo, P. *Malformations of the nervous system,* p. 98 (Elsevier, 2008).

16. Yokota, O., et al. Alcoholic cerebellar degeneration: a clinicopathological study of six Japanese autopsy cases and proposed potential progression pattern in the cerebellar lesion. *Neuropathology* 27, 99–113 (2007).

17. Takahashi, S. O. *Neurovascular imaging: MRI & microangiography* (Springer, 2010).

18. Kelly, P. J., et al. Functional recovery after rehabilitation for cerebellar stroke. *Stroke* 32, 530–534 (2001).

19. Apps, R. & Hawkes, R. Cerebellar cortical organization: a one-map hypothesis. *Nat Rev Neurosci* 10, 670–681 (2009).

20. Dietrichs, E. Clinical manifestation of focal cerebellar disease as related to the organization of neural pathways. *Acta Neurol Scand,* Suppl. (188) 186–111 (2008).

21. Nakanishi, S. Synaptic mechanisms of the cerebellar cortical network. *Trends Neurosci* 28, 93–100 (2005).

22. Strick, P. L., Dum, R. P. & Fiez, J. A. Cerebellum and nonmotor function. *Annu Rev Neurosci* 32, 413–434 (2009).

23. Huang, C. M. & Huang, R. H. Ethanol inhibits the sensory responses of cerebellar granule cells in anesthetized cats. *Alcohol Clin Exp Res* 31, 336–344 (2007).

24. Melillo, R. & Leisman, G. *Neurobehavioral disorders of childhood: an evolutionary perspective,* p. 55 (Kluwer Academic/Plenum Publishers, 2004).

16

Cerebral Gray Matter

Cerebral Hemisphere—Lateral Face

Cerebral Hemisphere—Medial Face

Cerebral Hemisphere—Inferior Face

The Insula (Advanced)

Cerebral Cytoarchitecture (Advanced)

Brodmann Areas

Know-It Points

Cerebral Hemisphere—Lateral Face

- The area anterior to the central sulcus is the frontal lobe.
- Posterior to the lateral parietotemporal line lies the occipital lobe.
- Superior to the temporo-occipital line lies the parietal lobe, and inferior to it lies the temporal lobe.
- The limbic lobe is present only on the brain's inferior and medial surfaces.

- The precentral gyrus lies in between the precentral sulcus and the central sulcus; it is the primary motor area.
- The postcentral gyrus lies in between the postcentral sulcus and the central sulcus; it is the primary sensory area.

Cerebral Hemisphere—Medial Face

- The cingulate sulcus and collateral sulcus delineate the bulk of the limbic lobe.
- The frontal lobe lies anterior to the central sulcus.
- The parieto-occipital sulcus separates the parietal lobe, anteriorly, from the occipital lobe, posteriorly.
- The subparietal sulcus demarcates the boundary between the parietal and limbic lobes.

- The temporal lobe lies anterior to the basal parietotemporal line.
- The cuneus lies superior to the calcarine sulcus.
- The parahippocampal gyrus lies superior to the collateral sulcus.
- The fusiform gyrus lies in between the collateral and occipitotemporal sulci.

Cerebral Hemisphere—Inferior Face

- The frontal pole lies at the anterior end of the frontal lobe.
- The temporal pole lies at the anterior end of the temporal lobe.
- The occipital pole lies at the posterior end of the occipital lobe.

- The Sylvian fissure runs in between the frontal and temporal lobes and ascends much of the lateral aspect of the brain.

The Insula (*Advanced*)

- The insula underlies the cerebral opercula.
- The circular sulcus circumscribes the insula.
- The central sulcus extends through the insula and divides the insula into anterior and posterior lobules.
- The orbital operculum lies inferior to the anterior horizontal ramus of the Sylvian fissure.

- The frontal operculum lies in between the anterior horizontal and anterior ascending Sylvian fissure rami.
- The parietal operculum lies in between the anterior ascending and posterior Sylvian fissure rami.
- The temporal operculum lies inferior to the posterior ramus of the Sylvian fissure.

Cerebral Cytoarchitecture (*Advanced*)

- Three different histologic patterns of cerebral cortex exist: neocortex, allocortex, and mesocortex.
- Neocortex (aka isocortex) is the phylogenetically newest cortical cytoarchitecture and comprises six layers.
- Allocortex is phylogenetically older and comprises from three to five layers.
- Mesocortex represents transitional cortex between neocortex and allocortex.
- A prominent example of a pyramidal cell are the Betz cells, which lie primarily within the primary motor cortex.
- The six cytoarchitectural layers of the neocortex, from outside to inside, are the molecular, external granular, external pyramidal, internal granular layer, internal pyramidal, and multiform layers.

Brodmann Areas

- Areas 3, 1, 2 lie within the postcentral and posterior paracentral gyri; they constitute the primary sensory area.
- Area 4 lies within the precentral and anterior paracentral gyri; it is the primary motor area.
- Area 8 lies in front of area 6; it contains the human homologue to the rhesus monkey frontal eye fields.
- Area 44 lies in the pars opercularis of the inferior frontal gyrus and area 45 lies in the pars triangularis of the inferior frontal gyrus; together, they make up Broca's area—the speech output area.
- Areas 41 and 42 lie in the transverse temporal gyri (Heschl's gyri); they make up the primary auditory cortex.
- Area 22 lies in the superior temporal gyrus and, posteriorly, it contains Wernicke's area—the language reception area.
- Area 17 lies on the banks of the calcarine sulcus and is the primary visual cortex.

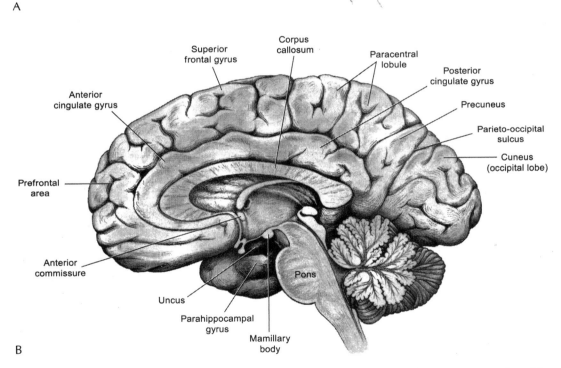

FIGURE 16-1 **Lateral and medial cerebral surfaces.** Used with permission from Devinsky, Orrin, and Mark D'Esposito. *Neurology of Cognitive and Behavioral Disorders*, Contemporary Neurology Series. Oxford; New York: Oxford University Press, 2004.

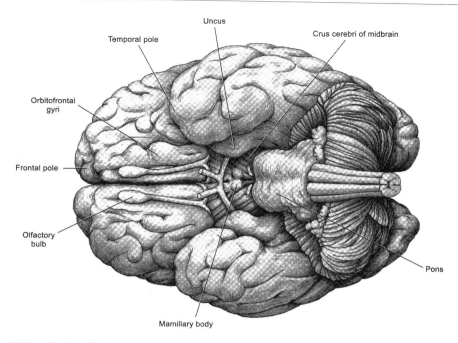

FIGURE 16-2 **Inferior cerebral surface.** Used with permission from Devinsky, Orrin, and Mark D'Esposito. *Neurology of Cognitive and Behavioral Disorders*, Contemporary Neurology Series. Oxford; New York: Oxford University Press, 2004.

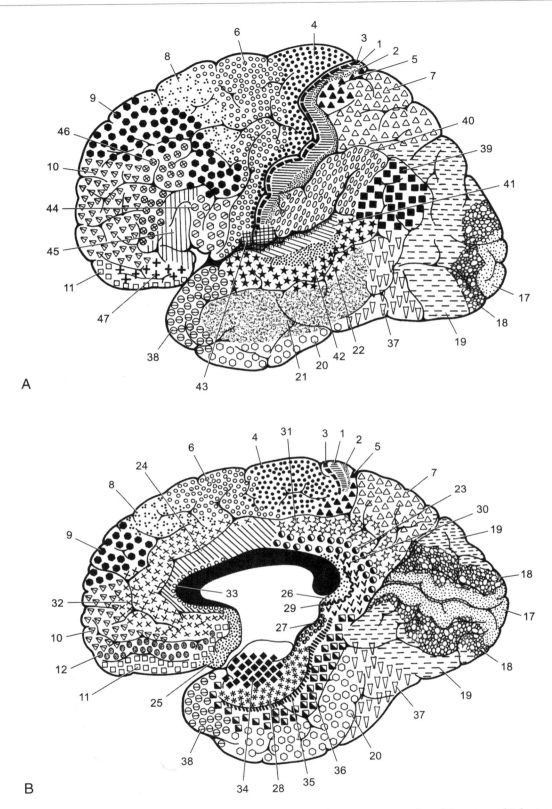

FIGURE 16-3 **Brodmann areas.** Used with permission from Devinsky, Orrin, and Mark D'Esposito. *Neurology of Cognitive and Behavioral Disorders*, Contemporary Neurology Series. Oxford; New York: Oxford University Press, 2004.

Cerebral Hemisphere—Lateral Face

Here, we will draw the lateral face of the cerebrum. First, draw the lateral aspect of a cerebral hemisphere and show the Sylvian fissure (aka the lateral sulcus) along a diagonal. Then, draw the central sulcus from the top of the brain to the Sylvian fissure. Label the area anterior to the central sulcus as the frontal lobe. Next, label the pre-occipital notch along the posterior undersurface of the brain and then the parieto-occipital sulcus along the superior convexity of the brain; note that the parieto-occipital sulcus terminates abruptly in the superolateral convexity—on the contrary, the parieto-occipital sulcus is prominent on the medial surface of the brain. Now, dot a vertical line from the termination of the parieto-occipital sulcus to the pre-occipital notch and label it as the lateral parietotemporal line. Posterior to this imaginary line, label the occipital lobe. Next, dot a roughly horizontal line from the posterior end of the Sylvian fissure to the middle of the anterior border of the occipital lobe and label this line as the temporo-occipital line. Superior to this line, label the parietal lobe, and inferior to it, label the temporal lobe. We have now drawn the four cerebral lobes visible on the lateral surface of the brain; the fifth lobe, the limbic lobe, is present only on the brain's inferior and medial surfaces.

Next, let's draw the gyri and sulci of the lateral surface of the brain. Redraw a lateral hemisphere and include the central sulcus and Sylvian fissure. Divide the anterior frontal lobe into three horizontally distributed gyri using two parallel sulci. Label the top sulcus as the superior frontal sulcus and the bottom sulcus as the inferior frontal sulcus. Then, indicate that the superior frontal gyrus lies above the superior frontal sulcus; that the middle frontal gyrus lies in between the superior and inferior frontal sulci; and that the inferior frontal gyrus lies in between the inferior frontal sulcus and the inferior border of the frontal lobe. Note that the inferior frontal gyrus is triangular, and it contains pars orbitalis, pars triangularis, and pars opercularis divisions.

Now, let's draw the gyri and sulci of the lateral temporal lobe. Again draw two sulci—label the top sulcus as the superior temporal sulcus and the bottom sulcus as the inferior temporal sulcus. Then, label the superior temporal gyrus above the superior temporal sulcus; the middle temporal gyrus in between the superior and middle temporal sulci; and the inferior temporal gyrus below the inferior temporal sulcus.

Next, let's draw a similar arrangement for the occipital gyri of the lateral surface of the brain. Draw the superior occipital sulcus (aka the intraoccipital sulcus), which follows the path of the intraparietal sulcus (drawn later), and then draw the inferior occipital sulcus, which follows the path of the inferior temporal sulcus. Above the superior occipital sulcus, label the superior occipital gyrus; in between the superior and inferior occipital sulci, label the middle occipital gyrus (aka the lateral occipital gyrus); and below the inferior occipital sulcus, label the inferior occipital gyrus. The middle occipital gyrus is the largest of the occipital gyri on the lateral surface of the brain, and it is sometimes subdivided into superior and inferior gyri.

Now, label the basal, anterior surface of the frontal lobe as the orbitofrontal cortex. Then, in the posterior aspect of the frontal lobe, draw the precentral sulcus, and in between it and the central sulcus, label the precentral gyrus, which is the primary motor area.

Next, let's draw the gyri and sulci of the parietal lobe. First, draw the postcentral sulcus, and in between it and the central sulcus, label the postcentral gyrus, which is the primary sensory area. Then, draw the intraparietal sulcus, and show that it divides the remainder of the parietal lobe into the superior parietal lobule, superiorly, and the inferior parietal lobule, inferiorly—the inferior parietal lobule divides into the supramarginal gyrus and angular gyrus. The supramarginal gyrus caps the posterior end of the Sylvian fissure and the angular gyrus caps the posterior end of the superior temporal sulcus.[1-6]

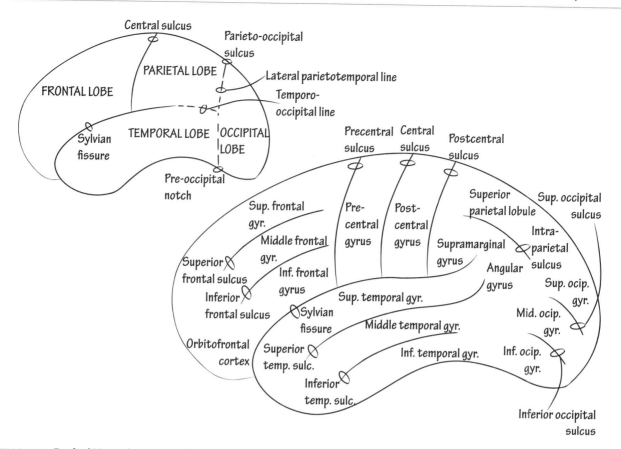

DRAWING 16-1 **Cerebral Hemisphere—Lateral Face**

Cerebral Hemisphere—Medial Face

Here, we will draw the lobes, gyri, and sulci of the medial face of the cerebrum. Draw an outline of the medial face of a cerebral hemisphere. Label the cingulate sulcus above and in parallel to the corpus callosum. Then, label the collateral sulcus in the temporal region in parallel to the brain's inferior border. Indicate that these sulci delineate the limbic lobe. Next, draw the central sulcus, and anterior to it, label the frontal lobe. Now, draw the parieto-occipital sulcus, and show that it separates the parietal lobe, anteriorly, from the occipital lobe, posteriorly. Next, use the subparietal sulcus to demarcate the boundary between the parietal and limbic lobes. Now, to separate the temporal and occipital lobes, dot a line between the pre-occipital notch and the parieto-occipital sulcus, and label the line as the basal parietotemporal line. The temporal lobe lies anterior to this line. Note that the basal parietotemporal line is alternatively drawn from the pre-occipital notch to the anterior end of the anterior calcarine sulcus (drawn later).

Now, let's draw the gyri and sulci of the medial surface of the cerebral hemisphere. First, redraw the hemisphere—include the corpus callosum and thalamus. Along the outer contour of the corpus callosum, label the callosal sulcus, and in parallel to it, draw the cingulate sulcus. In between these sulci, label the cingulate gyrus.

Next, in the central, superior hemisphere, draw the central sulcus, and anterior to it, draw the paracentral sulcus. Between these two sulci, draw the anterior paracentral gyrus—the medial extension of the precentral gyrus. Anterior to the paracentral sulcus label the superior frontal gyrus (aka the medial frontal gyrus). Then, posterior to the central sulcus, continue the cingulate sulcus as the pars marginalis (the marginal branch of the cingulate sulcus), and between it and the central sulcus,

label the posterior paracentral gyrus—the medial extension of the postcentral gyrus. Note that together the anterior and posterior paracentral gyri are referred to as the paracentral lobule.

Now, posterior to the pars marginalis, draw the parieto-occipital sulcus, and in between these two sulci, label the precuneus gyrus. Then, show that the subparietal sulcus separates the precuneus from the cingulate gyrus. Next, show that the calcarine sulcus extends directly posterior from the inferior tip of the parieto-occipital sulcus, and then indicate that the anterior calcarine sulcus extends anteriorly from the inferior tip of the parieto-occipital sulcus to underneath the posterior corpus callosum (the splenium). Within the occipital lobe, superior to the calcarine sulcus, label the cuneus, and inferior to it, label the lingual gyrus. Now, along the path of the anterior calcarine sulcus, draw the collateral sulcus, and superior to it, label the parahippocampal gyrus. Then, inferior and in parallel to the collateral sulcus, label the occipitotemporal sulcus, and in between these two sulci, label the fusiform gyrus. Finally, inferolateral to the fusiform gyrus, label the inferior temporal gyrus.

Note that there are substantial variations in the definitions of the anatomy of the inferomedial temporal and occipital gyri and substantially differing semantics used to describe these areas. For instance, the lingual gyrus is sometimes referred to as the medial occipitotemporal gyrus and the fusiform gyrus is sometimes referred to as the lateral occipitotemporal gyrus. The fusiform gyrus is also sometimes referred to as the combined medial and lateral occipitotemporal gyri or as a subportion of the occipitotemporal gyrus. Also, the collateral sulcus is alternatively referred to as the medial occipitotemporal sulcus and the occipitotemporal sulcus is sometimes called the lateral occipitotemporal sulcus.[1-6]

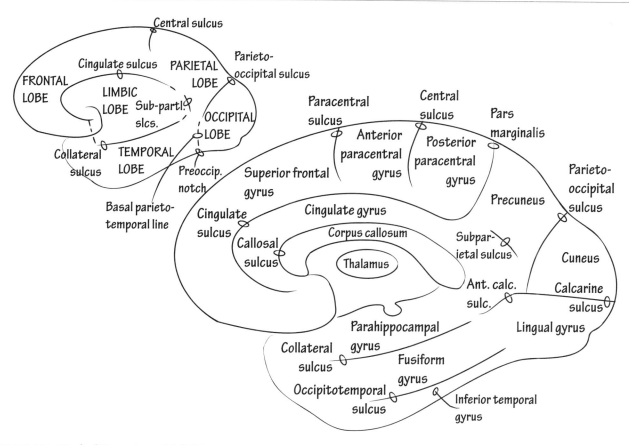

DRAWING 16-2 Cerebral Hemisphere—Medial Face

Cerebral Hemisphere—Inferior Face

Here, we will draw the lobes, gyri, and sulci of the inferior surface of the brain and we will also learn the anatomy of the Sylvian fissure. Draw the undersurface of the brain, but on one side, leave out the anterior end of the temporal lobe. Include the following anatomic landmarks: the optic chiasm and neighboring pituitary body and mammillary bodies, the midbrain, and cerebellum. Next, in the anterior one third of the hemisphere, label the frontal lobe. Then, in the posterior one third of the hemisphere, draw the basal parietotemporal line; anterior to it, label the temporal lobe, and posterior to it, label the occipital lobe. Finally, include the collateral sulcus and label the limbic lobe medial to it.

Now, on the opposite side of the brain, let's draw the gyri and sulci. First, within the medial frontal lobe, label the olfactory sulcus. Medial to it, label the gyrus rectus, and lateral to it, label the orbital gyri and orbital sulci. Now, on the medial aspect of the occipital lobe, label the lingual gyrus, and on the lateral aspect, label the inferior occipital gyrus. Next, within the temporal lobe, draw the collateral and occipitotemporal sulci. Medial to the collateral sulcus, label the parahippocampal gyrus, and in between the collateral and occipitotemporal sulci, label the fusiform gyrus. Then, lateral to the fusiform gyrus, label the inferior temporal gyrus. Next, at the anterior end of the collateral sulcus, label the rhinal sulcus—the collateral sulcus either merges with this sulcus or runs in parallel to it (see Drawing 21-3). Now, show that the parahippocampal gyrus doubles back onto itself as the uncus; this is, generally, the first portion of the brain to herniate over the tentorium cerebellum during uncal herniation.

Next, let's draw the anatomic poles of the brain: label the frontal pole at the anterior end of the frontal lobe; label the temporal pole at the anterior end of the temporal lobe; and label the occipital pole at the posterior end of the occipital lobe.

Now, we will draw the Sylvian fissure. First, further define the region surrounding the optic chiasm as the anterior perforated substance, which is perforated by short branches of the proximal middle cerebral artery. Next, label the internal carotid artery just lateral to the optic chiasm. Then, show that the proximal middle cerebral artery (the M1 branch) originates from the internal carotid artery within the cistern of the vallecula cerebri (aka the carotid cistern) and passes laterally within this cistern through the deep (or basal) portion of the Sylvian fissure between the frontal and temporal lobes. As the Sylvian fissure wraps around to the lateral convexity of the brain, the related cisternal space becomes the cistern of the lateral cerebral fossa; exactly where this cisternal transition occurs is inconsistently defined.[1,7–11]

Now, let's continue with the lateral face of the Sylvian fissure. Draw an outline of the lateral cerebral hemisphere and include the central sulcus for orientational purposes. First, draw the anterior-inferior division of the Sylvian fissure; then, at its midpoint, draw a "V" for the rami extensions from the Sylvian fissure. Label the lower arm of the "V" as the anterior horizontal ramus and the upper arm as the anterior ascending ramus: the anterior horizontal ramus runs roughly horizontally and the anterior ascending ramus runs roughly vertically. These rami subdivide the inferior frontal gyrus as follows: beneath the anterior horizontal ramus, label the pars orbitalis; then, in between the two rami, label the triangular-shaped pars triangularis; and lastly, posterior to the anterior ascending ramus, label the pars opercularis.

Next, let's draw the posterior-superior division of the Sylvian fissure. At the distal end of the central sulcus, draw the horizontally directed posterior horizontal ramus and then complete the Sylvian fissure with the posterior ascending ramus. The supramarginal gyrus caps this ramus. Note that a posterior descending ramus also exists, which lies along the vertical plane of the posterior ascending ramus (we leave it out for simplicity).[1–6]

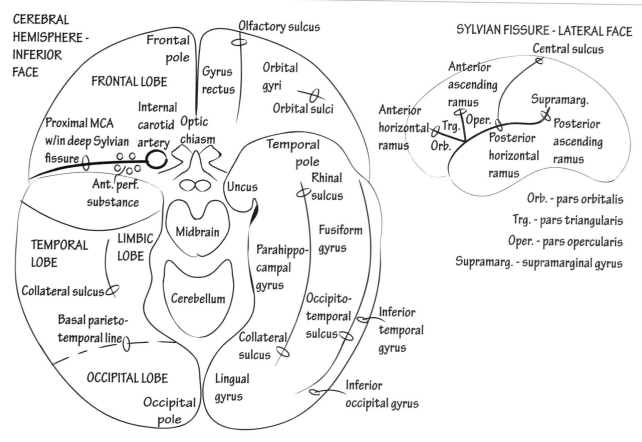

CEREBRAL HEMISPHERE - INFERIOR FACE

FRONTAL LOBE

Frontal pole

Olfactory sulcus

Gyrus rectus

Orbital gyri

Orbital sulci

Internal carotid artery

Optic chiasm

Proximal MCA w/in deep Sylvian fissure

Ant. perf. substance

Uncus

Temporal pole

Rhinal sulcus

Fusiform gyrus

Midbrain

LIMBIC LOBE

TEMPORAL LOBE

Parahippo-campal gyrus

Collateral sulcus

Cerebellum

Basal parieto-temporal line

Occipito-temporal sulcus

Inferior temporal gyrus

Collateral sulcus

OCCIPITAL LOBE

Lingual gyrus

Inferior occipital gyrus

Occipital pole

SYLVIAN FISSURE - LATERAL FACE

Central sulcus

Anterior ascending ramus

Supramarg.

Anterior horizontal ramus

Trg.

Oper.

Orb.

Posterior horizontal ramus

Posterior ascending ramus

Orb. - pars orbitalis

Trg. - pars triangularis

Oper. - pars opercularis

Supramarg. - supramarginal gyrus

DRAWING 16-3 **Cerebral Hemisphere—Inferior Face**

The Insula (*Advanced*)

Here, we will draw the insula (aka the island of Reil), which underlies the cerebral opercula. First, draw a lateral hemisphere. Then, carve out the center of the hemisphere and indicate that the circular sulcus circumscribes the insula (except in the antero-inferior region at the limen insulae—the insular apex). Next, show that the central sulcus extends through the insula and divides it into anterior and posterior lobules. Then, indicate that the anterior lobule contains three short insular gyri and that the posterior lobule contains two long insular gyri.

Within the anterior lobule, draw the precentral sulcus, and anterior to it, draw the short insular sulcus. In between the precentral and central sulci, label the posterior short insular gyrus; in between the precentral and short insular sulci, label the middle short insular gyrus; and finally, anterior to the short insular sulcus, label the anterior short insular gyrus.

Now, within the posterior lobule, draw the postcentral sulcus, and in between it and the central sulcus, label the anterior long insular gyrus, and posterior to it, label the posterior long insular gyrus.

Next, draw a coronal view of the insula so we can, at least partially, draw its different opercular coverings. In accordance with Nieuwenhuys' description, label the orbital operculum, which lies inferior to the anterior horizontal ramus of the Sylvian fissure; next, label the frontal operculum, which lies in between the anterior horizontal and anterior ascending Sylvian fissure rami; then, label the parietal operculum, which lies in between the anterior ascending and posterior Sylvian fissure rami; and finally, label the temporal operculum, which lies inferior to the posterior ramus of the Sylvian fissure. Indicate that the temporal operculum is formed from both the superior temporal gyrus and transverse temporal gyri (Heschl's gyri).

The insula has widespread intracortical connectivity, including connections to the hypothalamus, thalamus, cortical sensory association areas, auditory cortex, and limbic system. It has been shown to play a role in pain modulation, appetite, awareness of visceral sensation, anxiety and emotion, socialization, auditory processing, and much more.[4–6,9,12–14]

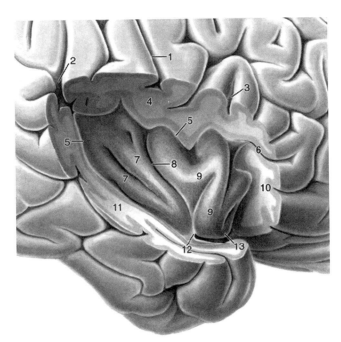

1 Central sulcus
2 Lateral sulcus, posterior branch
3 Lateral sulcus, ascending branch
4 Frontoparietal operculum
5 Circular sulcus of the insula
6 Lateral sulcus, anterior branch
7 Long gyrus of the insula
8 Central sulcus of the insula
9 Short gyri of the insula
10 Frontal operculum
11 Temporal operculum
12 Limen insulae
13 Anterior pole of the insula

FIGURE 16-4 Insular cortex. Used with permission from Nieuwenhuys, Rudolf, Christiaan Huijzen, Jan Voogd, and SpringerLink (Online service). "The Human Central Nervous System." Berlin, Heidelberg: Springer Berlin Heidelberg, 2008.

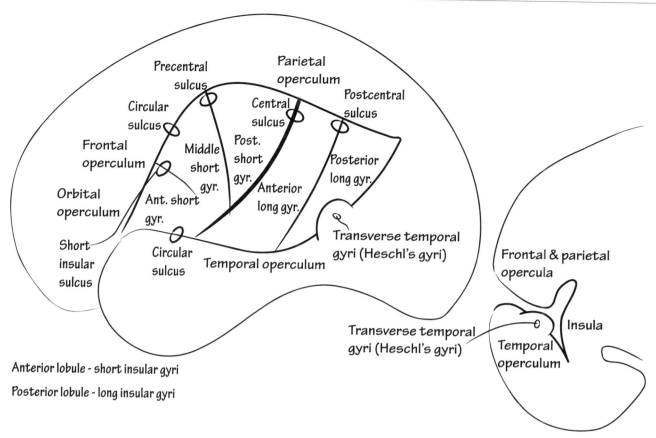

Anterior lobule - short insular gyri

Posterior lobule - long insular gyri

DRAWING 16-4 **The Insula**

Cerebral Cytoarchitecture (*Advanced*)

Here, we will draw the cytoarchitecture of the cerebral cortex. First, indicate that three different histologic patterns of cerebral cortex exist: neocortex, allocortex, and mesocortex. Neocortex (aka isocortex) is the phylogenetically newest cortical cytoarchitecture; it constitutes roughly 90% of the cerebral cortex and comprises six histologically distinct layers. Allocortex is phylogenetically older and comprises from three to five layers (the actual number is inconsistently defined). Allocortex subdivides into paleocortex and archicortex. The most prominent example of paleocortex is the olfactory cortex and the most prominent example of archicortex is the hippocampus. Mesocortex represents transitional cortex between neocortex and allocortex and it subdivides into periallocortex and proisocortex. Periallocortex further subdivides into peripaleocortex and periarchicortex.

Now, in order to learn the six histologic layers of the neocortex, let's discuss the neocortical cell populations, themselves. The cerebral cortex contains roughly 50 billion neurons, which are commonly divided into pyramidal and non-pyramidal cells. Indicate that pyramidal cells are 10 to 80 micrometers (μm) in diameter and are shaped like a flask with a single thick, cortically oriented apical dendrite and multiple basal dendrites. Indicate that one important pyramidal cell type is the Betz cell; by at least one commonly held definition, Betz cells lie primarily within the primary motor cortex but also extend, to a lesser extent, into the premotor cortex—note that select authors instead define Betz cells as being solely confined to the primary motor cortex. Then, indicate that the non-pyramidal cells are much smaller: they are 5 to 15 μm in diameter. The most notable non-pyramidal cell type is the stellate (or granule) cell. Other non-pyramidal cell types include the basket, fusiform, horizontal, Martinotti, and neurogliaform cells.[15–17]

Next, let's label the six cytoarchitectural layers of the neocortex from outside to inside. Label the outermost cytoarchitectural layer as layer I, the molecular (or plexiform) layer; indicate that it is primarily a nerve fiber layer, meaning that it is cell sparse and predominantly comprises axons and dendritic processes. Then, show that the next innermost layer is layer II, the external granular layer; indicate that it predominantly contains non-pyramidal cells and much fewer small pyramidal cells. Next, label layer III, the external pyramidal layer; indicate that it predominantly contains pyramidal cells of varying sizes. Also, layer III is sparsely populated with non-pyramidal cells. Now, label layer IV, the internal granular layer; indicate that it is densely packed with non-pyramidal cells. Layer IV is the narrowest cellular layer and it contains the horizontally oriented external band of Baillarger, which is a prominent thalamocortical nerve fiber layer. In the primary visual cortex, this nerve fiber band is called the line of Gennari. Next, label layer V, the internal pyramidal (or ganglionic) layer; indicate that it contains the largest pyramidal cells, most notably the Betz cells which are the major cortical motor neurons. The horizontally oriented internal band of Baillarger lies deep within this layer. Now, label layer VI, the multiform (or fusiform) layer; indicate that it contains a wide variety of pyramidal and non-pyramidal cells. Layer VI blends into the underlying white matter.[10,18]

Although the specific cellular constitution and nerve fiber density of each histologic layer varies across the cerebral cortex, certain areas of similarity exist. In 1909, Korbinian Brodmann published the most widely recognized cytoarchitectural maps of the human brain, which distinguish 52 different cytoarchitectural areas. Each area or group of areas subserves a unique function. In the next diagram, we will draw select, fundamental Brodmann areas and learn their significance.

CORTICAL CLASSIFICATION

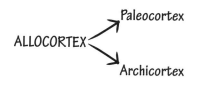

NEOCORTEX
(Isocortex)

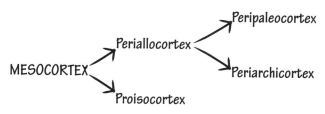

CELL NOMENCLATURE

Pyramidal cells - 10 to 80 μm; example - Betz cell

Non-pyramidal cells - 5 to 15 μm; example - stellate cells

DRAWING 16-5 **Cerebral Cytoarchitecture**

NEOCORTICAL CYTOARCHITECTURE

LAYER	HISTOLOGY
I. Molecular	Cell sparse, primarily axons & dendrites
II. External granular	Non-pyramidal & few small pyramidal cells
III. External pyramidal	Pyramidal cells of varying sizes
IV. Internal granular	Non-pyramidal cells & external band of Baillarger
V. Internal pyramidal	Large pyramidal cells & internal band of Baillarger
VI. Multiform	Multitude of cell types, blends into underlying white matter

Brodmann Areas

Here, we will draw select, fundamental Brodmann areas. First, draw lateral and medial surfaces of the cerebrum. Next, include certain key sulci. On the lateral hemispheric face, include the precentral, central, and postcentral sulci, and then the Sylvian fissure with its anterior horizontal and anterior ascending rami, and also include the lateral parietotemporal line. On the medial face, include the corpus callosum, cingulate sulcus, and pars marginalis, and then the paracentral, central, parieto-occipital, and calcarine sulci.

Now, within the postcentral and posterior paracentral gyri, from anterior to posterior, label Brodmann areas 3, 1, 2; they constitute the primary sensory area. Then, within the precentral and anterior paracentral gyri, label area 4, which is the primary motor area. Within the primary motor and sensory areas, cortical representation of the face and body is somatotopically arranged in what is referred to as the homunculus (see Drawing 19-4).

Now, in front of area 4, label area 6. On the lateral hemisphere, area 6 is called the premotor area, and it lies in the anterior precentral gyrus and posterior superior and middle frontal gyri. On the medial hemisphere, area 6 is called the supplementary motor area, and it lies in the medial aspect of the superior frontal gyrus. The premotor and supplementary motor areas help assemble complex motor programs.[19]

Next, in front of area 6, label area 8. The most notable feature of area 8 is that on its lateral surface it contains the human homologue to the rhesus monkey frontal eye fields—the animal model for human eye movements. In humans, however, volitional control of eye movements is derived from the anterior wall of the precentral sulcus and portions of many additional disparate Brodmann areas, including areas 4, 6, 8, and 9.[14,20,21]

Now, label area 44 in the pars opercularis and area 45 in the pars triangularis of the inferior frontal gyrus. Areas 44 and 45 make up Broca's area—the speech output area.

Next, peel back the superior temporal gyrus and label areas 41 and 42 in the transverse temporal gyri (Heschl's gyri); these gyri form the primary auditory cortex. Then, label the superior temporal gyrus as area 22. Wernicke's area, the language reception area, lies in the posterior portion of area 22 (and it also extends into the angular gyrus, Brodmann area 39 [not drawn]).[22]

Next, antero-inferior to area 8, along the surface of the lateral and medial faces of the cerebrum, from superior to inferior, label areas 9, 10, and 11; then, in between area 45 and area 10, label area 46; then, beneath area 46, label area 47; and finally, in the anterior cingulate gyrus, label area 24. These areas form the prefrontal cortex, which is subdivided into dorsolateral prefrontal, orbitofrontal, and anterior cingulate (medial frontal) cortices; each subdivision governs a discrete cognitive domain. Although the exact anatomy of these divisions is inconsistently defined, there is consensus regarding their functions. Indicate that, generally, the dorsolateral prefrontal cortex encompasses areas 9, 46, and a portion of area 10; the orbitofrontal cortex comprises areas 11, 47, and a portion of area 10; and the anterior cingulate cortex comprises area 24. Indicate that dorsolateral prefrontal cortex mediates executive function and task sequencing—injury here results in organizational deficits; that orbitofrontal cortex governs social behavior—damage here results in impulsivity; and that anterior cingulate (medial frontal) cortex mediates motivation—injury here results in a lack of motivation (abulia).[23,24]

Finally, within the occipital lobe, label the visual cortex. On the medial surface, indicate that area 17, the primary visual cortex, lies on the banks of the calcarine sulcus; and then show that area 18, the secondary visual cortex, lies above and below area 17; and then that area 19, the tertiary visual cortex, lies above and below area 18. On the lateral surface, show that area 17 lies at the occipital pole, that area 18 lies anterior to area 17, and that area 19 lies anterior to area 18.[25,26]

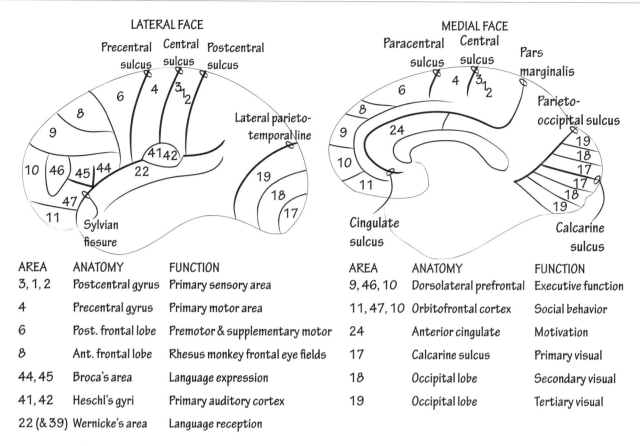

LATERAL FACE

Precentral sulcus   Central sulcus   Postcentral sulcus

Lateral parieto-temporal line

Sylvian fissure

MEDIAL FACE

Paracentral sulcus   Central sulcus   Pars marginalis

Parieto-occipital sulcus

Cingulate sulcus

Calcarine sulcus

AREA	ANATOMY	FUNCTION
3, 1, 2	Postcentral gyrus	Primary sensory area
4	Precentral gyrus	Primary motor area
6	Post. frontal lobe	Premotor & supplementary motor
8	Ant. frontal lobe	Rhesus monkey frontal eye fields
44, 45	Broca's area	Language expression
41, 42	Heschl's gyri	Primary auditory cortex
22 (& 39)	Wernicke's area	Language reception

AREA	ANATOMY	FUNCTION
9, 46, 10	Dorsolateral prefrontal	Executive function
11, 47, 10	Orbitofrontal cortex	Social behavior
24	Anterior cingulate	Motivation
17	Calcarine sulcus	Primary visual
18	Occipital lobe	Secondary visual
19	Occipital lobe	Tertiary visual

DRAWING 16-6 **Brodmann Areas**

References

1. Stippich, C. & Blatow, M. *Clinical functional MRI: presurgical functional neuroimaging,* p. 242 (Springer, 2007).

2. Ono, M., Kubik, S. & Abernathey, C. D. *Atlas of the cerebral sulci* (G. Thieme Verlag; New York: Thieme Medical Publishers, 1990).

3. Duvernoy, H. M. & Bourgouin, P. *The human brain: surface, three-dimensional sectional anatomy with MRI, and blood supply,* 2nd completely rev. and enl. ed. (Springer, 1999).

4. Bruni, J. E. & Montemurro, D. G. *Human neuroanatomy: a text, brain atlas, and laboratory dissection guide* (Oxford University Press, 2009).

5. Mai, J. K., Voss, T. & Paxinos, G. *Atlas of the human brain,* 3rd ed. (Elsevier/Academic Press, 2008).

6. Rhoton, A. L., Jr. The cerebrum. Anatomy. *Neurosurgery* 61, 37–118; discussion 118–119 (2007).

7. Seeger, W. *Endoscopic and microsurgical anatomy of the upper basal cisterns* (Springer, 2008).

8. Nieuwenhuys, R., Voogd, J. & Huijzen, C. V. *The human central nervous system,* 4th ed. (Springer, 2008).

9. Kulkarni, N. V. *Clinical anatomy for students: problem solving approach,* p. 949 (Jaypee, 2006).

10. Kretschmann, H.-J. & Weinrich, W. *Cranial neuroimaging and clinical neuroanatomy: atlas of MIR imaging and computed tomography,* 3rd ed. (Georg Thieme Verlag; Thieme Medical Publishers, 2004).

11. Fossett, D. T. & Caputy, A. J. *Operative neurosurgical anatomy,* p. 23 (Thieme, 2002).

12. Halim, A. *Human anatomy: volume III: Head, neck and brain* (I.K. International Publishing House Pvt. Ltd., 2009).

13. Govaert, P. & De Vries, L. S. *An atlas of neonatal brain sonography,* 2nd ed., pp. 18–19 (Mac Keith Press, 2010).

14. Clark, D. L., Boutros, N. N. & Mendez, M. F. *The brain and behavior: an introduction to behavioral neuroanatomy,* 3rd ed., p. 50 (Cambridge University Press, 2010).

15. Pritchard, T. *Medical neuroscience* (Fence Creek Publishing, LLC, 1999).

16. Krause, W. J. *Krause's essential human histology for medical students,* 3rd ed., p. 320 (Universal Publishers, 2005).

17. Jacobson, S. & Marcus, E. M. *Neuroanatomy for the neuroscientist,* pp. 158–161 (Springer, 2008).

18. Dambska, M. & Wisniewski, K. E. *Normal and pathologic development of the human brain and spinal cord* (John Libbey, 1999).

19. Wyllie, E., Gupta, A. & Lachhwani, D. K. *The treatment of epilepsy: principles & practice,* 4th ed. (Lippincott Williams & Wilkins, 2006).

20. Leigh, R. J. & Zee, D. S. *The neurology of eye movements* (Oxford University Press, 2006).

21. Büttner-Ennever, J. A. *Neuroanatomy of the oculomotor system* (Elsevier, 1988).

22. Afifi, A. K. & Bergman, R. A. *Functional neuroanatomy: text and atlas,* 2nd ed. (Lange Medical Books/McGraw-Hill, 2005).

23. Salloway, S., Malloy, P. & Duffy, J. D. *The frontal lobes and neuropsychiatric illness,* 1st ed. (American Psychiatric Press, 2001).

24. Cummings, J. L. & Mega, M. S. *Neuropsychiatry and behavioral neuroscience,* Chapter 18 (Oxford University Press, 2003).

25. Grill-Spector, K. & Malach, R. The human visual cortex. *Annu Rev Neurosci* 27, 649–677 (2004).

26. Rajimehr, R. & Tootell, R. Organization of human visual cortex. In *The senses: a comprehensive reference* (ed. A. I. Basbaum) (Elsevier Inc., 2008).

Cerebral White Matter

Know-It Points

Cerebral White Matter—Overview

- Association fibers connect areas within a hemisphere.
- Striatal fibers provide communication between the cerebral cortex and the basal ganglia.
- Cord fibers either directly connect areas on opposite sides of the neuroaxis or provide an important step in that cross-axis connection.
- Cord fibers subdivide into commissural and subcortical fiber bundles.

- Subcortical projection fibers divide into the thalamic bundle and the pontine bundle.
- The deep white matter region between the cortex and the diencephalon is anatomically divided into the centrum semiovale and the corona radiata.
- The centrum semiovale lies above the level of the lateral ventricles and the corona radiata lies at their level.

Long Association Fibers (*Advanced*)

- The superior longitudinal fasciculus connects the parietal and frontal cortices.
- The arcuate fasciculus originates in the posterior superior temporal area and passes forward to the frontal lobe; it is classically considered the language conduction pathway.
- The cingulum is the main white matter bundle of the limbic system.
- The middle longitudinal fasciculus spans from the posterior end of the superior temporal gyrus to the temporal pole.

- The inferior longitudinal fasciculus is the major white matter bundle of the ventral occipitotemporal visual pathway, the so-called "what" pathway.
- The fronto-occipital fasciculus transmits visual spatial information to the frontal motor areas to guide movement via the "where" pathway.

Internal Capsule

- The internal capsule fills a V-shaped wedge within the conglomeration of the basal ganglia and thalamus.
- The anterior limb of the internal capsule lies in between the head of the caudate and the lentiform nucleus.
- The genu of the internal capsule is the bend; it lies along the medial-lateral plane of the anterior thalamus.

- The posterior limb of the internal capsule lies in between the thalamus and the lentiform nucleus.
- Both the sublenticular and retrolenticular limbs lie posterior to the posterior limb.
- Infarction to the genu and posterior limb of the internal capsule produces a classic and common pure motor stroke.

Commissures & Disconnections (*Advanced*)

- Commissural fibers connect corresponding areas of the cerebrum; the two main commissural bundles are the anterior commissure and the corpus callosum.
- The corpus callosum lies superior to the anterior commissure and connects dorsal cortical areas, whereas the anterior commissure connects ventral areas.
- The anterior commissure connects the bilateral ventral posterior frontal lobes and also the bilateral anterior temporal lobes.
- The corpus callosum connects the bilateral hemispheres from the frontal to the occipital poles.

- The anterior-inferior portion of the corpus callosum is the rostrum; the anterior-superior portion is the genu; the length of the corpus callosum is the body; and the posterior portion is the splenium.
- In alexia without agraphia, there is injury to the medial left posterior occipital lobe and also to the right visual projection fibers after they have crossed midline within the splenium of the corpus callosum.
- Alien hand syndrome has three forms: the callosal variant, which manifests with intermanual conflict; the frontal variant, which manifests with involuntary grasping; and the sensory variant, which manifests with limb ataxia.

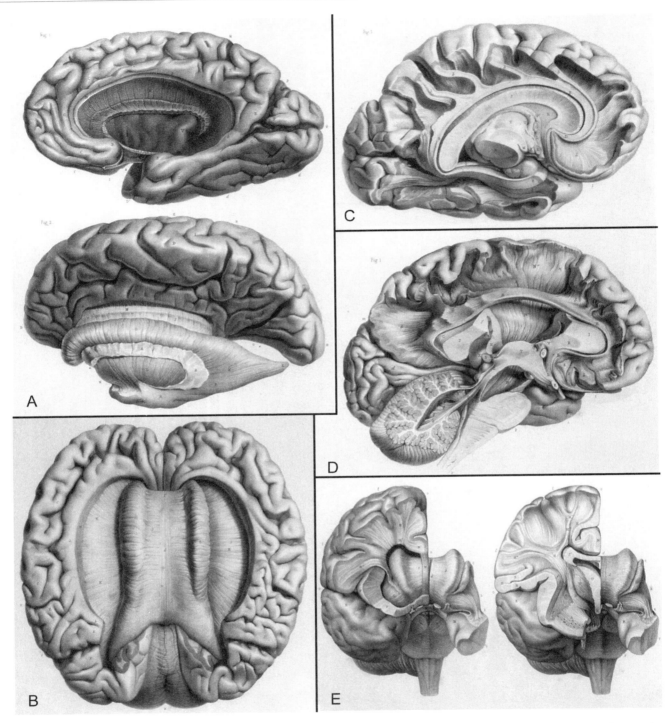

FIGURE 17-1 Achille-Louis Foville's illustrations of white matter, 1844. Used with permission from Schmahmann, Jeremy D., and Deepak N. Pandya. *Fiber Pathways of the Brain.* New York: Oxford University Press, 2006.

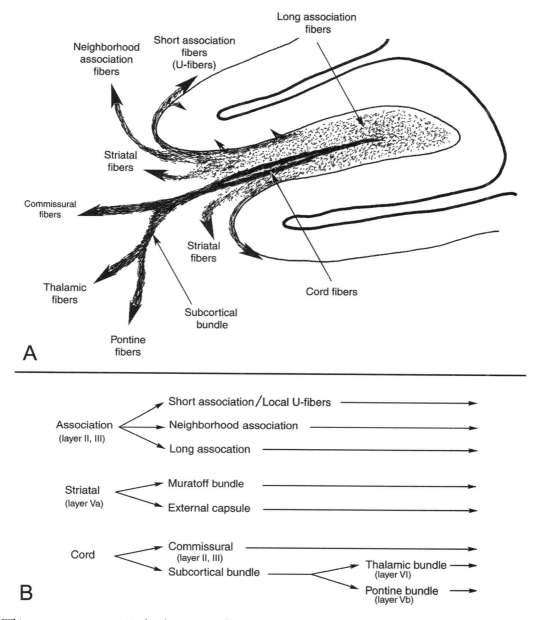

FIGURE 17-2 White matter organization. Used with permission from Schmahmann, Jeremy D., and Deepak N. Pandya. *Fiber Pathways of the Brain.* New York: Oxford University Press, 2006.

Cerebral White Matter—Overview

Here, we will draw an overview of the white matter pathways in accordance with the organization described in the 2006 white matter textbook *Fiber Pathways of the Brain*. Begin with a coronal section through the brain, brainstem, and upper spinal cord. Include a sulcal indentation on the surface of the cerebral cortex as a point of reference and also include a thalamus and head of the caudate. Three white matter pathway types exist: association fibers, which connect areas within a hemisphere; cord fibers, which either directly connect areas on opposite sides of the neuroaxis or provide an important step in that cross-axis connection; and striatal fibers, which provide communication between the cerebral cortex and the basal ganglia.

First, we will draw the association fibers, which are subdivided in accordance with the distance they travel. Begin with a short association fiber (aka U-fiber or arcuate bundle). Short association fibers travel between gyri just underneath the innermost cerebral cortical gray matter layer (layer 6). Certain white matter diseases, such as subtypes of multiple sclerosis, spare the short association fibers. Next, draw a mid-range association fiber, called a neighborhood association fiber. Neighborhood association fibers extend into the deep white matter to connect areas a mid-distance away from one another. Finally, draw a long-distance association fiber, called a long association fiber. Long association fibers extend deep into the brain and connect distant ipsihemispheric regions. Note that we will draw the specific, named long association fibers in our sagittal diagram, separately.

Next, draw a prototypical striatal fiber projection from the cerebral cortex to the basal ganglia. Projections from throughout the cortex synapse in the basal ganglia and are evidentiary of the widespread role of the basal ganglia in behavioral as well as motor functions.

Indicate that the two types of striatal fiber bundles are the Muratoff bundle (aka subcallosal fasciculus) and the external capsule.

Now, we will draw the cord fibers, which connect opposite sides of the nervous system: they subdivide into commissural and subcortical fiber bundles and they form the dense aggregate of deep white matter underneath the cortical gray matter. Draw a transverse-oriented commissural fiber connection from one side of the cortex to the other. The key commissural fibers are the anterior commissure and corpus callosum—the latter contains roughly 300 million myelinated axons.[1] Next, draw two vertically oriented representative subcortical projection fibers: an ascending one from the thalamus to the cortex, called the thalamic bundle, and a descending one from the cortex to the opposite side of the brainstem, called the pontine bundle. The thalamic bundle encompasses such pathways as the somatosensory afferents from the spinal cord and the cerebellar projections of the corticopontocerebellar pathway; these pathways relay in the thalamus in their ascent to the cerebral cortex. The pontine bundle encompasses such pathways as the corticospinal tract, which descends through the internal capsule and pons, and the corticopontine tract, which synapses in the pons. Note that although the thalamic bundle and the corticopontine tract are actually ipsihemispheric projections, they both are steps in larger pathways that connect opposite sides of the neuroaxis.

The cord fibers form the deep white matter region between the cortex and the diencephalon, which is anatomically divided into the centrum semiovale and corona radiata. The name corona radiata stands for "radiating crown"; however, its radiating appearance is appreciable only in detailed anatomic dissection. Indicate that the centrum semiovale lies above the level of the lateral ventricles and that the corona radiata lies at their level.[2–8]

GENERAL ORGANIZATION - CORONAL VIEW

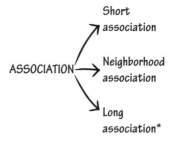

Short
association
fiber

Neighborhood
association
fiber

Long
association
fiber*

Striatal
fibers

Subcortical
cord bundles

Thalamic
bundle

Commissural
cord fibers

Pontine
bundle

CENTRUM SEMIOVALE & CORONA RADIATA
Centrum semiovale - above lateral ventricles
Corona radiata - at level of the lateral ventricles

GENERAL ORGANIZATION - NOMENCLATURE

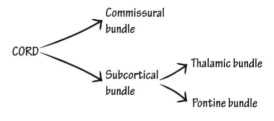

ASSOCIATION → Short association
→ Neighborhood association
→ Long association*

CORD → Commissural bundle
→ Subcortical bundle → Thalamic bundle
→ Pontine bundle

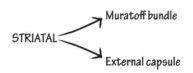

STRIATAL → Muratoff bundle
→ External capsule

*Trajectory best viewed
in sagittal section

DRAWING 17-1 **Cerebral White Matter—Overview**

Long Association Fibers (*Advanced*)

Here, we will draw the long association fibers. Begin with a sagittal section through a cerebral hemisphere. The first fibers we will draw are the superior longitudinal fasciculus and the arcuate fasciculus. Note that historically and commonly these fibers are classified either synonymously or as part of a single system. First, show that the superior longitudinal fasciculus is a bidirectional pathway that connects the parietal and frontal cortices—classically it is more broadly defined as involving the temporal and occipital cortices, as well. The superior longitudinal fasciculus is further subcategorized into three different fasciculi, which, roughly, from rostral to caudal are SLF I, II, and III. In accordance with its broad anatomy, the superior longitudinal fasciculus is involved in a wide variety of cognitive functions, but indicate that, notably, it communicates spatial information between the frontal and parietal lobes.

Next, show that the arcuate fasciculus originates in the posterior superior temporal area and passes forward to the frontal lobe. The ability to repeat language, which is called language conduction, has historically been assigned to the arcuate fasciculus (and still commonly is). Language conduction requires the transmission of language from the superior temporal reception area to the frontal motor speech output area. Despite its historical assignment to the arcuate fasciculus, evidence suggests that the arcuate fasciculus is actually more generally involved in the spatial orientation of sound and that the superior longitudinal fasciculus (specifically, SLF III), the middle longitudinal fasciculus, and the extreme capsule, instead, transmit language conduction.

Now, draw the uncinate fasciculus, which connects the orbital prefrontal cortex and anterior cingulate gyrus with the anterior temporal lobe. Indicate that the uncinate fasciculus combines processed somatosensory information (auditory, visual, gustatory) with emotional response regulation to assist in decision-making processes.

Next, we will draw the cingulum, which is the main white matter bundle of the limbic system. Show that the cingulum projects bidirectionally through the limbic lobe: from the cingulate gyrus around the posterior end of the corpus callosum back forward through the parahippocampal gyrus. Indicate that the cingulum plays an important role in emotional processing. Interestingly, cingulotomy (ie, cingulum fiber transection) was unsuccessfully used to treat psychosis in the mid-twentieth century and was abandoned, but is now sometimes used for the treatment of obsessive-compulsive disorder and intractable pain.

Now, draw the middle longitudinal fasciculus from the posterior end of the superior temporal gyrus to the temporal pole (note that this is not the *medial* longitudinal fasciculus, which lies in the brainstem and transmits eye movements). Indicate that the middle longitudinal fasciculus connects paralimbic, associative, and prefrontal cortices.

Next, draw the inferior longitudinal fasciculus from the antero-inferior temporal lobe to the parieto-occipital lobe. The inferior longitudinal fasciculus is the major white matter bundle of the ventral occipitotemporal visual pathway, which is responsible for object recognition and identification—the so-called "what" pathway. Next, draw the fronto-occipital fasciculus in the superior cortex from the parieto-occipital area to the prefrontal area. The fronto-occipital pathway is the "where" pathway corollary to the ventral occipitotemporal "what" pathway; it transmits visual spatial information to the frontal motor areas to guide movement.

Lastly, show that the extreme capsule spans from the middle temporal area to the ventral prefrontal cortex. It is discretely situated between the claustrum and the insula (as opposed to the external capsule, which is situated between the claustrum and the putamen) and is most easily viewed on coronal radiographic imaging. Indicate that the extreme capsule plays a role in language, specifically in syntax and grammar, and as discussed previously, conduction aphasia may at least partially be due to dysfunction within this white matter bundle.[3-8]

ABBREVIATION	FIBER BUNDLE	FUNCTION
SLF	Superior longitudinal fasciculus	Spatial awareness
AF	Arcuate fasciculus	Classic view - language conduction Modern view - sound orientation
UF	Uncinate fasciculus	Connects somatosensation & emotion for decision-making
CB	Cingulum bundle	Emotional processing
MLF	Middle longitudinal fasciculus	Associative, paralimbic, prefrontal communication
ILF	Inferior longitudinal fasciculus	"What" visual pathway
FOF	Fronto-occipital fasciculus	"Where" visual pathway
EC	Extreme capsule	Language syntax & grammar

LONG ASSOCIATION FIBER BUNDLES - SAGITTAL VIEW

DRAWING 17-2 **Long Association Fibers**

Internal Capsule

Here, we will draw the anatomy of the internal capsule in both axial and sagittal views. The internal capsule comprises fiber bundles that originate from widespread brain regions and it carries fibers of many disparate functional modalities, including motor, sensory, cognitive, and emotional fiber pathways. We will begin by drawing an axial view of the key basal ganglia structures (and the thalamus) because the internal capsule forms a wedge in between them. For orientational purposes, first draw the posterior aspect of the lateral ventricle and then the frontal horn of the lateral ventricle. Next, draw the head of the caudate; then, the thalamus; and next, the globus pallidus and putamen, which together form the lentiform nucleus. Now, show that the internal capsule fills the V-shaped wedge in between these nuclei.

Next, re-draw an axial view of the internal capsule so we can label its individual limbs. Indicate that the anterior portion, between the head of the caudate and the lentiform nucleus, is called the anterior limb; then, show that the middle (bend) of the internal capsule, which occurs along the medial–lateral plane of the anterior thalamus, is called the genu; next, indicate that the portion of internal capsule between the thalamus and the lentiform nucleus is called the posterior limb; then, show that the retrolenticular limb lies posterior to the posterior limb—its fibers run posterior to the lentiform nucleus; and finally, label the sublenticular limb in parentheses—its fibers run underneath the lentiform nucleus and lie inferior to the plane of this diagram. Note that the relative anterior–posterior positions of the sublenticular and retrolenticular limbs are inconsistently defined; therefore, we consider them both together as lying posterior to the posterior limb.

In sagittal view, we will now show the position of a few fiber bundles that pass through the internal capsule; bear in mind that the fibers we will draw represent only a few key clinical highlights. Most important to clinical neurology is the position of the motor fibers because infarction of the genu and posterior limb of the internal capsule produces a classic and common pure motor stroke. The motor fibers are arranged somatotopically, meaning the facial fibers pass through the genu, the arm fibers lie posterior to the facial fibers in the anterior portion of the posterior limb, and the leg fibers descend posterior to the arm fibers in the posterior portion of the posterior limb. Importantly, the motor fibers crowd together inferiorly within the internal capsule; thus, the more inferior the infarct, the more broad the motor deficit relative to the size of the infarct.

Draw a sagittal view of the internal capsule as a broad-based triangle sitting on a pointed edge; the internal capsule gradually dips down along the anterior–posterior course of the anterior limb and then rises again along the anterior–posterior course of the posterior limb. From anterior to posterior, label the anterior limb, genu, posterior limb, and sublenticular and retrolenticular limbs. Indicate that the anterior limb consists of fibers from the prefrontal cortex, predominantly anterior thalamic radiation fibers that connect the frontal cortex with the thalamus and also frontopontine fibers. Then, show that the genu and posterior limbs comprise the motor fibers. We commonly associate the facial fibers purely with the genu, but show that the facial fibers actually begin in the anterior limb, descend through the genu, and enter the posterior limb. Next, show that the arm fibers descend through the anterior portion of the posterior limb. Then, show that the leg fibers originate posterior to the arm fibers and pass anteriorly during their descent through the posterior limb. Finally, indicate that the sublenticular limb carries auditory fibers from the medial geniculate body, and then show that both the sublenticular and retrolenticular limbs carry visual projection fibers.[3–9]

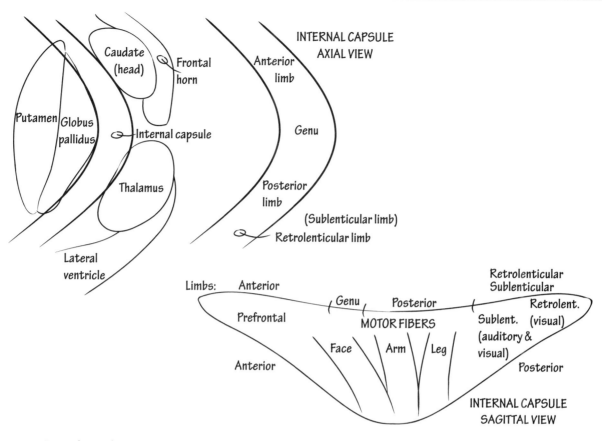

DRAWING 17-3 **Internal Capsule**

Commissures & Disconnections (*Advanced*)

Here, we will draw the commissural fibers and learn about the major disconnection syndromes. Commissural fibers connect corresponding areas of the cerebrum; the two main commissural bundles are the anterior commissure and the corpus callosum. The corpus callosum lies superior to the anterior commissure and connects dorsal cortical areas, whereas the anterior commissure connects ventral areas. First, let's use an axial plane through the inferior surface of the brain. Hash the anterior commissure bundle, which connects the bilateral ventral posterior frontal lobes and also the bilateral anterior temporal lobes. Then, draw the corpus callosum fibers, which connect the bilateral hemispheres from the frontal to the occipital poles. Indicate that the frontal fibers are called the anterior forceps (aka forceps minor, frontal forceps) and that the occipital fibers are called the posterior forceps (aka forceps major, occipital forceps).

Next, let's draw a sagittal view of the corpus callosum to show its four regions. Label the anterior-inferior portion of the corpus callosum as the rostrum; the anterior-superior portion as the genu, which is the anterior bend; the length of the corpus callosum as the body; and the posterior portion as the splenium. Indicate that the pre-frontal fibers run through the rostrum and genu; the frontal fibers run through the anterior body; the temporo-parietal fibers run through the posterior body; and the temporo-occipital fibers run through the splenium. Now, return to our axial diagram and indicate that the genu fibers correspond to the anterior forceps; the splenial fibers correspond to the posterior forceps; and the body fibers correspond to the midportion of the callosum. The rostral fibers run beneath the genu and are inferior to the plane of this axial section.

Additional smaller commissural fiber pathways exist, including the hippocampal commissure, which lies inferior to the splenium of the corpus callosum and connects the bilateral hippocampal formations, and the posterior, habenular, and supraoptic commissures.

The function of the commissural fibers has aroused great interest throughout the past several centuries, and although the commissural fibers have long been understood to provide interhemispheric communication, the full extent of their function is still not known. Functional analysis of the corpus callosum suggests a role for it in both sensory integration and high-level cognitive processing. Much of what is known about the commissural bundles, however, comes from callosal resection surgeries, which are still done today to prevent the transmission of epileptic activity between the cerebral hemispheres (ie, to stem the propagation of seizures), and also from commissural fiber disruption injuries, which can result in disconnection syndromes.

Here, we will address two major disconnection syndromes: pure alexia without agraphia and alien hand syndrome. In 1892, Dejerine memorably described the syndrome of pure alexia without agraphia, which is a syndrome in which patients are unable to read but are still able to write. To illustrate the anatomic underpinnings of alexia without agraphia, draw an anatomic axial section through a mid-height of the cerebrum. Then, label the language center in the left superior temporal gyrus. Next, label the left visual cortex and show that it directly communicates with the language center. Then, draw the right visual cortex and then the splenium of the corpus callosum. Indicate that the right visual cortex projects to the language center through the splenium of the corpus callosum. Now, show that in pure alexia without agraphia, there is a posterior cerebral lesion that affects the medial left posterior occipital lobe and the related visual projection fibers, and indicate that the lesion also involves the right visual projection fibers after they have crossed midline within the splenium of the corpus callosum. From this lesion, the left visual center is directly cut off from the language center and the communication between the right visual center and the language center is disrupted from the injury to the corpus callosum.

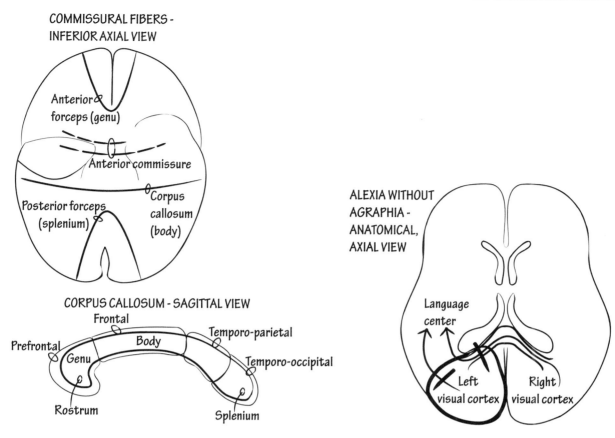

COMMISSURAL FIBERS - INFERIOR AXIAL VIEW

Anterior forceps (genu)

Anterior commissure

Corpus callosum (body)

Posterior forceps (splenium)

CORPUS CALLOSUM - SAGITTAL VIEW

Frontal

Body

Temporo-parietal

Prefrontal

Temporo-occipital

Genu

Rostrum

Splenium

ALEXIA WITHOUT AGRAPHIA - ANATOMICAL, AXIAL VIEW

Language center

Left visual cortex

Right visual cortex

DRAWING 17-4 **Commissures & Disconnections—Partial**

Commissures & Disconnections (*Advanced*) (Cont.)

Left posterior cerebral artery infarction is a common cause of alexia without agraphia. Note that a coincident right homonymous hemianopia often occurs in this syndrome due to the left posterior occipital injury, and also note that our diagram is an anatomic drawing, in which the left side of the brain is on the left-hand side of the page; radiographic images have the opposite orientation (see Drawing 1-2).[10]

Another disconnection syndrome that receives attention from both neurologists and Hollywood, alike, is called alien hand syndrome (aka alien limb sign). It was cinematized most memorably in Stanley Kubrick's *Dr. Strangelove.* Three forms of alien hand syndrome exist, each with a discrete anatomic localization; however, patients commonly present with overlapping symptoms. Across the top of the page, label variant, manifestation, localization, and dominance. First, label the callosal variant, which manifests with intermanual conflict or so-called self-oppositional behavior. In this alien hand syndrome variant, one hand is in direct conflict with the other, most commonly the left with the right. To show yourself what is meant by self-oppositional behavior, open a desk drawer with your right hand and then immediately slam it shut with your left. Indicate that this variant is most commonly caused by a lesion in the anterior corpus callosum and that the nondominant hand (ie, the left hand) is most commonly affected, meaning the left hand opposes the actions of the right.

Next, label the frontal variant, which manifests with involuntary grasping, groping, or manipulation of objects. To demonstrate what happens in this syndrome, with one hand involuntarily grasp at an object. Indicate that this variant is due to a lesion to the medial frontal lobe. The lesion is most commonly in the dominant hemisphere and the dominant hand (ie, the right hand)

is most commonly affected. Left anterior cerebral artery infarction is a notable cause of this variant of alien hand syndrome.[11-13]

Finally, label the sensory variant, which manifests with limb ataxia. To demonstrate the sensory variant of alien hand syndrome, let your hand dangle out away from your body and try to forget its existence. Patients with the sensory variant are generally unaware of their limb or even frankly deny that it's their own. Indicate that parieto-occipital lobe lesions cause this iteration of alien hand syndrome and that the nondominant hemisphere and hand are most commonly affected. Corticobasal degeneration, a neurodegenerative cause of dementia, can cause this alien hand syndrome variant.[11-13]

Other important clinical aspects regarding the corpus callosum are the frequency with which it fails to develop and the wide range of diseases that affect it. Congenital failure of the corpus callosum to fully develop is known as callosal agenesis and it occurs either in isolation or as part of a more complex syndrome, such as the Arnold-Chiari, Dandy-Walker, or Aicardi syndromes. Acquired forms of corpus callosum abnormalities occur from a wide range of causes, including demyelinating disorders, such as multiple sclerosis, and head trauma. Also, certain tumors characteristically invade the corpus callosum, such as glial tumors—most commonly glioblastoma multiforme, lymphomas, and lipomas. Lastly, metabolic disorders can also affect the corpus callosum, such as Marchiafava-Bignami, which is a rare cause of necrotic layering of the corpus callosum. Marchiafava-Bignami was originally described from the autopsies of three Italian men known to have been heavy red wine drinkers but has subsequently been found in both alcoholics and non-alcoholics, alike, and is ascribed to vitamin B complex deficiency.[3,14-18]

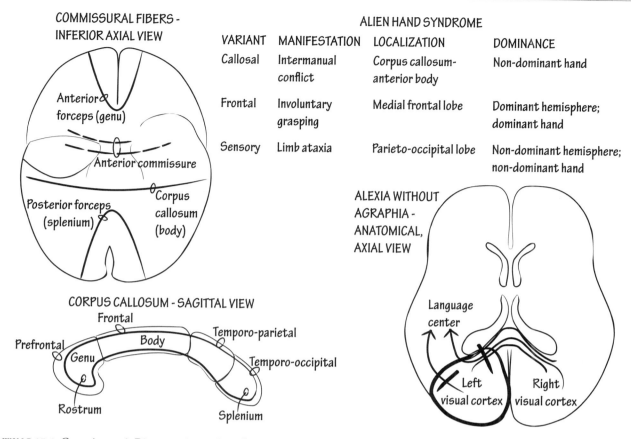

COMMISSURAL FIBERS - INFERIOR AXIAL VIEW

Anterior forceps (genu)

Anterior commissure

Posterior forceps (splenium)

Corpus callosum (body)

ALIEN HAND SYNDROME

VARIANT	MANIFESTATION	LOCALIZATION	DOMINANCE
Callosal	Intermanual conflict	Corpus callosum-anterior body	Non-dominant hand
Frontal	Involuntary grasping	Medial frontal lobe	Dominant hemisphere; dominant hand
Sensory	Limb ataxia	Parieto-occipital lobe	Non-dominant hemisphere; non-dominant hand

CORPUS CALLOSUM - SAGITTAL VIEW

Frontal

Prefrontal

Genu

Body

Temporo-parietal

Temporo-occipital

Rostrum

Splenium

ALEXIA WITHOUT AGRAPHIA - ANATOMICAL, AXIAL VIEW

Language center

Left visual cortex

Right visual cortex

DRAWING 17-5 **Commissures & Disconnections—Complete**

References

1. Filley, C. M. *The behavioral neurology of white matter,* Chapter 2 (Oxford University Press, 2001).

2. Joyce, C. *Diagnostic imaging in critical care: a problem based approach* (Churchill Livingstone Elsevier, 2010).

3. Schmahmann, J. D. & Pandya, D. N. *Fiber pathways of the brain* (Oxford University Press, 2006).

4. Jones, D. K. *Diffusion MRI: theory, methods, and application,* pp. 20–22 (Oxford University Press, 2011).

5. Moritani, T., Ekholm, S. & Westesson, P.-L. *Diffusion-weighted MR imaging of the brain,* 2nd ed., Chapter 2 (Springer, 2009).

6. Haines, D. E. & Ard, M. D. *Fundamental neuroscience: for basic and clinical applications,* 3rd ed. (Churchill Livingstone Elsevier, 2006).

7. Mendoza, J. E. & Foundas, A. L. *Clinical neuroanatomy: a neurobehavioral approach* (Springer, 2008).

8. Jacobson, S. & Marcus, E. M. *Neuroanatomy for the neuroscientist,* pp. 158–161 (Springer, 2008).

9. Chowdhury, F., Haque, M., Sarkar, M., Ara, S. & Islam, M. White fiber dissection of brain; the internal capsule: a cadaveric study. *Turk Neurosurg* 20, 314–322 (2010).

10. Festa, J. R. & Lazar, R. M. *Neurovascular neuropsychology,* pp. 32–33 (Springer, 2009).

11. Biran, I. & Chatterjee, A. Alien hand syndrome. *Arch Neurol* 61, 292–294 (2004).

12. Biller, J., Fleck, J. D. & Pascuzzi, R. M. *Practical neurology DVD review,* pp. 43–44 (Lippincott Williams & Wilkins, 2005).

13. Bogousslavsky, J. & Caplan, L. R. *Stroke syndromes,* 2nd ed., pp. 319–321 (Cambridge University Press, 2001).

14. Arbelaez, A., Pajon, A. & Castillo, M. Acute Marchiafava-Bignami disease: MR findings in two patients. *AJNR Am J Neuroradiol* 24, 1955–1957 (2003).

15. Jinkins, R. *Atlas of neuroradiologic embryology, anatomy, and variants* (Lippincott Williams & Wilkins, 2000).

16. Dobbs, M. R. *Clinical neurotoxicology: syndromes, substances, environments,* 1st ed., p. 93 (Saunders/Elsevier, 2009).

17. Mahmut Gazi Yaşargil, C. D. A. *Microsurgery of CNS tumors,* pp. 297–298 (Thieme, 1996).

18. Prabhakar Rajiah, A. G. S. S. *Paediatric radiology: clinical cases,* Case 5.15 (PasTest, 2008).

18

Basal Ganglia

.

Know-It Points

Basal Ganglia: Anatomy

- The caudate nucleus lies along the lateral wall of the lateral ventricle.
- The lens-shaped lentiform nucleus subdivides into the putamen, laterally, and the globus pallidus, medially.
- The internal capsule lies in between the lentiform nucleus and the head of the caudate, anteriorly, and the lentiform nucleus and the thalamus, posteriorly.

- The putamen and head of the caudate are connected at the nucleus accumbens.
- The lateral medullary lamina separates the putamen and the globus pallidus.
- The medial medullary lamina subdivides the globus pallidus into an internal (or medial) segment and an external (or lateral) segment.

Basal Ganglia: Nomenclature

- The term *corpus striatum* comprises the caudate, putamen, and globus pallidus.
- The caudate nucleus divides into a head, body, and tail.
- Striations connect the caudate and the putamen; thus, collectively, they are the striatum.

- The pale appearance of the globus pallidus gives it its name: pallidum.
- The subthalamic nucleus and substantia nigra are functionally but not developmentally associated with the basal ganglia.

Direct & Indirect Pathways: Anatomy *(Advanced)*

- Field H lies medial to the subthalamic nucleus and inferior to the zona incerta.
- Field H1 lies in between the thalamus and zona incerta.
- Field H2 lies lateral to the zona incerta and medial to the internal capsule.
- The ansa lenticularis originates in the globus pallidus internal segment, projects inferomedially, passes beneath the subthalamic nucleus, and then passes through Field H and Field H1 to enter the thalamus.

- The lenticular fasciculus projects from the internal segment of the globus pallidus through Fields H2, H, and H1 to enter the thalamus.
- Where the ansa lenticularis and the lenticular fasciculus run together in Field H1, they are collectively called the thalamic fasciculus.
- The subthalamic fasciculus refers to projections between the globus pallidus and subthalamic nucleus.

Direct & Indirect Pathways: Circuitry

- The direct pathway:
  - The cortex excites the striatum
  - The striatum inhibits the combined globus pallidus internal segment and the substantia nigra reticulata (GPi/STNr)
  - The GPi/STNr inhibits the thalamus (the thalamus excites the cerebral cortex)
  - The direct pathway is overall excitatory
- The indirect pathway:
  - The cortex excites the striatum
  - The striatum inhibits the globus pallidus external segment
  - The globus pallidus external segment inhibits the GPi/STNr
    - The GPi/STNr inhibits the thalamus (the thalamus excites the cerebral cortex)
    - The indirect pathway is overall inhibitory
    - A parallel circuit also exists within the indirect pathway that passes through the subthalamic nucleus in which the globus pallidus external segment inhibits the subthalamic nucleus and the subthalamic nucleus excites the GPi/STNr
    - This parallel indirect pathway through the subthalamic nucleus is also overall inhibitory
- Dopamine from the substantia nigra compacta excites the direct pathway (via dopamine 1 receptors) and inhibits the indirect pathway (via dopamine 2 receptors); both of these effects promote movement.

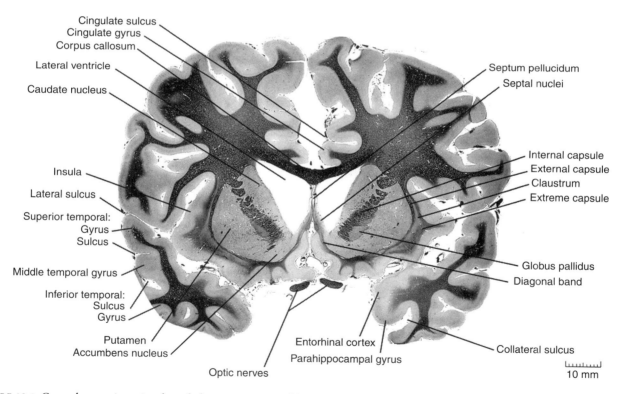

FIGURE 18-1 Coronal anatomic section through the anterior region of the basal ganglia. Used with permission from the Michigan State University: Brain Biodiversity Bank. https://www.msu.edu/~brains/

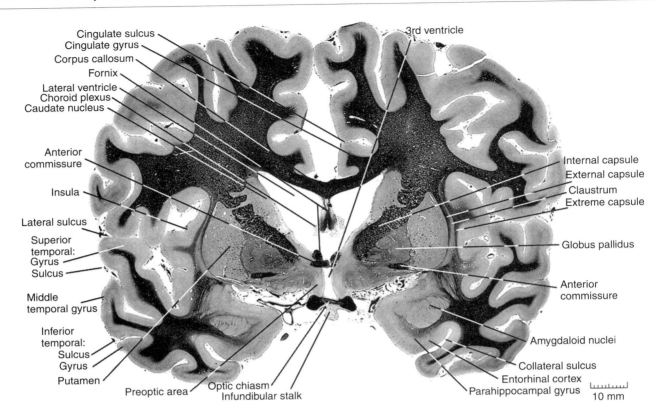

FIGURE 18-2 Coronal anatomic section through the middle region of the basal ganglia. Used with permission from the Michigan State University: Brain Biodiversity Bank. https://www.msu.edu/~brains/

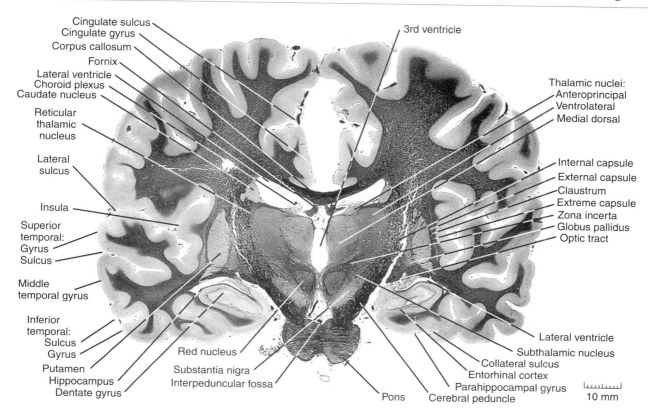

FIGURE 18-3 **Coronal anatomic section through the posterior region of the basal ganglia. Used with permission from the Michigan State University: Brain Biodiversity Bank. https://www.msu.edu/~brains/**

Basal Ganglia: Anatomy

Here, we will draw the basal ganglia and its related structures in axial, coronal, and sagittal views. Note that we will not be able to show all of the structures in each view; however, through the combined views we will draw the fundamental anatomy of the basal ganglia. Also, note that the basal ganglia are more correctly referred to as the basal nuclei because by definition a ganglion is a neuronal aggregation within the peripheral nervous system and the basal nuclei lie within the central nervous system. Begin with an axial view. First, draw a few orientational landmarks: along the medial aspect of the diagram, anteriorly, draw the frontal horn of the lateral ventricle; then, posteriorly, draw the body of the lateral ventricle and the thalamus; next, along the lateral edge of the diagram, draw the insula and then medial to it, draw the claustrum.

Next, let's include a few key basal ganglia structures. Along the lateral wall of the frontal horn of the lateral ventricle, label the head of the caudate. Then, at the postero-lateral tip of the thalamus in the lateral wall of the body of the lateral ventricle, draw the tail of the caudate. Note that the body of the caudate is not visible at this axial height. Now, in the center of the diagram, draw the lens-shaped lentiform nucleus and subdivide it into the putamen, laterally, and the globus pallidus, medially. Early in development, the globus pallidus migrates into the medial wall of the putamen—we can envision the lentiform nucleus as a globus pallidus core surrounded by a putaminal shell. Next, in between the lentiform nucleus and the head of the caudate and thalamus, label the internal capsule. Then, in between the putamen and the claustrum, label the external capsule, and in between the claustrum and the insula, label the extreme capsule.

Now, let's draw a coronal view through the anterior aspect of the basal ganglia. At the inferomedial aspect of the diagram, draw the optic chiasm; then, along the superior aspect of the diagram, draw the corpus callosum; just below it, draw the frontal horn of the lateral ventricle. Next, draw the combined putamen and head of the caudate and show that they are connected at the base by the nucleus accumbens. The nucleus accumbens is the bridge that persists between the head of the caudate and putamen after the anterior limb of the internal capsule separates the head of the caudate from the putamen. Now, beneath the nucleus accumbens, draw the basal forebrain.

Next, draw another coronal view just posterior to the previous section. To establish the anterior-posterior plane of this diagram, inferiorly, draw the optic tract and third ventricle; the hypothalamus immediately surrounds the third ventricle. Next, draw the corpus callosum and frontal horn of the lateral ventricle. Along the lateral wall of the frontal horn, draw the head of the caudate. Then, draw the putamen, and medial to it, draw the globus pallidus; show that the lateral medullary lamina separates them. Note that the medial medullary lamina subdivides the globus pallidus into an internal (or medial) segment and an external (or lateral) segment. Next, in between the lentiform nucleus and the caudate, draw the internal capsule. Now, beneath the globus pallidus, draw the basal forebrain and then draw the horizontally oriented anterior commissure in between them. Note that the globus pallidus actually extends beneath the anterior commissure as the ventral pallidum (see Drawing 18-2).

Lastly, let's draw the basal ganglia in sagittal view. First, draw the corpus callosum and the subjacent lateral ventricular system: label the frontal horn, atrium, and temporal horn divisions of the ventricular system. Next, draw the caudate and label the head and body. Note that the tail is not visible in this section. Then, anteriorly, draw the putamen and, posteriorly, draw the thalamus. In between these structures, label the internal capsule, and show that it funnels, inferiorly, into the cerebral peduncle.

BASAL GANGLIA & RELATED STRUCTURES

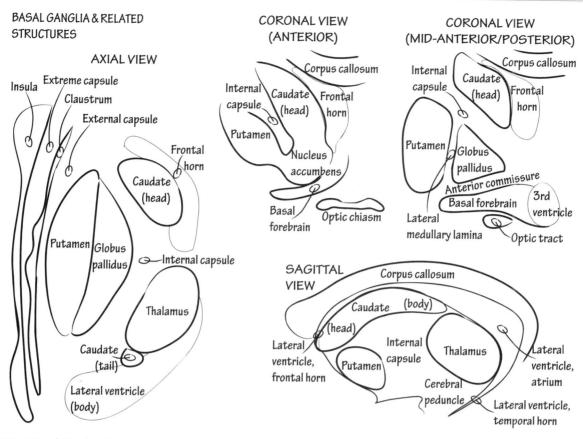

DRAWING 18-1 **Basal Ganglia: Anatomy**

Basal Ganglia: Nomenclature

Here, we will draw a flow diagram for the nomenclature of the basal ganglia. Begin with the term *corpus striatum*, which comprises the caudate, putamen, and globus pallidus. Indicate that the caudate nucleus, itself, is divided into a head, body, and tail and that the globus pallidus is divided into external (lateral) and internal (medial) segments. Striations connect the caudate and the putamen, which are collectively known as the striatum. The striatum is further subdivided into dorsal and ventral divisions. The dorsal striatum comprises the bulk of the caudate and putamen, whereas the ventral striatum is limited to only the ventromedial caudate and putamen, but the ventral striatum also encompasses the nucleus accumbens and select basal forebrain structures. The dorsal striatum is involved in a wide array of processes, including the sensorimotor circuits, whereas the ventral striatum associates principally with the limbic system and is primarily involved in emotional and behavioral processes.

Now, indicate that together the globus pallidus and putamen are called the lentiform nucleus, due to their collective lens-shaped appearance. Bundles of myelinated fibers traverse the globus pallidus, giving it a pale appearance, so the globus pallidus is also commonly called the pallidum. Just as the striatum divides dorsally and ventrally, so the pallidum is further subdivided into a dorsal pallidum and ventral pallidum. Similar to the striatum, the dorsal pallidum refers to the bulk of the globus pallidus, whereas the ventral pallidum refers to the anteromedial portion of the globus pallidus that lies below the anterior commissure. However, although we consider the ventral striatum and ventral pallidum to be divisions of the striatum and pallidum, here, certain texts distinguish these ventral structures as entirely separate nuclei (ie, they distinguish the ventral pallidum from the pallidum, itself). Also, note that because the globus pallidus is derived from the phylogenetically older portion of the brain—the diencephalon, and the caudate and putamen are derived from the phylogenetically newer part of the brain—the telencephalon, the pallidum is sometimes referred to as the paleostriatum, whereas the caudate and putamen are sometimes collectively referred to as the neostriatum.

The corpus striatum also encompasses several fiber pathways that pass between the globus pallidus and the subthalamic nucleus and thalamus: the ansa lenticularis, lenticular fasciculus, subthalamic fasciculus, and thalamic fasciculus. These fibers comprise a considerable portion of the white matter region inferolateral to the thalamus, which is called the fields of Forel (aka prerubral fields or Forel's Field H).

As a final note, the subthalamic nucleus and substantia nigra are functionally but not developmentally associated with the basal ganglia; therefore, although they are variably included as part of the basal ganglia, we do not include them in our definition of the basal ganglia, here, in accordance with the *Terminologia Anatomica*.

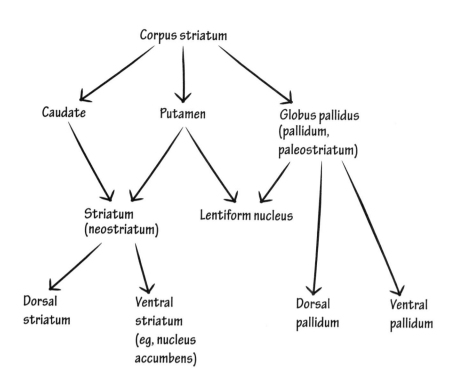

Caudate nucleus
1. head
2. body
3. tail

Globus pallidus
1. external (lateral) segment
2. internal (medial) segment

Basal ganglia-diencephalic white matter connections
1. ansa lenticularis
2. lenticular fasciculus
3. subthalamic fasciculus
4. thalamic fasciculus

DRAWING 18-2 **Basal Ganglia: Nomenclature**

Direct & Indirect Pathways: Anatomy (*Advanced*)

Here, in coronal view, we will draw the anatomy of the direct and indirect pathways and the anatomy of the fields of Forel. Note that we exclude the related corticostriatal projections. First, draw the lentiform nucleus and divide it into the putamen and globus pallidus; then, further subdivide the globus pallidus into its internal and external segments. Next, draw the thalamus, and inferolateral to it, draw the zona incerta. Then, inferior to the zona incerta, draw the subthalamic nucleus, and then inferior to it, draw the substantia nigra. Finally, through the middle of the diagram draw the posterior limb of the internal capsule and indicate that it becomes the cerebral peduncle as it descends through the brainstem.

Now, we are able to label the individual fields of Forel, which are Fields H, H1, and H2. First, indicate that Field H lies medial to the subthalamic nucleus and inferior to the zona incerta; then, show that Field H1 lies in between the thalamus and zona incerta (medial to the zona incerta and inferolateral to the thalamus); and finally, indicate that Field H2 lies lateral to the zona incerta and medial to the internal capsule.

Next, we will draw the direct pathway fibers, which comprise the pallidothalamic pathways, and which emanate from the internal segment of the globus pallidus. Start with the ansa lenticularis. Show that it projects inferomedially from the globus pallidus internal segment, courses beneath the subthalamic nucleus, then turns superiorly to pass through Field H and Field H1 to enter the thalamus. Next, show that the lenticular fasciculus projects from the internal segment of the globus pallidus across the internal capsule, through Field H2 and then Field H, and then show that it courses superiorly through Field H1 to enter the thalamus. Now, indicate that where the ansa lenticularis and the lenticular fasciculus run together in Field H1, they are collectively called the thalamic fasciculus; note that this is the most limited

definition of the thalamic fasciculus. Additional fiber pathways pass through Field H and H1 in their ascent into the thalamus; they include the cerebellothalamic fibers from the corticopontocerebellar pathway, the medial lemniscus, the nigrothalamic fibers, and the spinothalamic fibers of the anterolateral system pathway. The term *thalamic fasciculus* is sometimes broadened to include the cerebellothalamic fibers and it is also sometimes used synonymously with the term *Field H1*, just as the term *lenticular fasciculus* is sometimes used synonymously with term *Field H2*. Finally, note that the thalamic fasciculus projects to multiple thalamic nuclei, including the ventroanterior nucleus, which most notably communicates with the globus pallidus; the ventrolateral nucleus, which most notably communicates with the cerebellum; the dorsomedial nucleus, which most notably communicates with the prefrontal cortex and basal ganglia; and the centromedian and parafascicular nuclei (the main intralaminar nuclei), which most notably communicate with the striatum and frontal lobes.

Now, we will draw the globus pallidus external segment projections, which subserve the indirect pathway, and which involve the subthalamic nucleus and substantia nigra. First, show that the external segment of the globus pallidus projects to the subthalamic nucleus, and then show that the subthalamic nucleus projects back to the external segment of the globus pallidus and also to the internal segment of the globus pallidus. Indicate that the reciprocal pallidosubthalamic and subthalamopallidal projections are collectively called the subthalamic fasciculus. Next, show that the subthalamic nucleus also projects to the substantia nigra and that the substantia nigra projects back to the subthalamic nucleus. Finally, show that the globus pallidus external segment projects to the substantia nigra and then that the substantia nigra projects fibers through Fields H and H1 that enter the thalamus.

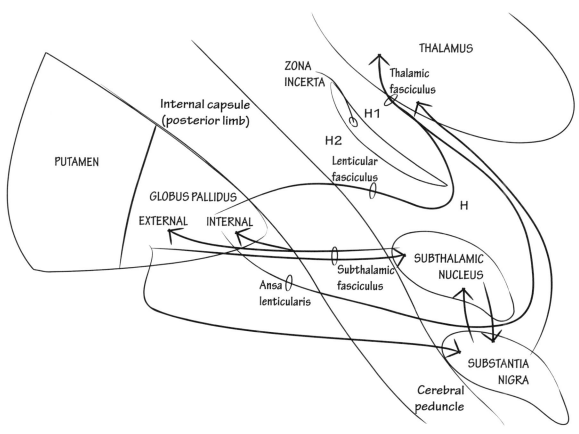

DRAWING 18-3 **Direct & Indirect Pathways: Anatomy**

Direct & Indirect Pathways: Circuitry

Here, we will draw a flow diagram for the circuitry of the direct and indirect pathways; they involve medium spiny neuron projections from the striatum to the globus pallidus and substantia nigra. The direct and indirect pathways are the best described of the numerous frontal-subcortical pathways that project through the basal ganglia. First, label the cerebral cortex, thalamus, and motor neurons. Then, show that the thalamus excites the cerebral cortex, which stimulates the motor neurons. Next, we will draw the direct pathway. Label the striatum—the combined caudate and putamen. Now, show that the cortex excites the striatum. Within the striatum, the sensorimotor cortex primarily targets the putamen; the putamen is the primary source of the direct and indirect pathways. Next, label the combined globus pallidus internal segment and the substantia nigra reticulata; they comprise the final output nuclei of the basal ganglia—hereafter, we consider them as a single functional entity: GPi/STNr. Next, show that the striatum inhibits the GPi/STNr and then show that the GPi/STNr inhibits the thalamus. Thus, indicate that the direct pathway is overall excitatory.

Now, we will draw the indirect pathway. First, include the globus pallidus external segment; show that it is inhibited by the striatum and then show that the globus pallidus external segment inhibits the GPi/STNr—thus, indicate that the indirect pathway is overall inhibitory. A parallel circuit also exists within the indirect pathway that passes through the subthalamic nucleus. So, now, add the subthalamic nucleus and show that it excites the GPi/STNr; then, show that the globus pallidus external segment inhibits the subthalamic nucleus. Therefore, whether it is because of the globus pallidus external segment inhibition of the GPi/STNr or because of the globus pallidus external segment inhibition of the subthalamic nucleus, through both means, the end result of the indirect pathway is that it is overall inhibitory. As a clinical corollary, when the subthalamic nucleus is selectively injured, patients develop wild ballistic, flinging movements, called hemiballismus, on the side contralateral to the subthalamic nucleus lesion due to a loss of motor inhibition.

Lastly, we need to account for the role of the substantia nigra compacta in the direct and indirect pathways. Parkinson's disease results from loss of dopaminergic cells within the substantia nigra compacta, and in Parkinson's disease, there is muscle rigidity, stiffness, difficulty with initiation of movement, and slowness and decomposition of rapid alternating movements. In our flow diagram, near the striatum, label the substantia nigra compacta, and indicate that it releases dopamine. If dopamine acted equally on both the direct and indirect pathways, the two pathways would equalize one another and the net effect would be nil. So, now, show that the two most prominent striatal dopamine receptors are the dopamine 1 receptor, which is part of the direct pathway and is excited by dopamine, and the dopamine 2 receptor, which is part of the indirect pathway and is inhibited by dopamine. Thus, dopamine from the substantia nigra compacta excites the direct pathway and inhibits the indirect pathway—both of these effects promote movement.

Note that many frontal-subcortical pathways project through the basal ganglia in addition to the motor pathways we have drawn; these pathways help drive a multitude of processes, including emotional, behavioral, somatosensory, and cognitive functional modalities. Through the corticostriatal fibers—the Muratoff bundle and the external capsule—the cerebral cortex targets the striatum in a topographic manner. For instance, the prefrontal cortex acts through innervation of the head and body of the caudate nucleus; the parietal lobes act through innervation of both the putamen and caudate; the primary auditory cortex projects to the caudoventral putamen and tail of the caudate; and the visual cortices project primarily to the nearest portion of the caudate nucleus.

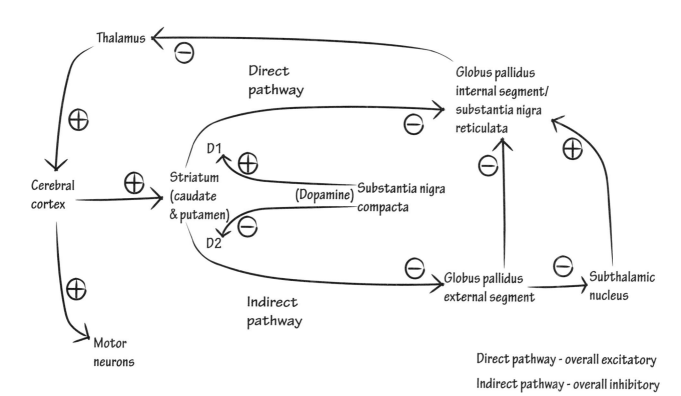

Direct pathway

Indirect pathway

Direct pathway - overall excitatory

Indirect pathway - overall inhibitory

DRAWING 18-4   Direct & Indirect Pathways: Circuitry

References

1. Afifi, A. K. & Bergman, R. A. *Functional neuroanatomy: text and atlas,* 2nd ed. (Lange Medical Books/McGraw-Hill, 2005).

2. Brodal, P. *The central nervous system: structure and function,* 4th ed. (Oxford University Press, 2010).

3. Campbell, W. W., DeJong, R. N. & Haerer, A. F. *DeJong's the neurologic examination: incorporating the fundamentals of neuroanatomy and neurophysiology,* 6th ed. (Lippincott Williams & Wilkins, 2005).

4. DeLong, M. R. & Wichmann, T. Circuits and circuit disorders of the basal ganglia. *Arch Neurol* 64, 20–24 (2007).

5. Haines, D. E. & Ard, M. D. *Fundamental neuroscience: for basic and clinical applications.* 3rd ed. (Churchill Livingstone Elsevier, 2006).

6. Hallett, M. & Poewe, W. *Therapeutics of Parkinson's disease and other movement disorders,* Chapter 3 (Wiley-Blackwell, 2008).

7. Heilman, K. M. & Valenstein, E. *Clinical neuropsychology,* 4th ed. (Oxford University Press, 2003).

8. Hirsch, M. C. *Dictionary of human neuroanatomy,* p. 149 (Springer, 2000).

9. Kiernan, J. A. & Barr, M. L. *Barr's the human nervous system: an anatomical viewpoint,* 9th ed. (Wolters Kluwer/Lippincott, Williams & Wilkins, 2009).

10. Koob, G. F. & Volkow, N. D. Neurocircuitry of addiction. *Neuropsychopharmacology* 35, 217–238 (2010).

11. Kopell, B. H. & Greenberg, B. D. Anatomy and physiology of the basal ganglia: implications for DBS in psychiatry. *Neurosci Biobehav Rev* 32, 408–422 (2008).

12. Nieuwenhuys, R., Voogd, J. & Huijzen, C. V. *The human central nervous system,* 4th ed. (Springer, 2008).

13. Noback, C. R. *The human nervous system: structure and function,* 6th ed. (Humana Press, 2005).

14. Patestas, M. A. & Gartner, L. P. *A textbook of neuroanatomy* (Blackwell Pub., 2006).

15. Paxinos, G. & Mai, J. K. *The human nervous system,* 2nd ed., Chapter 21 (Elsevier Academic Press, 2004).

16. Steiner, H. & Tseng, K.-Y. *Handbook of basal ganglia structure and function,* Chapter 24 (Elsevier/Academic Press, 2010).

17. Wieser, H. G. & Zumsteg, D. *Subthalamic and thalamic stereotactic recordings and stimulations in patients with intractable epilepsy,* pp. 30–31 (John Libbey Eurotext, 2008).

19

Arterial Supply

The Circle of Willis

Leptomeningeal Cerebral Arteries

Deep Cerebral Arteries (Advanced)

Arterial Borderzones

Brainstem Arteries (Advanced)

Cerebellar Arteries

Spinal Cord Arteries (Advanced)

Thalamic Arteries (Advanced)

Know-It Points

The Circle of Willis

- Two main arterial systems exist: an anterior-lying internal carotid artery system and a posterior-lying vertebral-basilar arterial system.
- The middle cerebral arteries originate from the internal carotid arteries and extend laterally.
- The anterior cerebral arteries branch anteriorly from the internal carotid arteries.

- The two vertebral arteries join to form the basilar artery.
- The basilar artery ascends the brainstem and bifurcates, superiorly, into the posterolaterally directed posterior cerebral arteries.

Leptomeningeal Cerebral Arteries

- The anterior cerebral artery supplies the medial one third of the mid/upper cerebrum.
- The middle cerebral artery supplies the lateral two thirds of the cerebrum.

- The posterior cerebral artery supplies the posterior portion of the mid/lower cerebrum.
- The superficial portion of the anterior choroidal artery supplies the medial temporal lobe.

Deep Cerebral Arteries (*Advanced*)

- The perforating branches of the middle cerebral artery supply the anterior-superior-lateral basal ganglia region.
- The perforating branches of the anterior cerebral artery supply the anterior-inferior-medial basal ganglia region.

- The perforating branches of the internal carotid artery supply the genu of the internal capsule and the area that immediately surrounds it.
- The perforating branches of the anterior choroidal artery supply the posterior-inferior-medial basal ganglia region.

Arterial Borderzones

- Infarcts in the borderzones in between the superficial, leptomeningeal arteries and the deep, perforating arteries are called "end-zone infarcts."
- Infarcts in the borderzones in between the superficial, leptomeningeal arteries are called "watershed infarcts."

- The somatotopic organization of the homunculus, from inferolateral to superomedial, is as follows: the tongue, face, hand, arm, and hip; and hanging over the medial face of the hemisphere are the leg and foot.

Brainstem Arteries (*Advanced*)

- The key medullary arteries are the anterior spinal artery and the posterior inferior cerebellar arteries.
- The common source for the key medullary arteries is the vertebral arteries.
- Most pontine arterial supply comes from circumferential arteries: the pontine paramedian arteries, short pontine circumferential arteries, and long pontine circumferential arteries.
- The common source for the circumferential arteries is the basilar artery.
- The key arteries that supply the midbrain are the paramedian mesencephalic and thalamoperforating arteries and the collicular, posteromedial choroidal, and superior cerebellar arteries.
- The common source for the key midbrain arteries is the posterior cerebral arteries (or distal basilar artery).

Cerebellar Arteries

- The posterior inferior cerebellar artery divides into lateral and medial branches, which supply the lateral and medial regions of the inferior cerebellum, respectively.
- The superior cerebellar artery divides into lateral and medial branches, which supply the lateral and medial superior cerebellum, respectively.
- The middle cerebellum is supplied by all three cerebellar arteries: the anterior inferior cerebellar artery supplies the anterior middle cerebellum; the posterior inferior cerebellar artery supplies the posterior middle cerebellum, inferiorly, and the superior cerebellar artery supplies the posterior middle cerebellum, superiorly.
- The anterior inferior cerebellar artery supplies much of the middle cerebellar peduncle and commonly gives off the internal auditory artery.

Spinal Cord Arteries (*Advanced*)

- The anterior spinal artery supplies the anterior two thirds of the spinal cord.
- The posterior spinal arteries supply the posterior one third of the spinal cord.
- Segmental arteries help supply the anterior and posterior spinal arteries throughout their descent.
- The pial network is a ring of arterial supply that surrounds the spinal cord; it has longitudinal connections that form an arterial meshwork around the spinal cord.
- The most important radiculomedullary artery is the artery of Adamkiewicz, which in the majority of people arises from T9 to T12 and from the left side of the body.
- The intrinsic arterial territories divide into the centrifugal and centripetal systems.

Thalamic Arteries (*Advanced*)

- The thalamotuberal artery supplies the anterior thalamus.
- The medial posterior choroidal artery supplies the medial posterior thalamus.
- The lateral posterior choroidal artery supplies the posterior thalamus.
- The thalamoperforating arteries supply the medial thalamus.
- The thalamogeniculate arteries supply the lateral thalamus.

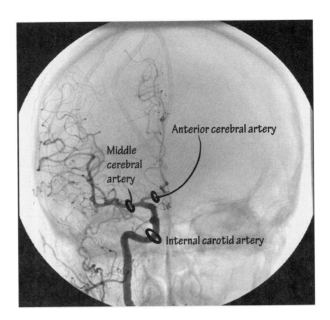

FIGURE 19-1 Cerebral angiography of internal carotid system, which supplies the anterior circulation.

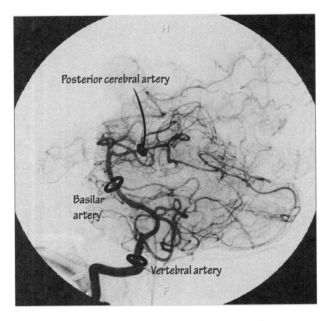

FIGURE 19-2 Cerebral angiography of vertebrobasilar system, which supplies the posterior circulation.

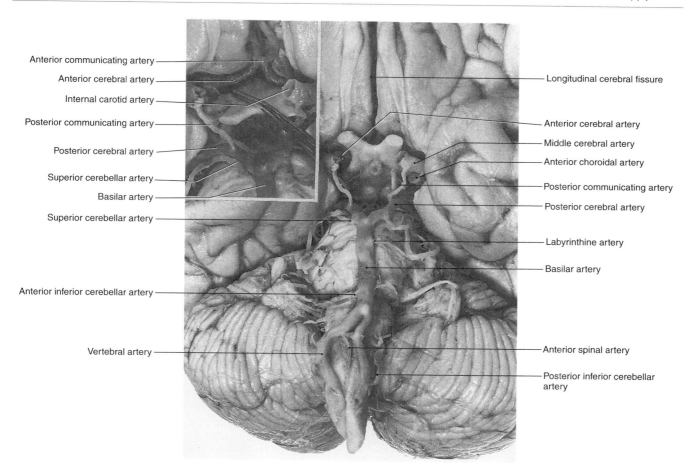

Anterior communicating artery

Anterior cerebral artery

Internal carotid artery

Posterior communicating artery

Posterior cerebral artery

Superior cerebellar artery

Basilar artery

Superior cerebellar artery

Anterior inferior cerebellar artery

Vertebral artery

Longitudinal cerebral fissure

Anterior cerebral artery

Middle cerebral artery

Anterior choroidal artery

Posterior communicating artery

Posterior cerebral artery

Labyrinthine artery

Basilar artery

Anterior spinal artery

Posterior inferior cerebellar artery

FIGURE 19-3 **Arteries of the base of the brain.** Used with permission from Bruni, J. E. & Montemurro, D. G. *Human Neuroanatomy: A Text, Brain Atlas, and Laboratory Dissection Guide.* New York: Oxford University Press, 2009.

The Circle of Willis

Here, we will draw the circle of Willis, which Thomas Willis first described in 1664. Let's stage our diagram so that we learn the most commonly discussed arteries first and then add the more advanced vasculature. As we learn the details of the cerebral vasculature, keep in mind that two main arterial systems exist: an anterior-lying internal carotid artery system and a posterior-lying vertebral-basilar system. Start our diagram with the anterior-lying internal carotid arteries; show axial sections through them. Next, show that the middle cerebral arteries originate from the internal carotid arteries and extend laterally. Then, indicate that the anterior cerebral arteries branch anteriorly from the internal carotids. Next, at the bottom of the diagram, show that the two vertebral arteries join to form the basilar artery, and then show that the basilar artery ascends the brainstem. At its apex, show that the basilar bifurcates into the posterolaterally directed posterior cerebral arteries. Now, show that branches of the vertebral arteries combine inferiorly to form the anterior spinal artery. Next, connect the internal carotid and posterior cerebral arteries with the posterior communicating arteries. Then, show that the anterior communicating artery connects the two anterior cerebral arteries. Next, on one side of the diagram, we will draw the cerebellar vessels from inferior to superior. First, draw the posterior inferior cerebellar artery off the vertebral artery; then, the anterior inferior cerebellar artery off the inferior portion of the basilar artery; and lastly, the superior cerebellar artery off the superior portion of the basilar artery. Now, draw the lenticulostriate branches of the middle cerebral artery; then, draw the anterior choroidal branch of the internal carotid artery. Finally, draw the basilar perforators: the pontine paramedian arteries, the short pontine circumferential arteries, and the long pontine circumferential arteries.[1-3]

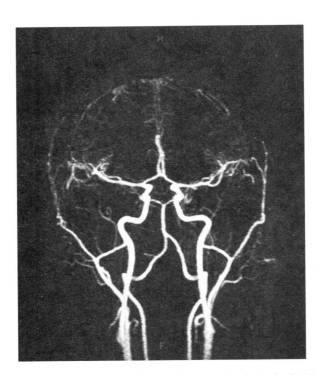

FIGURE 19-4 **Magnetic resonance angiography of the cerebral arterial system demonstrating the circle of Willis.**

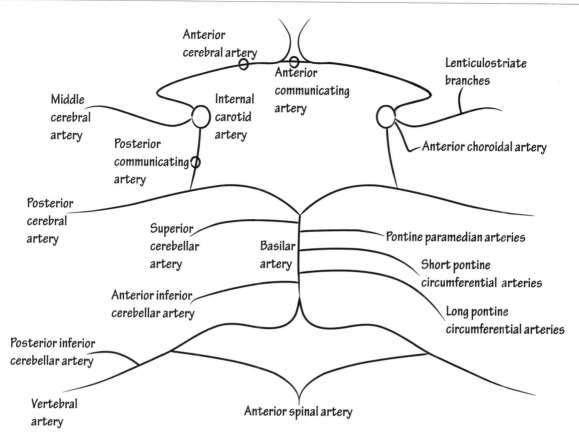

DRAWING 19-1 **The Circle of Willis**

Leptomeningeal Cerebral Arteries

We divide the arterial supply of the cerebral hemispheres into the superficial, leptomeningeal arterial branches and the deep, perforating arterial branches. Here, we will address the vascular territories of the leptomeningeal branches, which emanate from the anterior, middle, and posterior cerebral arteries, and we will also address the anterior choroidal artery. Note that because there is vast interpatient variability in the vascular territories, we should pay closer attention to the general vascular territory of each vessel than its specific territorial borders.

Begin with axial sections through the cerebrum at three different vertical heights: superior, middle, and inferior. To denote the mid-vertical cerebrum, include the lateral ventricles at the level of the body of the caudate nucleus, and to denote the inferior cerebrum, include the midbrain. First, at the superior level, show that the anterior cerebral artery (ACA) supplies the medial one third of the superior cerebrum and that the middle cerebral artery (MCA) supplies the lateral two thirds. For reference, indicate that the superior frontal sulcus separates the MCA and ACA supply. Next, at the mid-vertical level, show that the ACA supplies the medial one third of the hemisphere and that the MCA supplies the lateral two thirds, and also indicate that the

posterior cerebral artery (PCA) supplies a small portion of the posterior cerebral hemisphere. For reference, indicate that the parieto-occipital sulcus is the anterior boundary of the PCA. Now, indicate that at the inferior level, the ACA covers the medial one third of the cerebrum only as far posterior as the Sylvian fissure, and show that the MCA covers the lateral two thirds of the hemisphere—the MCA territory terminates just posterior to the medial-lateral axis of the posterior midbrain. Then, show that the PCA covers the posterior cerebrum. Lastly, indicate that the superficial portion of the anterior choroidal artery covers the medial temporal lobe.

Now, let's draw the arterial territories in sagittal view. Draw both the lateral and medial faces of the cerebrum. Show that the MCA supplies the majority of the lateral cerebral hemisphere, except for a strip of the antero-superior hemisphere, which the ACA supplies, and also a strip of the postero-inferior hemisphere, which the PCA supplies. Next, let's address the medial hemisphere; draw a diagonal line from the parieto-occipital sulcus to the anterior pole of the temporal lobe. Show that the ACA supplies the antero-superior hemisphere and that the PCA supplies the postero-inferior hemisphere, and also indicate that the anterior choroidal artery supplies the medial temporal lobe.[1,2,4–6]

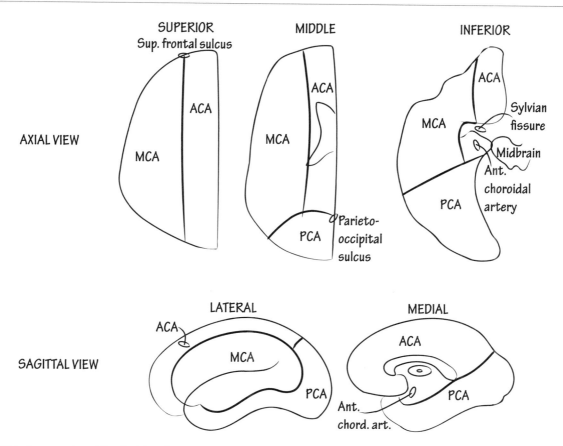

SUPERIOR
Sup. frontal sulcus

MIDDLE

INFERIOR

AXIAL VIEW

ACA

MCA

ACA

MCA

PCA

Parieto-
occipital
sulcus

ACA

MCA

Sylvian
fissure

Midbrain

Ant.
choroidal
artery

PCA

LATERAL

MEDIAL

SAGITTAL VIEW

ACA

MCA

PCA

ACA

PCA

Ant.
chord. art.

DRAWING 19-2 **Leptomeningeal Cerebral Arteries**

Deep Cerebral Arteries (*Advanced*)

Here, we will draw the deep, perforating cerebral arterial territories. Label the right-hand side of the page as the deep cerebral structures and the left-hand side as the perforating arterial territories. Note that an attempt to draw the exact vascular supply of each deep structure would be impractical due to the number of structures we would have to account for and the multiplicity of their arterialization. Instead, here, we will label only the vascularization of certain landmark structures. As we go through our vertically compressed axial diagram we must think in terms of three different axes. Draw the anterior–posterior and medial–lateral axes, now, and we will denote the superior–inferior variations in arterialization where appropriate in our diagram, itself.

First, draw the key anatomic landmarks. Indicate the hypothalamus, which lies in the anterior midline; it borders the third ventricle. Next, label the thalamus, which lies above the hypothalamus in midline. Then, anterior to the hypothalamus, draw the head of the caudate and then draw the lentiform nucleus, which is the globus pallidus and putamen combination. Sandwiched in between the aforementioned structures, draw the internal capsule and divide it into its central-lying genu and its anterior and posterior limbs.

Now, sketch this same arrangement on the arterial side of the page. Show that the perforating branches of the MCA, which are known as the lenticulostriate arteries, supply the anterior-superior-lateral basal ganglia region: they supply the putamen and lateral globus pallidus, superior internal capsule, the body of the caudate, and the superior caudate head. Then, show that the ACA perforating branches (including the recurrent artery of Heubner) supply the anterior-inferior-medial basal ganglia region: the anterior-inferior head of the caudate, anterior-inferior portion of the anterior limb of the internal capsule, and the medial lentiform nucleus. As we can

see, there is substantial overlap in the lenticulostriate and anterior cerebral artery vascularization of the basal ganglia. To distinguish the arterial supply of these vessels, denote that the lenticulostriate arteries supply the superior portion of the overlapping structures, whereas the ACAs supply the inferior portion.

Next, show that the perforating branches of the internal carotid artery supply the genu of the internal capsule and the areas that immediately surround it. Then, show that the anterior choroidal artery supplies the posterior-inferior-medial basal ganglia region: the lower posterior internal capsule, medial geniculate nucleus and related acoustic radiations, medial globus pallidus, and tail of the caudate. Now, show that the anterior communicating artery supplies the anterior hypothalamus and neighboring diencephalic structures. Then, show that the posterior communicating artery supplies the posterior hypothalamus, optic chiasm and mammillary bodies, and also the anterior thalamus via the thalamotuberal artery. Finally, show that many different thalamic arteries supply the remainder of the thalamus (see Drawing 19-8).

Next, let's consolidate this information into a single perforating artery–single structure/region list so we can simplify the aforementioned material. On the left-hand side, label the deep, perforating arteries, and on the right-hand side, label the single structure or region. Indicate that the lenticulostriate arteries supply the antero-supero-lateral basal ganglia; the ACA supplies the antero-infero-medial basal ganglia; the internal carotid artery supplies the genu of the internal capsule; the anterior communicating artery supplies the anterior hypothalamus; the posterior communicating artery supplies the posterior hypothalamus; the anterior choroidal artery supplies the posterior limb of the internal capsule; and the thalamic arteries supply the thalamus.[1,2,4–6]

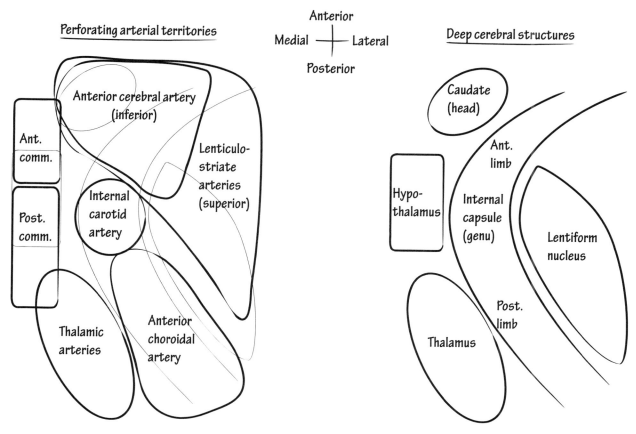

Perforating arterial territories

Anterior
Medial ─┼─ Lateral
Posterior

Deep cerebral structures

Ant.
comm.

Post.
comm.

Anterior cerebral artery
(inferior)

Lenticulo-
striate
arteries
(superior)

Internal
carotid
artery

Thalamic
arteries

Anterior
choroidal
artery

Caudate
(head)

Hypo-
thalamus

Ant.
limb

Internal
capsule
(genu)

Post.
limb

Lentiform
nucleus

Thalamus

DRAWING 19-3 **Deep Cerebral Arteries**

Arterial Borderzones

Here, let's use coronal slices through the cerebrum to draw the arterial borderzones. Vascular insufficiency within these arterial borders produces a clinically important form of cerebral infarction, called borderzone infarct. First, draw a coronal section through the cerebrum and label the general superficial, leptomeningeal arterial supply, and then label the deep, perforating arterial supply. The anastomoses (ie, collateralizations) that exist between the superficial, leptomeningeal arteries and the deep, perforating arteries are limited to capillary connections, which cannot sustain arterial perfusion in low-blood-flow states. Indicate that infarcts that occur within these borderzones are called "end-zone infarcts," so named because these arteries are essentially end arteries.

Now, draw another coronal section through the cerebrum. Here, we will focus on the borderzones that exist in between the superficial arterial territories. Indicate that the ACA supplies the supero-medial hemisphere, the PCA supplies the infero-medial hemisphere, and the MCA supplies the lateral two thirds of the cerebral hemisphere. Next, label the borderzones between these arteries. Again, the anastomoses that exist within these borderzones are insufficient to maintain cerebral perfusion in low-blood-flow states, resulting in stroke; infarcts to these borderzones are called "watershed infarcts."

Now, let's label the somatotopic cortical representation of the body, known as the homunculus. We do so in order to understand the clinical effect of an important type of watershed infarct—the MCA/ACA borderzone infarct, which produces the "man in a barrel" syndrome. The homunculus lies along the pre- and post-central gyri, laterally, and the paracentral gyri, medially. First, show that within the homunculus, the tongue lies inferiorly. Then, above it, show the face and then the hand above it. The tongue, face, and hand take up a disproportionately large area within the cortex relative to their actual size in the body. Now, continue counterclockwise around the convexity of the hemisphere, and include the arm and hip. Then, hanging over the medial face of the hemisphere, draw the leg and foot. Note that the foot terminates superior to the cingulate gyrus.

The somatotopic sensorimotor area that corresponds to the borderzone between the MCAs and ACAs encodes the proximal arms and legs. So when an ACA/MCA borderzone infarct occurs, patients have weakness of their proximal arms and legs with preservation of hand and feet strength; they act like a "man in a barrel." To demonstrate this clinical effect for yourself, sit with your arms at your side and wiggle your fingers and toes but be unable to raise your arms or your legs.[1,2,4–8]

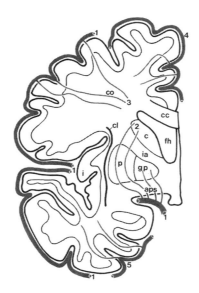

FIGURE 19-5 Coronal section of arterial borderzones. 1, middle cerebral artery; 2, perforating arteries; 3, medullary arteries; 4, anterior cerebral artery; 5, posterior cerebral artery. Used with permission from Bogousslavsky, J., and L. R. Caplan. *Stroke Syndromes,* 2nd ed. Cambridge and New York: Cambridge University Press, 2001.

CORONAL VIEW

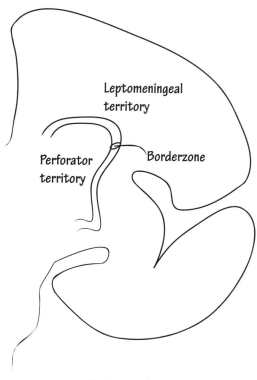

Leptomeningeal
territory

Perforator
territory

Borderzone

End-zone Infarct

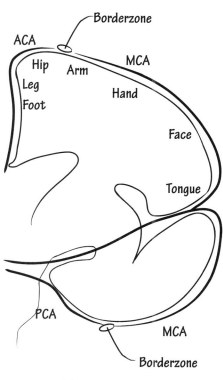

Borderzone

ACA

MCA

Hip   Arm

Leg

Foot   Hand

Face

Tongue

PCA

MCA

Borderzone

Watershed Infarct

DRAWING 19-4 **Arterial Borderzones**

Brainstem Arteries (*Advanced*)

Here, we will draw the brainstem arterial supply. We will begin with the four common brainstem arterial territories as originally defined in the 1960s by Gillian and Lazorthes. First, draw one half of an axial composite of the brainstem: a compression of all three brainstem levels. Then, designate the thin paramedian region as the anteromedial group. Now, divide the remainder of the brainstem from anterior to posterior into the anterolateral, lateral, and posterior groups.

Next, we will make a table of the specific vessels that supply the brainstem. Note that although our list will not be exhaustive, it will cover the major arteries. First, indicate that within the medulla, the anteromedial group is supplied by the anterior spinal artery and direct vertebral artery branches; the anterolateral group is supplied by the anterior spinal artery and the posterior inferior cerebellar arteries; the lateral group is supplied by the posterior inferior cerebellar arteries; and the posterior group is supplied by the posterior inferior cerebellar and posterior spinal arteries. Now, encircle the key medullary arterial vessels: the anterior spinal artery and the posterior inferior cerebellar arteries. Next, note that the common source for these arteries is the vertebral arteries. As a clinical corollary, ischemia to the posterior inferior cerebellar artery results in lateral medullary syndrome, called Wallenberg's syndrome.

Now, let's label the pontine arteries; the first three groups are supplied by basilar branches that travel progressively farther distances to their targets. Indicate that the anteromedial group is supplied by the pontine paramedian arteries; the anterolateral group is supplied by the short pontine circumferential arteries; the lateral group is supplied by the long pontine circumferential arteries and the anterior inferior cerebellar arteries; and,

lastly, the posterior group is supplied by the superior cerebellar arteries: note that the posterior group is found only in the upper pons—it is not present in the mid- or lower pons. Thus, most of the pontine arterial supply comes in the form of circumferential arteries that originate from the basilar and either travel a short distance (the pontine paramedian arteries), a mid-distance (the short pontine circumferential arteries), or a long distance (the long pontine circumferential arteries). The posterior portion of the pons receives additional supply from the anterior inferior cerebellar artery, inferiorly, and the superior cerebellar artery, superiorly. Note that the common source for these arteries is the basilar artery. Basilar ischemia can produce pontine basis strokes, which can cause locked-in syndrome.

Next, let's label the midbrain arteries. The anteromedial group is supplied by basilar tip and proximal PCA branches; indicate that from inferior to superior, these branches are called the inferior and superior paramedian mesencephalic arteries and the thalamoperforate arteries. Then, show that the anterolateral group is supplied by PCA branches: the collicular and posteromedial choroidal arteries. Next, indicate that the lateral and posterior groups are also supplied by the collicular and posteromedial choroidal arteries in concert with the superior cerebellar arteries. Now, let's encircle the key arteries that supply the midbrain: the paramedian mesencephalic and thalamoperforating arteries and the collicular, posteromedial choroidal, and superior cerebellar arteries. Note that the common source for these arteries is the PCAs or distal basilar artery. When basilar clot produces ischemia to the proximal PCAs, large midbrain strokes can occur and produce a so-called "top of the basilar" syndrome.[1-5]

BRAINSTEM ARTERIAL TERRITORIES: AXIAL VIEW

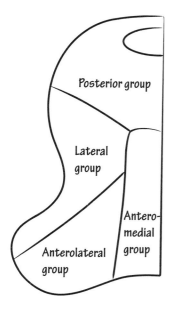

Posterior group

Lateral group

Antero-medial group

Anterolateral group

BRAINSTEM ARTERIAL SUPPLY

	MEDULLA	PONS	MIDBRAIN
ANTEROMEDIAL	Anterior spinal artery Vertebral artery	Pontine paramedian arteries	Paramedian mesen-cephalic & thalamo-perforating arteries
ANTEROLATERAL	Anterior spinal artery Posterior inferior cerebellar artery	Short pontine circum-ferential arteries	Collicular & Posteromedial choroidal arteries
LATERAL	Posterior inferior cerebellar artery	Long pontine circum-ferential arteries Anterior inferior cerebellar artery	Collicular, postero-medial choroidal, & superior cerebellar arteries
POSTERIOR	Posterior inferior cerebellar artery Posterior spinal artery	Superior cerebellar artery	Collicular, postero-medial choroidal, & superior cerebellar arteries
SOURCE	VERTEBRAL ARTERIES	BASILAR ARTERY	POSTERIOR CEREBRAL & DISTAL BASILAR ARTERIES

DRAWING 19-5 **Brainstem Arteries**

Cerebellar Arteries

Here, we will draw the cerebellar arterial supply. First, draw three axial sections through the cerebellum at different heights: inferior, middle, and superior. Next, associate each height with a brainstem level: the inferior cerebellum neighbors the medulla, the middle cerebellum borders the pons, and the superior cerebellum neighbors the midbrain. Three arteries supply the cerebellum: the posterior inferior cerebellar artery (PICA), the anterior inferior cerebellar artery (AICA), and the superior cerebellar artery (SCA). First, show that the PICA supplies the entire inferior cerebellum. Then, further indicate that it divides into lateral and medial branches, which supply the lateral and medial regions of the inferior cerebellum, respectively. Next, show that the SCA supplies the superior cerebellum. Then, further indicate that it divides into lateral and medial branches (similar to the PICA), which supply the lateral and medial superior cerebellum, respectively. Lastly, show that the middle cerebellum is supplied by all three cerebellar arteries: the AICA supplies the anterior, middle cerebellum; the PICA supplies the posterior, middle cerebellum, inferiorly; and the SCA supplies the posterior, middle cerebellum, superiorly. Note that the AICA supplies a large portion of the middle cerebellar peduncle, and also note that it commonly gives off the internal auditory artery, which supplies the inner ear.[1–4,9]

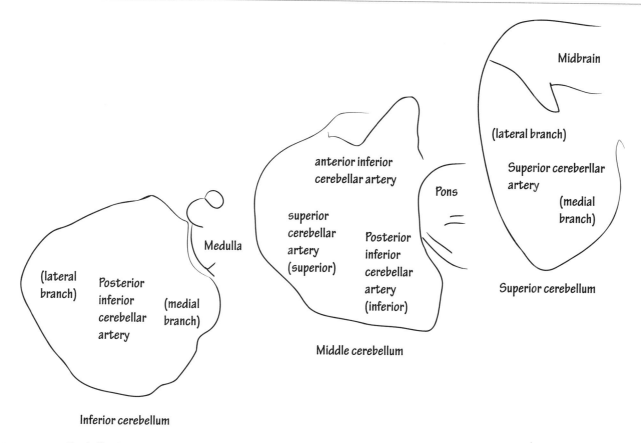

DRAWING 19-6 **Cerebellar Arteries**

Spinal Cord Arteries (*Advanced*)

Here, we will draw the arterial supply of the spinal cord. Begin with the extrinsic system: on one side of the page, draw an axial section through the spinal cord, and on the other, draw an oblique, coronal section. Indicate that a single anterior spinal artery descends the anterior median fissure and that a pair of posterior spinal arteries descends the posterior spinal cord. Next, in the axial cut, show that generally, the anterior spinal artery supplies the anterior two-thirds of the spinal cord and that the posterior arteries supply the posterior one-third. Now, on the coronal side of the diagram, draw the vertebral arteries. Show that near where they join as the basilar artery, vertebral artery branches also join to form the anterior spinal artery. Then, indicate that each vertebral artery produces a single posterior spinal artery. Note, however, that in many instances, the posterior spinal arteries originate from the PICAs, instead. Also, note that in addition to these posterolaterally situated arteries, posteromedial spinal arteries can also exist.

Segmental arteries help supply the anterior and posterior spinal arteries throughout their descent. In our axial diagram, show a source artery and an attached segmental artery. The source arteries and segmental arteries vary along the superior–inferior length of the spinal canal. Throughout the cervical spinal cord, the source artery is the subclavian artery. The segmental arteries in the upper cervical spinal cord are the spinal segmental branches of the vertebral arteries, and in the lower cervical spinal cord, they are the ascending cervical artery (from the thyrocervical trunk) and the deep cervical artery (from the costocervical trunk). In the thoracic and lumbar spinal cord, the descending aorta is the source artery. The segmental branches in the thoracic cord are the posterior intercostal arteries; in the lumbar cord, they are the lumbar arteries. Finally, in the sacral spinal cord, the source artery is the internal iliac artery, most commonly, and the segmental arteries are the lateral sacral arteries.

Next, indicate that where the segmental artery divides into ventral and dorsal branches, the dorsal branch is called the dorsospinal artery, and it forms three types of radicular arteries. Show that the radicular arteries (proper)—anterior and posterior—supply the nerve roots; the radiculomedullary arteries supply the anterior spinal artery; and the radiculopial arteries supply the posterior spinal arteries and also the pial network. Indicate that the pial network is a ring of arterial supply that surrounds the spinal cord; it has superior–inferior interconnections that form an arterial meshwork around the cord. Note that the most important radiculomedullary artery is the artery of Adamkiewicz, which in the majority of people arises from T9 to T12 but which can originate anywhere from T8 to L3; it most commonly originates from the left side of the body. Injury to this artery can lead to paraplegia. At the C5 to C7 level, another notable radiculomedullary artery exists—the artery of the cervical enlargement.

Now, let's draw the intrinsic arterial territories in axial view. They divide into the centrifugal and centripetal systems. Show that the centrifugal system comprises sulcal arteries from the anterior spinal artery, which supply the spinal cord from central to peripheral; they primarily supply the gray matter horns. Then, indicate that the centripetal system comprises vasocoronal perforating arteries from the pial arterial network, which supply the spinal cord from peripheral to central; they primarily supply the white matter funiculi.

We will not address the spinal cord venous system, here, except to note that extensive venous anastomoses exist that communicate with surrounding venous plexuses. The low-pressure state and valveless chambers of the spinal venous system expose the spinal canal to intrathoracic or intra-abdominal abscesses and neoplastic metastases.[2,10,11]

EXTRINSIC ARTERIAL SYSTEM

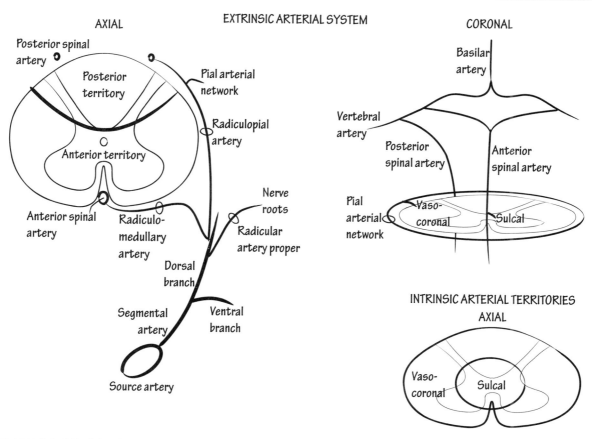

DRAWING 19-7 **Spinal Cord Arteries**

Thalamic Arteries (*Advanced*)

In this diagram, we will draw the thalamic arterial supply. First, on the left-hand side of the page, draw two outlines of the thalamus: we will use these outlines to show the arterial territories of the thalamus. Label one as dorsal and the other as ventral to distinguish the variation in thalamic arterial supply at different heights. Also, include the anterior–posterior and medial–lateral planes of orientation.

On the right-hand side of the page, we will draw the arteries, themselves. First, draw the basilar artery and show that it bifurcates into the bilateral PCAs. Next, draw an axial cut through the left internal carotid artery. Then, connect the left internal carotid artery and left PCA with the posterior communicating artery.

Now, let's show the vessels that supply the thalamus. Emanating from the posterior communicating artery, draw the thalamotuberal artery. The thalamotuberal artery has a few alternate names, which although cumbersome help us to understand its arterial distribution; they include the following: the anterior thalamoperforating artery, premammillary artery, and polar artery. Indicate that within the thalamus, both dorsally as well as ventrally, the thalamotuberal artery supplies the anterior thalamus: specifically, it supplies the ventroanterior nucleus, ventrolateral nucleus, and the anterior portion of the medial thalamic nuclei.

Next, we will draw the medial branch of the posterior choroidal artery. Show that it emerges from the PCA lateral to the posterior communicating artery. The medial posterior choroidal artery supplies the medial thalamus: most notably, the medial posterior pulvinar and medial geniculate body (of the metathalamus). Indicate that dorsally, its arterial supply extends anteriorly, whereas ventrally, its distribution is restricted to being more posterior.

Now, lateral to the medial posterior choroidal artery, draw the lateral posterior choroidal artery, which supplies the lateral pulvinar, dorsomedial thalamic nucleus, and lateral geniculate body (of the metathalamus). Show that dorsally its supply is restricted to the medial posterior thalamus, whereas ventrally its supply extends out laterally.

Next, show that the thalamoperforating arteries emanate from the PCA medial to the posterior communicating artery. Like the thalamotuberal artery, the thalamoperforating arteries have several alternate names; they include the following: the thalamic-subthalamic arteries, paramedian arteries, posterior inferior optic arteries, and deep interpeduncular profunda arteries. The thalamoperforating arteries supply the medial portion of the thalamus. Show that dorsally, the medial extent of their supply ends at the medial posterior choroidal artery territory, whereas ventrally, their supply extends to the medial edge of the thalamus. Much attention is given to the anatomic variant wherein a common stem, the artery of Percheron, emanates from one PCA and provides thalamoperforating branches to the bilateral medial thalamic and extra-thalamic thalamoperforating territories.

Now, in between the posterior choroidal arteries, draw the thalamogeniculate arteries, which supply the lateral thalamus and help supply the geniculate bodies. Dorsally, show that their supply extends posteriorly, whereas ventrally, show that it extends anteriorly.

In addition to supplying the thalamus and metathalamus, the thalamic arteries also help supply many other diencephalic structures, such as the hypothalamus, subthalamus, optic tracts, and internal capsule; they also help supply certain upper brainstem structures, as well as the choroid plexus and hippocampus.[2,4,12–16]

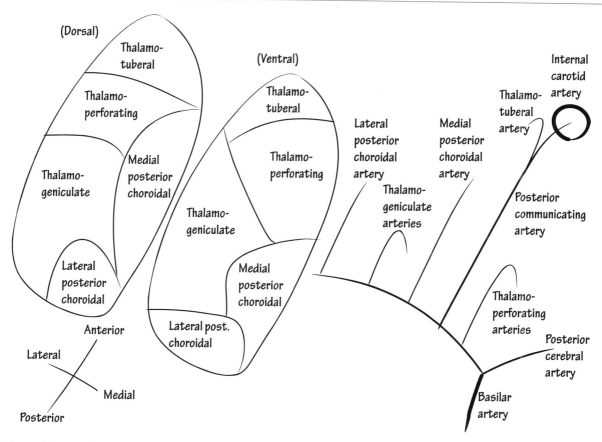

DRAWING 19-8 **Thalamic Arteries**

References

1. Naidich, T. P. & Duvernoy, H. M. *Duvernoy's atlas of the human brain stem and cerebellum: high-field MRI: surface anatomy, internal structure, vascularization and 3D sectional anatomy* (Springer, 2009).

2. Takahashi, S. O. *Neurovascular imaging: MRI & microangiography* (Springer, 2010).

3. Tatu, L., Moulin, T., Bogousslavsky, J. & Duvernoy, H. Arterial territories of human brain: brainstem and cerebellum. *Neurology* 47, 1125–1135 (1996).

4. Bogousslavsky, J. & Caplan, L. R. *Stroke syndromes,* 2nd ed. (Cambridge University Press, 2001).

5. Mai, J. K., Voss, T. & Paxinos, G. *Atlas of the human brain,* 3rd ed. (Elsevier/Academic Press, 2008).

6. Tatu, L., Moulin, T., Bogousslavsky, J. & Duvernoy, H. Arterial territories of the human brain: cerebral hemispheres. *Neurology* 50, 1699–1708 (1998).

7. Roach, E. S., Toole, J. F., Bettermann, K. & Biller, J. *Toole's cerebrovascular disorders,* 6th ed. (Cambridge University Press, 2010).

8. Von Kummer, R., Back, T. & Ay, H. *Magnetic resonance imaging in ischemic stroke* (Springer, 2006).

9. Kelly, P. J., et al. Functional recovery after rehabilitation for cerebellar stroke. *Stroke* 32, 530–534 (2001).

10. Kudo, K., et al. Anterior spinal artery and artery of Adamkiewicz detected by using multi-detector row CT. *AJNR Am J Neuroradiol* 24, 13–17 (2003).

11. Shimizu, S., et al. Origins of the segmental arteries in the aorta: an anatomic study for selective catheterization with spinal arteriography. *AJNR Am J Neuroradiol* 26, 922–928 (2005).

12. Bogousslavsky, J., Regli, F. & Assal, G. The syndrome of unilateral tuberothalamic artery territory infarction. *Stroke* 17, 434–441 (1986).

13. Carrera, E. & Bogousslavsky, J. The thalamus and behavior: effects of anatomically distinct strokes. *Neurology* 66, 1817–1823 (2006).

14. Perren, F., Clarke, S. & Bogousslavsky, J. The syndrome of combined polar and paramedian thalamic infarction. *Arch Neurol* 62, 1212–1216 (2005).

15. Schmahmann, J. D. Vascular syndromes of the thalamus. *Stroke* 34, 2264–2278 (2003).

16. Donkelaar, H. J. *Clinical neuroanatomy* (Springer, 2011).

20

Diencephalon

Know-It Points

The Diencephalon

- The thalamus contains numerous thalamic nuclei and related fiber tracts.
- The metathalamus comprises the medial and lateral geniculate nuclei.
- The subthalamus comprises the subthalamic nucleus, zona incerta, and the nuclei of the fields of Forel.
- The hypothalamus contains numerous hypothalamic nuclei and related fiber tracts, and it also contains the mammillary bodies, and neurohypophysis.

- The epithalamus comprises the habenula, pineal gland, and the pretectal structures.
- Major white matter bundles that pass through the diencephalon are the column of the fornix, stria medullaris thalami, and the anterior, posterior, and habenular commissures.

Thalamus: Anatomy & Function

- The internal medullary lamina separates the medial and lateral thalamic groups.
- The anterior group nuclei communicate with the limbic system.
- The medial group nuclei (the most prominent of which is the dorsomedial nucleus) connect with the prefrontal cortex.
- The lateral group nuclei divide into ventral and dorsal subgroups.
- The ventroanterior nucleus connects with the basal ganglia.
- The ventrolateral nucleus connects primarily with the cerebellum.
- The ventroposterior lateral nucleus receives sensory afferents from the body.
- The ventroposterior medial nucleus receives sensory afferents from the face.

- The dorsolateral nucleus communicates with the limbic system.
- The pulvinar is important for visual attention.
- The medial geniculate nucleus is part of the auditory system.
- The lateral geniculate nucleus is part of the visual system.
- The most notable function of the posterior group nuclei is nociceptive sensory processing.
- The intralaminar group helps form the ascending arousal system for wakefulness.
- The midline group nuclei function in limbic-related processes.
- The thalamic reticular nucleus modulates thalamic output.

Hypothalamus: Nuclei

- Within the hypothalamus, from medial to lateral, are the periventricular, intermediate, and lateral zones.
- Both the periventricular and intermediate zones are highly cellular whereas the lateral zone contains a high degree of white matter fibers.
- The anteromedial hypothalamus is involved in parasympathetic activity whereas the posterolateral hypothalamus is involved in sympathetic activity.

- The anterior (aka chiasmatic) group encompasses the region above and anterior to the optic chiasm and optic tract.
- The middle (aka tuberal) group encompasses the region between the optic chiasm and mammillary bodies (ie, the region above the tuber cinereum).
- The posterior (aka mammillary) group encompasses the mammillary bodies and the region above them.

Hypothalamus: Tracts

- The magnocellular neurons of the paraventricular and supraoptic nuclei project to the capillary plexus of the neurohypophysis via the hypothalamohypophysial tract.
- The paraventricular and supraoptic nuclei release the hormones vasopressin (aka antidiuretic hormone [ADH]) and oxytocin.
- The epithelial-cell–filled adenohypophysis releases the following hormones into the general circulation

via hypophysial veins: follicle-stimulating hormone, luteinizing hormone, adrenocorticotropic hormone, thyroid-stimulating hormone, prolactin, growth hormone, and melanocyte-stimulating hormone. The hypothalamus controls the release of the aforementioned hormones via a variety of parvocellular neurons, the most notable of which is the arcuate (aka infundibular) nucleus.

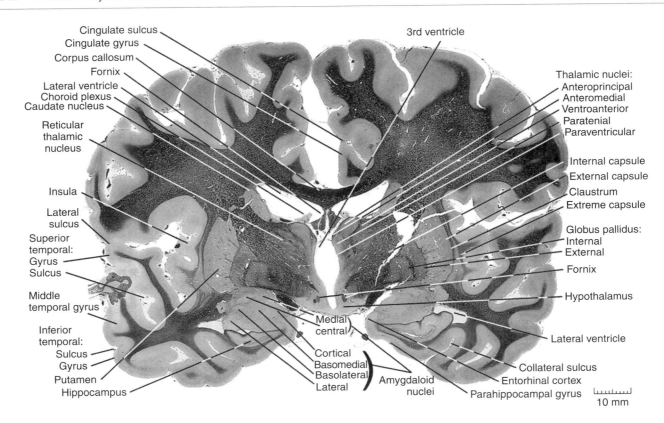

FIGURE 20-1 Coronal section through the diencephalon. Used with permission from the Michigan State University: Brain Biodiversity Bank. https://www.msu.edu/~brains/

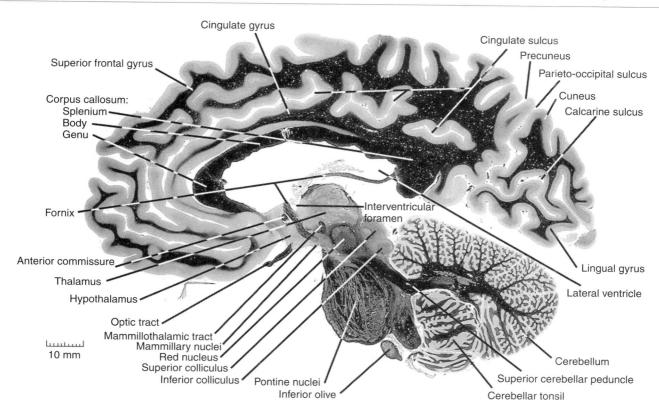

FIGURE 20-2 **Sagittal section through the diencephalon. Used with permission from the Michigan State University: Brain Biodiversity Bank.** https://www.msu.edu/~brains/

The Diencephalon

Here, we will draw the anatomy of the diencephalon. First, list the major groups of diencephalic structures: the thalamus, metathalamus, subthalamus, hypothalamus, and epithalamus. Now, include the major structures categorized within these groups. Indicate that the thalamus contains numerous thalamic nuclei and related fiber tracts; the metathalamus comprises the medial and lateral geniculate nuclei; the subthalamus comprises the subthalamic nucleus, zona incerta, and the nuclei of the fields of Forel; then, show that the hypothalamus contains numerous hypothalamic nuclei and related fiber tracts, and also contains the mammillary bodies, and neurohypophysis, which is the posterior lobe of the pituitary body and which subdivides into a neural lobe and infundibulum; then, show that the epithalamus comprises the habenula, pineal gland, and the pretectal structures, which include the pretectal area, pretectal nuclei, posterior commissure, and subcommissural organ. Finally, let's list some of the major white matter bundles that pass through the diencephalon: the column of the fornix, stria medullaris thalami, and the anterior, posterior, and habenular commissures.

Now, let's draw the diencephalon in sagittal view. First, label the central portion of the diagram as the hypothalamus and then define its borders. Draw the lamina terminalis as the anterior border of the hypothalamus; it separates the hypothalamus from the subcallosal region of the limbic lobe and it is variably considered either a diencephalic or telencephalic structure. Indicate that the lamina terminalis spans from the anterior commissure, superiorly, to the optic chiasm, inferiorly.[1-3] Next, draw the tuber cinereum as the inferior border of the hypothalamus. Show that it ends, posteriorly, at the mammillary bodies.

Next, antero-inferiorly, draw the funnel-shaped dip in the tuber cinereum called the median eminence; attach to it the infundibulum (the pituitary stalk); and attach to the infundibulum, the pituitary gland. Label the posterior part of the pituitary gland as the neural lobe; it is neurally connected to the hypothalamus via the hypothalamohypophysial tract. Then, label the anterior lobe of the pituitary gland as the adenohypophysis; it forms from Rathke's pouch—an outgrowth of the roof of the mouth, and therefore, it is not a diencephalic structure. The adenohypophysis is linked to the hypothalamus via the hypothalamohypophysial venous portal system.[4,5]

Now, for anatomic reference, include the midbrain and its superior and inferior colliculi. Then, draw the epithalamic structures: first, above the colliculi, draw the pineal gland; anterior to it, draw the pretectal structures; and then above them, draw the habenula and habenular commissure. Next, anterior to the epithalamus, draw the egg-shaped thalamus. Then, indicate that the stria medullaris thalami passes from the habenula along the dorsomedial thalamus to the septal nuclei, which lie above the anterior commissure (they are part of the limbic system). Finally, show that the column of the fornix descends through the hypothalamus and connects with the mammillary bodies.

Next, we will draw the central diencephalon in coronal view. For anatomic reference, superiorly, include the corpus callosum, body of the fornix, body of the lateral ventricle; then, laterally, include the internal capsule, which becomes the cerebral peduncle as it descends through the brainstem; next, inferiorly, draw the pons; in midline, lying medial to the cerebral peduncle, draw the interpeduncular cistern; and above it, draw the third ventricle. Now let's draw the major diencephalic structures visible in this section: superiorly, draw the thalamus; ventrolateral to it, draw the subthalamus; and ventromedial to it, along the lateral wall of the third ventricle, draw the hypothalamus and include its infero-lying mammillary bodies. Finally, show that the supramammillary commissure stretches across midline above the mammillary bodies.[6-8]

Diencephalon structures

thalamus
    thalamic nuclei
    thalamic fiber tracts

metathalamus
    medial geniculate nucleus
    lateral geniculate nucleus

subthalamus
    subthalamic nucleus
    zona incerta
    Forel's fields nuclei

hypothalamus
    hypothalamic nuclei
    hypothalamic fiber tracts
    mammillary bodies
    neurohypophysis
        neural lobe
        infundibulum

epithalamus
    habenula
    pineal gland
    pretectal structures
        pretectal area
        pretectal nuclei
        posterior commissure
        subcommissural organ

Major white matter bundles
column of fornix
stria medullaris thalami
commissures
    anterior
    posterior
    habenular

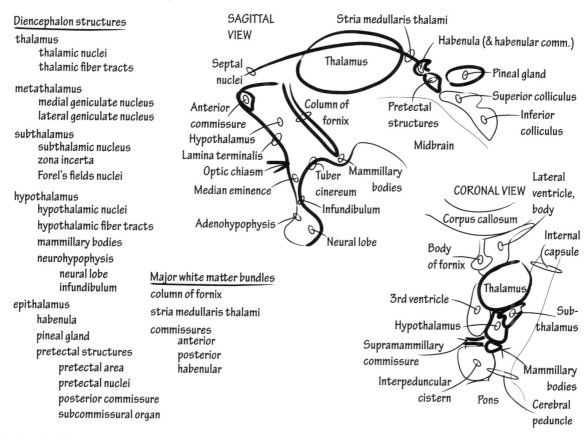

SAGITTAL VIEW

Stria medullaris thalami
Habenula (& habenular comm.)
Thalamus
Septal nuclei
Pineal gland
Anterior commissure
Column of fornix
Pretectal structures
Superior colliculus
Hypothalamus
Inferior colliculus
Lamina terminalis
Optic chiasm
Midbrain
Median eminence
Tuber cinereum
Mammillary bodies
Adenohypophysis
Infundibulum
Neural lobe

CORONAL VIEW
Lateral ventricle, body
Corpus callosum
Internal capsule
Body of fornix
Thalamus
3rd ventricle
Sub-thalamus
Hypothalamus
Supramammillary commissure
Mammillary bodies
Interpeduncular cistern
Pons
Cerebral peduncle

DRAWING 20-1 The Diencephalon

The Thalamus, Part 1 (*Advanced*)

Here, in two separate parts, we will create a table to organize the many different thalamic and metathalamic nuclei into several anatomic groups and briefly discuss their functional roles. Across the top of the page, write group, nucleus, function/connections. First, label the anterior nuclear group. Indicate that it comprises the principal anterior and anterodorsal nuclei; in nonhuman species, the principal anterior nucleus is subdivided into the anteromedial and anteroventral nuclei.[9] Show that the anterior nuclear group communicates with the mammillary bodies and cingulate gyrus as part of the Papez circuit.

Now, label the medial nuclear group. Indicate that the dorsomedial nucleus is the most prominent nucleus within this group, and show that it has important connections with the prefrontal cortex.

Next, label the lateral nuclear group, which divides into dorsal and ventral subgroups. Indicate that the dorsal subgroup comprises the dorsolateral, lateral posterior, and pulvinar nuclei. Then, show that the dorsolateral nucleus bundles functionally with the anterior nuclear group and communicates with the limbic system. Next, indicate that the lateral posterior and pulvinar nuclei collectively form the pulvinar–lateral posterior complex, which is involved in visual attention. The pulvinar relays visual input from the superior colliculus to the visual cortex as part of the extrageniculate visual pathway.

Now, show that the ventral subgroup of the lateral nuclear group comprises the ventroanterior, ventrolateral, and ventroposterior nuclei. Indicate that the ventroanterior nucleus receives projections from the basal ganglia, most notably, and that the ventrolateral nucleus receives cerebellar and red nucleus projections as part of the corticopontocerebellar pathway, most notably, but indicate that it also receives basal ganglia projections, as well. Both the ventroanterior and ventrolateral nuclei project to the motor cortex. Note that there is inconsistency in the literature regarding whether the ventroanterior nucleus projects to primary motor cortex as well as premotor cortex or simply premotor cortex and there is inconsistency as to whether its afferent fibers are primarily from the basal ganglia or cerebellum.[10]

Next, indicate that the ventroposterior nucleus subdivides into medial and lateral nuclei, and show that the ventroposterior medial nucleus receives sensory afferents from the face and that the ventroposterior lateral nucleus receives sensory afferents from the body. The ventroposterior inferior nucleus, a less commonly discussed nucleus, also exists. Sensory information in the thalamus has a very specific somatosensory map in which the fist is adjacent to the mouth. Small ventroposterior strokes in the lateral portion of the ventroposteromedial nucleus and medial portion of the ventroposterolateral nucleus result in the characteristic cheiro-oral syndrome in which there is loss of sensation around the mouth and in the fist contralateral to the side of the thalamic infarct.

Now, label the posterior nuclear group, which lies beneath the pulvinar and spans posteriorly from the caudal pole of the ventroposterior nucleus to the medial geniculate nucleus and also extends medial to the medial geniculate nucleus. Show that it comprises the posterior, limitans, and suprageniculate nuclei. The posterior nuclear group has broad cortical connections; here, simply denote the commonly cited secondary somatosensory cortical projections of the posterior nucleus, which are involved in nociceptive sensory processing.[3,8,11,12]

We complete the table, next.

THALAMUS (PART 1)

GROUP	NUCLEUS	FUNCTION/CONNECTIONS
Anterior nuclear	Principal anterior Anterodorsal	Papez circuit
Medial nuclear	Dorsomedial	Prefrontal cortex
Lateral nuclear		
Dorsal subgroup	Dorsolateral Lateral posterior Pulvinar	Limbic system Lateral posterior & pulvinar- subserve visual attention
Ventral subgroup	Ventroanterior Ventrolateral Ventroposterior	Basal ganglia Cerebellum, red nucleus (& basal ganglia)
	Medial Lateral	Facial sensory fibers Body sensory fibers
Posterior nuclear	Posterior Limitans Suprageniculate	Example: posterior nucleus- nociceptive sensation

DRAWING 20-2 **The Thalamus, Part 1**

The Thalamus, Part 2 (*Advanced*)

Now, label the intralaminar nuclear group, which divides into caudal and rostral subgroups. The caudal subgroup is the most notable; it comprises the centromedian and parafascicular nuclei. The rostral subgroup comprises a cluster of closely related nuclei: the central medial, paracentral, and central lateral nuclei. The intralaminar nuclei project to other thalamic nuclei, notably the ventroanterior and ventrolateral nuclei; they have key connections to the basal ganglia; and they project diffusely to other cortical and subcortical areas. The intralaminar nuclei play an important role in a wide range of processes; as an important example, indicate that they participate in the ascending arousal system, which is fundamental to wakefulness.[13,14]

Next, indicate the midline nuclear group, which, by at least one definition, comprises the rhomboid, parataenial, paraventricular, and reuniens nuclei—the reuniens nucleus lies immediately ventral to the interthalamic adhesion. Show that this group of nuclei is reportedly involved in limbic-related processes and that it has important hippocampal connections.[15]

Now, label the thalamic reticular nucleus, which lies along the rostral, ventral, and lateral aspects of the thalamus in between the thalamic external medullary lamina and the posterior limb of the internal capsule. Show that it contains GABAergic neurons, which modulate thalamic output. The external medullary lamina is a white matter layer that surrounds the lateral aspect of the thalamus.

Finally, indicate the metathalamus and show that it comprises the medial geniculate and lateral geniculate nuclei. Indicate that the medial geniculate nucleus forms an important step in the auditory system pathway; it receives afferents from the inferior colliculus, which it projects to the transverse temporal gyri (of Heschl). Then, show that the lateral geniculate nucleus forms an important step in the visual system pathway; it receives afferents from the optic tract, which it projects to the primary visual cortex.[8]

THALAMUS (PART 2)

GROUP	NUCLEUS	FUNCTION/CONNECTIONS
Intralaminar nuclear		
Caudal subgroup	Centromedian	Connects with other thalamic nuclei,
	Parafascicular	basal ganglia, and diffuse cortical/
Rostral subgroup	Central medial	subcortical areas; example function -
	Paracentral	ascending arousal system
	Central lateral	
Midline nuclear	Rhomboid	Limbic-related processes/
	Parataenial	hippocampal connections
	Paraventricular	
	Reuniens	
	Thalamic reticular	Modulates thalamic output

METATHALAMUS

NUCLEUS	FUNCTION/CONNECTIONS
Medial geniculate	Auditory system
Lateral geniculate	Visual system

DRAWING 20-3 **The Thalamus, Part 2**

Thalamus: Anatomy & Function

Here, we will draw the egg-shaped anatomy of the thalamus and metathalamus and review their functional highlights. First, draw the back end of the thalamus and then the front; we leave the thalamus open so we can label its interior nuclei. Now, draw the anterior–posterior and medial–lateral planes of orientation. Next, along the anterior–posterior axis of the thalamus, draw the internal medullary lamina. Show that anteriorly it bifurcates to envelop the anterior group nuclei; the length of the internal medullary lamina separates the medial and lateral thalamic groups. Now, indicate that the anterior group nuclei communicate with the limbic system. Then, label the medial group nuclei (the most prominent of which is the dorsomedial nucleus) and show that they connect with the prefrontal cortex.

Next, let's label the lateral group nuclei, which divide into ventral and dorsal subgroups. First, label the ventral subgroup nuclei: anteriorly, label the ventroanterior nucleus, which connects with the basal ganglia; in the middle, label the ventrolateral nucleus, which connects with the cerebellum, red nucleus, and, to a lesser extent, the basal ganglia; and posteriorly, label the ventroposterior nucleus. Show that the ventroposterior nucleus further divides into lateral and medial nuclei. Denote that the ventroposterior lateral nucleus receives sensory afferent projections from the body whereas the ventroposterior medial nucleus receives sensory afferents from the face; both nuclei then relay these sensory projections to the somatosensory cortex.

Next, let's label the dorsal subgroup of the lateral group nuclei. First, anteriorly, label the dorsolateral nucleus, which communicates with the limbic system along with the anterior group nuclei; in the middle, label the lateral posterior nucleus; and posteriorly, label

the pulvinar. Indicate that the pulvinar, which is part of the extrageniculate visual pathway, is important for visual attention (as is the lateral posterior nucleus).

Now, let's address the two metathalamic nuclei: draw the medial geniculate nucleus underneath the medial aspect of the pulvinar and the lateral geniculate nucleus underneath the lateral aspect of the pulvinar. Show that the medial geniculate nucleus is part of the auditory system and that the lateral geniculate nucleus is involved in the visual system.

Next, beneath the pulvinar, label the posterior group nuclei; they span posteriorly from the caudal pole of the ventroposterior nucleus to the medial geniculate nucleus and they also extend medial to the medial geniculate nucleus. The most notable function of the posterior group nuclei is nociceptive sensory processing. Although it is not easy to appreciate the following from this diagram, the pulvinar, which lies above the posterior group nuclei, actually extends farther posterior than any of the other thalamic nuclei or the metathalamic nuclei.

Next, in the center of the diagram, label the intralaminar group, which has widespread connectivity and is involved in multiple functional roles but most notably helps form the ascending arousal system for wakefulness. Now, draw the midline group nuclei along the ventromedial portion of the thalamus in the midline of the central nervous system; they function in limbic-related processes. Then, lastly, write out that the thalamic reticular nucleus forms a shell around the rostral/ventral/lateral thalamus, and indicate that it modulates thalamic output. The posterior limb of the internal capsule lies lateral to the reticular nucleus and the external medullary lamina lies in between the reticular nucleus and the lateral border of the thalamus.

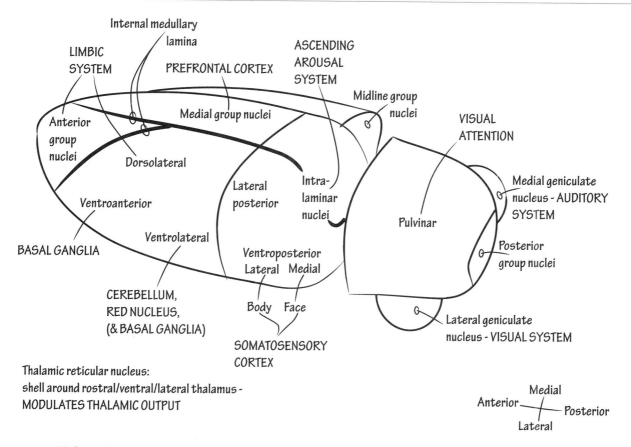

DRAWING 20-4 **Thalamus: Anatomy & Function**

Hypothalamus: Nuclei

Here, we will draw the hypothalamic zones, nuclear groups, and the most prominent hypothalamic nuclei. First, draw the hypothalamic zones in coronal section. Draw the third ventricle and the adjacent hypothalamus and above it label the thalamus. Next, from medial to lateral within the hypothalamus, label the periventricular, intermediate, and lateral zones. Indicate that the column of the fornix lies in between the intermediate and lateral zones and distinguishes them. Now, indicate that the periventricular and intermediate zones are often collectively referred to as the medial zone (as we will routinely refer to them, here); however, the medial zone is sometimes used to refer to the intermediate zone, only, instead. Both the periventricular and intermediate zones are highly cellular whereas the lateral zone contains a high degree of white matter fibers.

Now, we will draw hypothalamic nuclear groups. Draw a sagittal outline of the hypothalamus: along the inferior border, include the pituitary stalk and mammillary bodies and in between them label the tuber cinereum; then, label the anterior border of the hypothalamus as the lamina terminalis and antero-superiorly draw the anterior commissure and antero-inferiorly draw the optic chiasm. Next, although it is an oversimplification, include the following important physiologic principle: the anteromedial hypothalamus is involved in parasympathetic activity (eg, satiety, sleep, and heat dissipation to decrease body temperature) and the posterolateral hypothalamus is involved in sympathetic activity (hunger, wakefulness, and heat conservation to increase body temperature).[3,16] Now, label the anterior (aka chiasmatic) group as encompassing the region above and anterior to the optic chiasm and optic tract; then, label the middle (aka tuberal) group as encompassing the region between the optic chiasm and mammillary bodies (ie, the region above the tuber cinereum); and then, label the posterior (aka mammillary) group as encompassing the mammillary bodies and the region above them.

Next, let's draw the individual nuclei; begin with the hypothalamic nuclei of the medial zone (the collective periventricular and intermediate zones). First, draw the anterior (chiasmatic) group nuclei: from inferior to superior, starting just above the optic chiasm, draw the suprachiasmatic, anterior, and paraventricular nuclei. Next, in the preoptic region, label the medial preoptic nucleus in front of the anterior nucleus. The preoptic nucleus develops as part of the telencephalon but is anatomically and functionally related to the hypothalamus, so it is commonly included as part of the hypothalamus. Note that the preoptic region is often distinguished from the anterior group as its own nuclear group. Now, draw the middle (tuberal) group nuclei: from inferior to superior, starting along the tuber cinereum, draw the infundibular (aka arcuate) nucleus and then the ventromedial and dorsomedial nuclei. Next, draw the posterior (mammillary) group nuclei: first, within the mammillary body, draw the medial mammillary nucleus, and then above it, draw the posterior nucleus. Finally, extending through the inferior aspect of the middle (tuberal) and posterior (mammillary) groups, draw the medial aspect of the tuberomammillary nucleus.

Now, recreate a sagittal view of the hypothalamus so we can draw the lateral zone hypothalamic nuclei. First, anteriorly, in the preoptic region, draw the lateral preoptic nucleus. Then, above the optic tract, draw the supraoptic nucleus. Note that many texts list this nucleus as lying within the medial zone of the hypothalamus rather than the lateral zone. Next, draw the lateral aspect of the tuberomammillary nucleus along the inferior aspect of the hypothalamus extending through the middle and posterior groups. Now, draw a small nucleus in the posterior aspect of the tuberal region, called the lateral tuberal nucleus. Then, label the lateral mammillary nucleus. And finally, delineate the lateral hypothalamic area, which spans from the posterior optic chiasm to the posterior end of the hypothalamus; it, most notably, contains the medial forebrain bundle.[3,6–8,17–21]

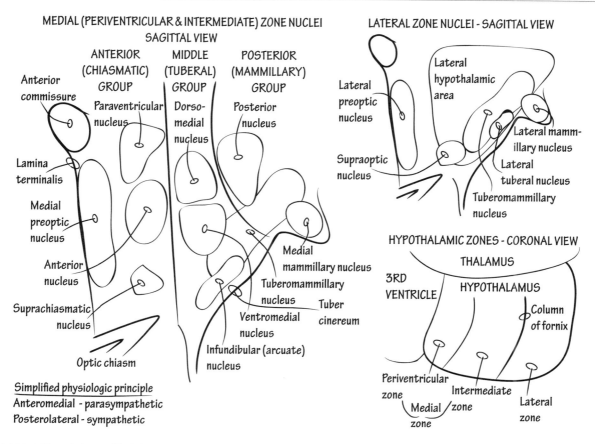

MEDIAL (PERIVENTRICULAR & INTERMEDIATE) ZONE NUCLEI
SAGITTAL VIEW

ANTERIOR (CHIASMATIC) GROUP
MIDDLE (TUBERAL) GROUP
POSTERIOR (MAMMILLARY) GROUP

Anterior commissure

Paraventricular nucleus

Dorso-medial nucleus

Posterior nucleus

Lamina terminalis

Medial preoptic nucleus

Anterior nucleus

Suprachiasmatic nucleus

Medial mammillary nucleus

Tuberomammillary nucleus

Tuber cinereum

Ventromedial nucleus

Infundibular (arcuate) nucleus

Optic chiasm

Simplified physiologic principle
Anteromedial - parasympathetic
Posterolateral - sympathetic

LATERAL ZONE NUCLEI - SAGITTAL VIEW

Lateral hypothalamic area

Lateral preoptic nucleus

Lateral mammillary nucleus

Supraoptic nucleus

Lateral tuberal nucleus

Tuberomammillary nucleus

HYPOTHALAMIC ZONES - CORONAL VIEW

THALAMUS

3RD VENTRICLE

HYPOTHALAMUS

Column of fornix

Periventricular zone

Intermediate zone

Lateral zone

Medial zone

DRAWING 20-5 **Hypothalamus: Nuclei**

Hypothalamus: Tracts

Here, we will draw the prominent pathways of the hypothalamus and in the process learn select highlights of its physiology. Draw a sagittal view of the hypothalamus and pituitary gland, midbrain, and thalamus. Then divide the pituitary gland into the adenohypophysis, anteriorly, and neurohypophysis, posteriorly. Next, label the paraventricular and supraoptic nuclei (a more accurate depiction of their anatomic positions is shown in Drawing 20-5). Now, within the neurohypophysis, draw a capillary plexus. Then, show that the magnocellular neurons of the paraventricular and supraoptic nuclei project to the capillary plexus of the neurohypophysis via the hypothalamohypophysial tract, and then show that the neurohypophysis releases hormones into the general circulation via the hypophysial veins. Indicate that through this pathway, the paraventricular and supraoptic nuclei release the hormones vasopressin (aka antidiuretic hormone [ADH]) and oxytocin. Vasopressin causes increased reabsorption of water in the collecting tubules of the kidneys. Oxytocin causes increased uterine and mammillary gland contraction. Note that the hypothalamohypophysial tract is also referred to as the combined supraopticohypophysial and paraventriculohypophysial tracts.

Now, within the median eminence of the hypothalamus, draw the primary capillary plexus. Then, within the adenohypophysis, draw the secondary capillary plexus. Next, connect the primary and secondary plexuses with the hypothalamohypophysial portal venous system. Then, show that the epithelial-cell–filled adenohypophysis releases the following hormones into the general circulation via hypophysial veins: follicle-stimulating hormone, luteinizing hormone, adrenocorticotropic hormone, thyroid-stimulating hormone, prolactin, growth hormone, and melanocyte-stimulating hormone. Note that the first five hormones form the quirky yet memorable acronym FLATPiG. The hypothalamus controls the release of these hormones via a variety of parvocellular neurons, which release chemicals (peptides, most notably) into the primary capillary plexus that serve as either releasing hormones or release-inhibiting hormones; the most notable source of these neurochemicals is the arcuate (aka infundibular) nucleus. Often the name of the releasing hormone contains the name of the hormone itself; for instance, growth hormone-releasing hormone promotes the release of growth hormone.[20,21] One clinically important release-inhibiting hormone is dopamine, which inhibits the release of prolactin; therefore, exogenous dopamine agonists, such as bromocriptine, are used to help control prolactin levels and reduce tumor size in prolactin-secreting pituitary tumors (prolactinomas).[22]

Now, let's show some additional hypothalamic tracts. Show that the amygdala, the emotional center, projects fibers that pass over the thalamus to the bed nucleus of the stria terminalis, septal nuclei, and hypothalamus via the stria terminalis.[23] Then, show that the fornix sends a descending column through the hypothalamus to the mammillary nuclei and that the mammillary nuclei project to the anterior thalamic nuclei via the mammillothalamic fasciculus; these two projections form a key portion of the Papez circuit, an important limbic system pathway for memory consolidation (see Drawing 21-4).

Next, indicate that the mammillary nuclei project via the mammillotegmental fasciculus to the brainstem tegmentum. Most texts indicate that the mammillotegmental fasciculus terminates in the midbrain, but select texts indicate that it also projects to the pons.[24,25] Then, show that the retino-hypothalamic pathway, which is fundamental for the regulation of the light–dark circadian cycle, synapses in the suprachiasmatic nuclei. Now, show that diffuse nuclei of the limbic system, including those of the septal nuclei and the olfactory and periamygdaloid areas, project through the lateral hypothalamus to the midbrain tegmentum as the medial forebrain bundle.[20,25] Finally, show that the dorsal longitudinal fasciculus projects from the hypothalamus into the brainstem; it coalesces most prominently in the periaqueductal gray area (in the midbrain).[6,7]

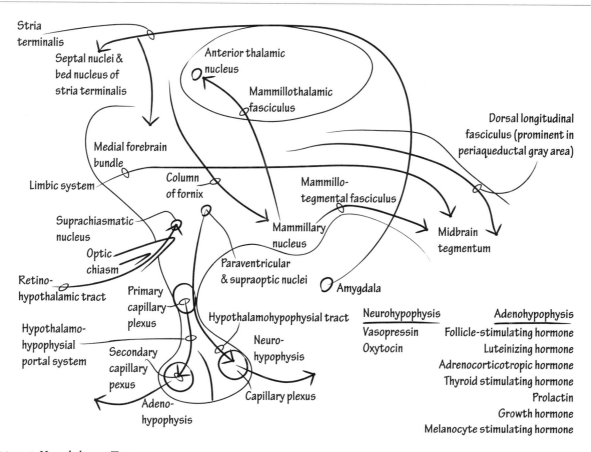

Stria terminalis

Septal nuclei & bed nucleus of stria terminalis

Anterior thalamic nucleus

Mammillothalamic fasciculus

Dorsal longitudinal fasciculus (prominent in periaqueductal gray area)

Medial forebrain bundle

Limbic system

Column of fornix

Mammillo-tegmental fasciculus

Suprachiasmatic nucleus

Optic chiasm

Retino-hypothalamic tract

Paraventricular & supraoptic nuclei

Mammillary nucleus

Midbrain tegmentum

Amygdala

Primary capillary plexus

Hypothalamohypophysial tract

Hypothalamo-hypophysial portal system

Secondary capillary pexus

Neuro-hypophysis

Adeno-hypophysis

Capillary plexus

Neurohypophysis	Adenohypophysis
Vasopressin	Follicle-stimulating hormone
Oxytocin	Luteinizing hormone
	Adrenocorticotropic hormone
	Thyroid stimulating hormone
	Prolactin
	Growth hormone
	Melanocyte stimulating hormone

DRAWING 20-6 **Hypothalamus: Tracts**

References

1. Upledger, J. E. *A brain is born: exploring the birth and development of the central nervous system,* 1st pbk. ed., pp. 149–150 (North Atlantic Books; Upledger Enterprises, 2010).

2. Badie, B. *Neurosurgical operative atlas. Neuro-oncology,* 2nd ed., pp. 42–44 (Thieme; American Association of Neurosurgeons, 2007).

3. Afifi, A. K. & Bergman, R. A. *Functional neuroanatomy: text and atlas,* 2nd ed., Chapter 21 (Lange Medical Books/McGraw-Hill, 2005).

4. Ramamurti, R. *Textbooks of operative neurosurgery,* Vol. 1, Chapter 41 (BI Publications Pvt. Ltd., 2005).

5. Akalan, N. Neuroendocrine research models. *Acta Neurochir Suppl* 83, 85–91 (2002).

6. Mai, J. K., Voss, T. & Paxinos, G. *Atlas of the human brain,* 3rd ed. (Elsevier/Academic Press, 2008).

7. Naidich, T. P. & Duvernoy, H. M. *Duvernoy's atlas of the human brain stem and cerebellum: high-field MRI: surface anatomy, internal structure, vascularization and 3D sectional anatomy* (Springer, 2009).

8. Nieuwenhuys, R., Voogd, J. & Huijzen, C. V. *The human central nervous system,* 4th ed. (Springer, 2008).

9. Butler, A. B. & Hodos, W. *Comparative vertebrate neuroanatomy: evolution and adaptation,* 2nd ed., p. 435 (Wiley-Interscience, 2005).

10. Citow, J. S. *Neuroanatomy and neurophysiology : a review,* p. 35 (Thieme, 2001).

11. Jacobson, S. & Marcus, E. M. *Neuroanatomy for the neuroscientist,* Chapters 6 & 7 (Springer, 2008).

12. Arslan, O. *Neuroanatomical basis of clinical neurology,* pp. 101–102 (Parthenon Pub. Group, 2001).

13. Mendoza, J. E. & Foundas, A. L. *Clinical neuroanatomy: a neurobehavioral approach,* p. 204 (Springer, 2008).

14. Steriade, M. *The intact and sliced brain,* p. 255 (MIT Press, 2001).

15. Dauber, W. & Feneis, H. *Pocket atlas of human anatomy,* 5th rev. ed., p. 364 (Thieme, 2007).

16. Biller, J. *The interface of neurology & internal medicine,* p. 466 (Wolters Kluwer Health/Lippincott Wiliams & Wilkins, 2008).

17. Haines, D. E. & Ard, M. D. *Fundamental neuroscience: for basic and clinical applications,* 3rd ed. (Churchill Livingstone Elsevier, 2006).

18. Standring, S. & Gray, H. *Gray's anatomy: the anatomical basis of clinical practice,* 40th ed., p. 318 (Churchill Livingstone/Elsevier, 2008).

19. Waxman, S. G. *Clinical neuroanatomy.* 25th ed., p. 127 (Lange Medical Books/McGraw-Hill, Medical Pub. Division, 2003).

20. Moore, S. P. & Psarros, T. G. *The definitive neurological surgery board review,* pp. 44–49 (Blackwell Pub., 2005).

21. Kiernan, J. A. & Barr, M. L. *Barr's the human nervous system: an anatomical viewpoint,* 9th ed. (Wolters Kluwer/Lippincott, Williams & Wilkins, 2009).

22. Becker, K. L. *Principles and practice of endocrinology and metabolism,* 3rd ed., p. 238 (Lippincott Williams & Wilkins, 2001).

23. Liddle, P. F. & Royal College of Psychiatrists. *Disordered mind and brain: the neural basis of mental symptoms,* p. 43 (Gaskell; Distributed in North America by American Psychiatric Press, 2001).

24. Martin, J. H. *Neuroanatomy: text and atlas,* 3rd ed., p. 499 (McGraw-Hill Companies, Inc., 2003).

25. Conn, M. *Neuroscience in Medicine,* 3rd ed., p. 389 (Humana Press, 2008).

21

Limbic and Olfactory Systems

Limbic System, Part 1

Limbic System, Part 2 (Advanced)

Hippocampus: Anatomy

Hippocampus: Circuitry

Olfactory System, Part 1

Olfactory System, Part 2 (Advanced)

Olfactory Cortex & Basal Forebrain, Part 1

Olfactory Cortex & Basal Forebrain, Part 2 (Advanced)

Know-It Points

Limbic System, Part 1

- The limbic system forms outer and inner rings around the diencephalon.
- The anterior cingulate gyrus is part of the anterior network of motivation, attention, and behavior and is associated with the amygdala.
- The posterior cingulate gyrus is part of the posterior network of learning and memory and is associated with the hippocampus.
- The parahippocampal gyrus forms the inferior aspect of the limbic gyrus; it channels information to and from the hippocampus to help in memory consolidation.
- The hippocampus lies along the anteroposterior length of the superior aspect of the parahippocampal gyrus; it is the center for memory processing.
- The amygdala divides into corticomedial and basolateral groups.
- The corticomedial group of the amygdala connects, most notably, to the olfactory system and hypothalamus for autonomic function.
- The basolateral group of the amygdala connects, most notably, to the thalamus and prefrontal cortex for such functions as sensory processing of visual, auditory, and somatosensory stimuli.

Limbic System, Part 2 (*Advanced*)

- The cingulum spans the cingulate and parahippocampal gyri.
- The cingulum, most notably, interconnects intracingulate areas and synapses in the hippocampus.
- Via the stria terminalis, the amygdala projects to the septal nuclei, bed nucleus of the stria terminalis, and hypothalamus.
- The fornix emerges from the hippocampus, wraps around the thalamus, and passes anteriorly in midline just below the corpus callosum.

Hippocampus: Anatomy

- The subdivisions of the cornu ammonis from the dentate gyrus to the subiculum are CA4, CA3, CA2, and CA1.
- CA1 forms the largest stretch of Ammon's horn and is distinctively susceptible to anoxic injury.
- The entorhinal and perirhinal cortices form the anterior parahippocampal gyrus.
- The posterior parahippocampal gyrus is referred to as the parahippocampal cortex and corresponds to Von Economo areas TF and TH.
- The uncus forms the anterior gyral thumb of the parahippocampal gyrus.

Hippocampus: Circuitry

- The Papez circuit (extrahippocampal circuitry):
  - The entorhinal cortex projects to the hippocampus.
  - The hippocampus projects to the mammillary nuclei.
  - The mammillary nuclei project to the anterior thalamic nuclei.
  - The anterior thalamic nuclei project to the cingulate gyrus.
  - The cingulate gyrus projects back to the entorhinal cortex.
- The Papez circuit is the cornerstone of memory consolidation.

- The perforant pathway (intrahippocampal circuitry):
  - The entorhinal cortex projects through the subiculum to the dentate gyrus.
  - The dentate gyrus projects to CA3.
  - CA3 projects to CA1 via Schaffer collaterals.
  - CA1 projects to the subiculum.
  - The subiculum projects along the alveus to the fimbria, which passes posteriorly and becomes the crus of the fornix.
  - The subiculum also projects back to the entorhinal cortex.

Olfactory System

- The olfactory neurons lie within the olfactory epithelium and project through the cribriform plate to innervate the olfactory bulb.
- The olfactory bulb and tract are telencephalic extensions of the cerebrum.
- The medial olfactory stria innervates the medial olfactory area in the subcallosal region.
- The lateral olfactory stria innervates the primary olfactory cortex in the basal frontal and anteromedial temporal lobes.

- Two principle classes of secondary olfactory neuron exist: tufted cells and mitral cells.
- Dendrites from secondary olfactory neurons communicate with the primary olfactory axons within the glomerular layer of the olfactory bulb.
- The olfactory system bypasses the thalamus in its projection to the cerebral cortex.

Olfactory Cortex & Basal Forebrain

- The basal forebrain structures with the most notable cholinergic properties are the medial septal nuclei, the diagonal band of Broca, and the basal nucleus of Meynert.
- The medial, intermediate, and primary (aka lateral) olfactory cortices are innervated by the medial, intermediate, and lateral olfactory striae, respectively.

- The medial olfactory cortex comprises, most notably, the subcallosal and paraterminal gyri.
- The intermediate stria terminates in the olfactory tubercle within the anterior perforated substance.
- The primary olfactory cortex comprises the piriform cortex, periamygdaloid cortex, corticomedial amygdala, and a small portion of the entorhinal cortex, anteriorly.

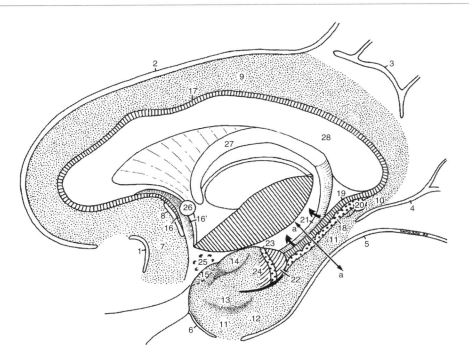

FIGURE 21-1 Drawing showing a sagittal section, right hemisphere. The limbic lobe is separated from the isocortex by the limbic fissure and may be divided into two gyri: the limbic and intralimbic gyri. The line a-a indicates the plane of the section on Figure 21.1. Bar, 7.7 mm Limbic fissure: 1, anterior paraolfactory sulcus (subcallosal sulcus); 2, cingulate sulcus; 3, subparietal sulcus; 4, anterior calcarine sulcus; 5, collateral sulcus; 6, rhinal sulcus. Limbic gyrus; 7, subcallosal gyrus; 8, posterior paraolfactory sulcus; 9, cingulate gyrus; 10, isthmus; 11', parahippocampal gyrus, posterior part; 11, parahippocampal gyrus, anterior part (piriform lobe). Piriform lobe; 12, entorhinal area; 13, ambient gyrus; 14, semilunar gyrus; 15, prepiriform cortex. Intralimbic gyrus; 16, prehippocampal rudiment; 16', paraterminal gyrus; 17, indusium griseum. Hippocampus; 18, gyrus dentatus; 19, cornu Ammonis; 20, gyri of Andreas Retzius; 21, fimbria (displaced upwards, arrows); 22, uncal apex; 23, band of Giacomini; 24, uncinate gyrus; 25, anterior perforated substance; 26, anterior commissure; 27, fornix; 28, corpus callosum. Used with permission from Duvernoy, Henri M. *The Human Hippocampus: Functional Anatomy, Vascularization and Serial Sections with MRI,* 3rd ed. Berlin; New York: Springer, 2005.

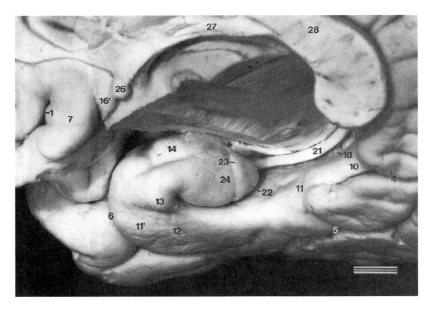

FIGURE 21-2 Dissection showing a sagittal section, right hemisphere. The limbic lobe is separated from the isocortex by the limbic fissure and may be divided into two gyri: the limbic and intralimbic gyri. Limbic fissure: 1, anterior paraolfactory sulcus (subcallosal sulcus); 2, cingulate sulcus; 3, subparietal sulcus; 4, anterior calcarine sulcus; 5, collateral sulcus; 6, rhinal sulcus. Limbic gyrus; 7, subcallosal gyrus; 8, posterior paraolfactory sulcus; 9, cingulate gyrus; 10, isthmus; 11', parahippocampal gyrus, posterior part; 11, parahippocampal gyrus, anterior part (piriform lobe). Piriform lobe; 12, entorhinal area; 13, ambient gyrus; 14, semilunar gyrus; 15, prepiriform cortex. Intralimbic gyrus; 16, prehippocampal rudiment; 16', paraterminal gyrus; 17, indusium griseum. Hippocampus; 18, gyrus dentatus; 19, cornu Ammonis; 20, gyri of Andreas Retzius; 21, fimbria (displaced upwards, arrows); 22, uncal apex; 23, band of Giacomini; 24, uncinate gyrus; 25, anterior perforated substance; 26, anterior commissure; 27, fornix; 28, corpus callosum. Used with permission from Duvernoy, Henri M. *The Human Hippocampus: Functional Anatomy, Vascularization and Serial Sections with MRI,* 3rd ed. Berlin; New York: Springer, 2005.

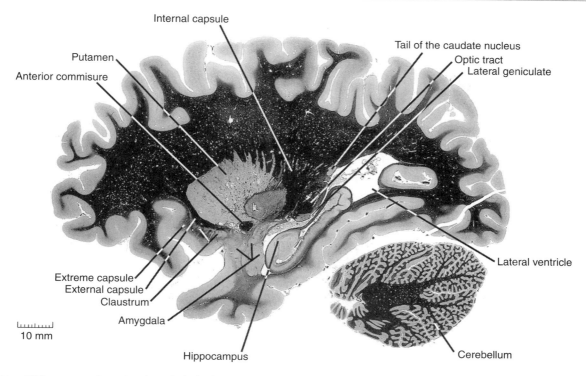

FIGURE 21-3 **Oblique anatomic section through the limbic system to highlight the length of the hippocampus. Used with permission from the Michigan State University: Brain Biodiversity Bank. https://www.msu.edu/~brains/**

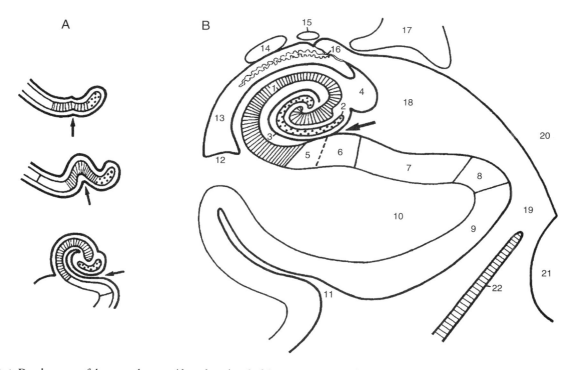

FIGURE 21-4 **Development of the gyrus dentatus (dotted area) and of the cornu Ammonis (hatched area) towards B their definitive desposition. Arrows indicate the hippocampal sulcus (superficial part). (Modified after Williams 1995) 1, cornu Ammonis; 2, gyrus dentatus; 3, hippocampal sulcus (deep or vestigial part); 4, fimbria; 5, prosubiculum, 6, subiculum proper; 7, presubiculum; 8, parasubiculum; 9, entorhinal area; 10, parahippocampal gyrus; 11, collateral sulcus; 12, collateral eminence; 13, temporal (inferior) horn of the lateral ventricle; 14, tail of caudate nucleus; 15, stria terminalis; 16, choroid fissure and choroid plexuses; 17, lateral geniculate body; 18, lateral part of the transverse fissure (wing of ambient cistern); 19, ambient cistern; 20, mesencephalon; 21, pons; 22, tentorium cerebelli. Used with permission from Williams, Peter. Gray's Anatomy. 38th edition. New York: Churchill Livingstone, 1995.**

Limbic System, Part 1

Here, we will draw the anatomy of the limbic system. Generally, the limbic system is meant to encompass the limbic lobe and functionally related structures, most notably the cingulate and parahippocampal gyri, hippocampus, and amygdala. First, we will draw a sagittal view of the major gray matter structures of the limbic system. The limbic system forms outer and inner rings around the diencephalon. Draw the following important anatomic landmarks: the corpus callosum, basal frontal lobe, thalamus, and the septum pellucidum. Next, draw the outer ring: the limbic gyrus. To do so, first, above the corpus callosum, label the cingulate gyrus. The cingulate gyrus is commonly divided into anterior and posterior divisions. The anterior cingulate gyrus is part of the anterior network of motivation, attention, and behavior and is associated with the amygdala, whereas the posterior cingulate gyrus is part of the posterior network of learning and memory and is associated with the hippocampus. Next, posterior to the rostrum of the corpus callosum and underneath the septum pellucidum, label the subcallosal area; show that it extends anteriorly directly underneath the corpus callosum—we draw this region in detail at the end. Then, show that the parahippocampal gyrus forms the inferior aspect of the limbic gyrus, and label the gyral fold at its anterior tip as the uncus. The parahippocampal gyrus channels information to and from the hippocampus to help in memory consolidation; an efficient parahippocampal gyrus is required for effective memory processing. Now, label the posterior transitional zone between the cingulate and parahippocampal gyri as the isthmus of the cingulate gyrus.

Next, let's draw the inner limbic ring: the intralimbic gyrus. Along the superior surface of the corpus callosum, beneath the cingulate gyrus, draw the indusium griseum (aka the supracallosal gyrus). The indusium griseum, along with the anatomically associated medial and longitudinal striae, are considered vestigial remnants of the hippocampal formation.[1] Now, along the bulk of the anteroposterior length of the superior aspect of the parahippocampal gyrus, draw the hippocampus. The hippocampus is the center for memory processing; we draw it in detail in Drawing 21-3. Next, just beneath the splenium of the corpus callosum, draw the fasciolar gyrus, which is the transitional zone between the hippocampus and the indusium griseum.

Now, just anterior to the hippocampus, deep to the posterior aspect of the uncus, draw the almond-shaped amygdala (aka amygdaloid body). The simplest way to understand the amygdala is to divide it into corticomedial and basolateral groups. Both groups connect to a wide variety of brain regions, but the corticomedial group connects, most notably, to the olfactory system and hypothalamus for autonomic function and the basolateral group connects, most notably, to the thalamus and prefrontal cortex for more conscious-related processes such as sensory processing of visual, auditory, and somatosensory stimuli.[2,3] Bilateral amygdala destruction results in Klüver Bucy syndrome, which involves, most prominently, social tameness and loss of avoidance manifesting with hypermetamorphosis (the incessant exploration of objects within the environment), hyperorality, visual agnosia, and hypersexuality. Klüver Bucy syndrome was first described from the effects of bilateral amygdala and hippocampal destruction in monkeys, but it is a rare complication of a variety of naturally occurring illnesses in humans, including herpes simplex encephalitis, frontotemporal lobar dementia, and anoxic-ischemic lesions in the bilateral anterior medial temporal lobes.[4]

Next, include the following diencephalic structures: the anterior nuclei of the thalamus and the mammillary body of the hypothalamus, both of which are fundamental to the Papez circuit. The mammillary bodies (along with other midline periventricular structures: the dorsomedial thalamus, periaqueductal region, and floor of the fourth ventricle) are affected in Wernicke-Korsakoff syndrome, which manifests with confusion, memory loss, ophthalmoplegia, and ataxia.[3,5–10]

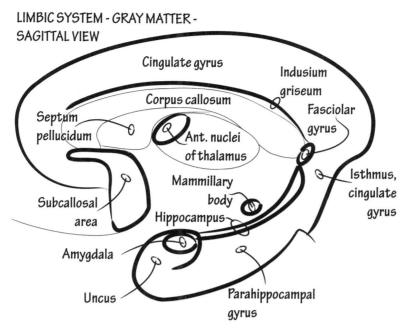

LIMBIC SYSTEM - GRAY MATTER -
SAGITTAL VIEW

DRAWING 21-1 **Limbic System, Part 1**

Limbic System, Part 2 (*Advanced*)

Now, let's return to the subcallosal region and draw a detailed view of its anatomy; include the anterior commissure for reference. Indicate that the anterior paraolfactory sulcus separates the subcallosal gyrus from the frontal lobe, anteriorly, and show that the posterior paraolfactory sulcus divides the subcallosal area into the subcallosal gyrus, anteriorly, and the paraterminal gyrus, posteriorly. Note that additional descriptors for this region include the terms the septal area and paraolfactory (or parolfactory) area. Also note that the nomenclature used to describe the subcallosal region displays extraordinary intertextual inconsistency and contradiction. Next, show that the septal nuclei lie, most notably, within the fibrous septum pellucidum above the anterior commissure, beneath the corpus callosum, posterior to the subcallosal area, and anterior to the fornix. Then, show that the bed nucleus of the stria terminalis sits just above the anterior commissure and below the septal nuclei.

Next, let's draw the limbic pathways in sagittal view. Draw an outline of a sagittal view of the limbic system gray matter, corpus callosum, and thalamus. Then, show that the cingulum spans the cingulate and parahippocampal gyri. Indicate that it interconnects intracingulate areas; synapses in the hippocampus (through the entorhinal cortex); and also projects to many additional areas, including most cortical regions, including the prefrontal, temporal, parietal, and occipital cortices. Next, show that the fornix emerges from the hippocampus, wraps around the thalamus, and passes anteriorly just below the corpus callosum. At the interventricular foramen of Monro it divides and descends as bilateral columns. Each column contains a small precommissural bundle that descends anterior to the anterior commissure and projects to diffuse areas, including the septal nuclei, frontal lobes, hypothalamus, and ventral striatum; and each column also contains a large postcommissural bundle, which originates solely within the subiculum of the hippocampus, projects posterior to the anterior

commissure, and synapses, most notably, in the mammillary bodies. Note that postcommissural fornix connections to the anterior thalamic nuclei and midbrain also exist. Next, show that the mammillothalamic fasciculus connects the mammillary body to the anterior thalamic nuclei. Note that the postcommissural fornix and the mammillothalamic fasciculus form key steps in the Papez circuit.

Now, show that via the stria terminalis, the amygdala projects along the dorsal aspect of the thalamus and terminates in the septal nuclei and bed nucleus of the stria terminalis and also in the hypothalamus. Finally, show that via the amygdalofugal tract, the amygdala projects to diffuse areas: most notably, the basal forebrain, prefrontal, temporal, occipital, and insular cortices; thalamus; hypothalamus; septal nuclei; and the autonomic and neurobehavioral substrate of the brainstem.[8]

Finally, because the stria terminalis and fornix follow such similar paths, let's draw a coronal view of the diencephalon to distinguish their trajectories; in this diagram, we will also show the position of the stria medullaris thalami, which is an important diencephalic pathway that travels near the fornix and stria terminalis. As anatomic landmarks, draw the corpus callosum, caudate, thalamus, lateral ventricle, and third ventricle. Now, show the body of the fornix underneath the midline of the corpus callosum; the fornix emerges from the hippocampus, wraps around the thalamus, and passes anteriorly in midline just below the corpus callosum. Next, draw the stria terminalis along the inferomedial aspect of the caudate (lateral to the body of the fornix); the stria terminalis emerges from the amygdala and passes along the inferomedial aspect of the caudate nucleus throughout most of its course along the lateral wall of the lateral ventricular system. Finally, in midline, along the dorsomedial aspect of the thalamus, draw the stria medullaris thalami, which spans from the habenula to the septal nuclei.[3,6–10]

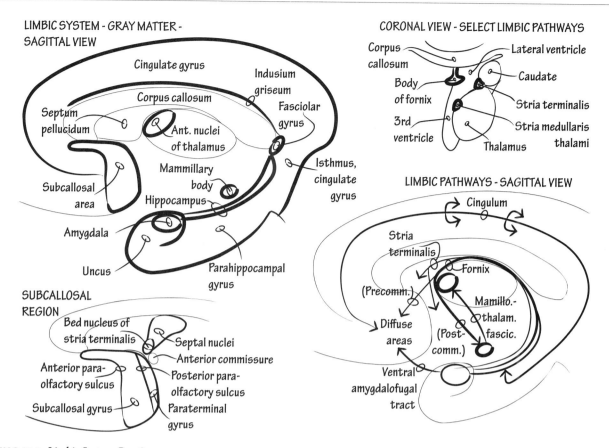

LIMBIC SYSTEM - GRAY MATTER - SAGITTAL VIEW

Cingulate gyrus

Indusium griseum

Corpus callosum

Fasciolar gyrus

Septum pellucidum

Ant. nuclei of thalamus

Isthmus, cingulate gyrus

Subcallosal area

Mammillary body

Hippocampus

Amygdala

Uncus

Parahippocampal gyrus

CORONAL VIEW - SELECT LIMBIC PATHWAYS

Corpus callosum

Lateral ventricle

Body of fornix

Caudate

Stria terminalis

3rd ventricle

Stria medullaris thalami

Thalamus

LIMBIC PATHWAYS - SAGITTAL VIEW

Cingulum

Stria terminalis

Fornix

(Precomm.)

Mamillo.-thalam. fascic.

Diffuse areas

(Post-comm.)

Ventral amygdalofugal tract

SUBCALLOSAL REGION

Bed nucleus of stria terminalis

Septal nuclei

Anterior commissure

Anterior para-olfactory sulcus

Posterior para-olfactory sulcus

Subcallosal gyrus

Paraterminal gyrus

DRAWING 21-2 **Limbic System, Part 2**

Hippocampus: Anatomy

Here, we will draw a coronal view of the medial temporal lobe (ie, the antero-inferior limbic lobe) to learn the anatomy of the hippocampus and anterior parahippocampal gyrus. Before we begin our diagram, draw a small coronal insert in the corner of the page of half of the brain and upper brainstem. Include the temporal horn of the lateral ventricle and the tentorium cerebelli, and encircle the medial temporal lobe—this is the region we will draw.

Next, begin our main diagram. Draw the pons and midbrain and extend our drawing along the basal forebrain. Then, include the temporal horn of the lateral ventricle. Next, use the choroid fissure to separate the temporal horn of the lateral ventricle from the neighboring subarachnoid space: the ambient cistern.

To draw the hippocampus, first draw a double-sided S. Then, divide the S into its superior turn, horizontal stretch, and inferior turn. As we will show, the cornu ammonis, which is Latin for "horn of the ram," and which is also known as Ammon's horn or the hippocampus proper, comprises the superior turn; the subicular complex forms the horizontal stretch; and the parahippocampal gyrus comprises the inferior turn. Internal to the superior turn, draw the C-shaped dentate gyrus, which cups the cornu ammonis. Next, label the subdivisions of the cornu ammonis: label CA4 adjacent to the dentate gyrus; label CA3 along the medial vertical; label CA2 along the top of the turn; and finally, label CA1 along the lateral vertical. CA1 forms the largest stretch of Ammon's horn and is distinctively susceptible to anoxic injury.

Now, label the horizontal stretch of our diagram as the subicular complex, and show that the hippocampal sulcus separates it from the dentate gyrus. From lateral to medial (ie, from CA1 to the ambient cistern), the subicular complex comprises the subiculum, presubiculum, and parasubiculum. The subiculum is the source of the postcommissural fornix fibers, which terminate in the mammillary nuclei and which form a key step in the Papez circuit. The *Terminologia Anatomica* lists the complete subicular complex as part of the hippocampus, whereas other sources list the subiculum, only, as part of the hippocampus and list the pre- and parasubiculum as part of the parahippocampal region.

Next, label the inferior turn as the entorhinal cortex, which forms the medial aspect of the anterior parahippocampal gyrus. Now, draw the perirhinal cortex and show that the rhinal sulcus separates the perirhinal and entorhinal cortices. Next, in the corner of the diagram, write out that the entorhinal and perirhinal cortices form the anterior parahippocampal gyrus. The posterior parahippocampal gyrus is referred to as the parahippocampal cortex and corresponds to Von Economo areas TF and TH.[11] Next, for anatomic context, show that the collateral sulcus distinguishes the fusiform gyrus, laterally, from the parahippocampal gyrus, medially.

Now, let's discuss the uncus, which, simply put, forms the anterior gyral thumb of the parahippocampal gyrus. Anteriorly, the uncus encompasses the amygdala, and posteriorly, it forms the anterior portion of the hippocampus, which complicates the simple definition of the uncus as listed, here. The term "uncal herniation" is used to describe medial temporal lobe herniation over the tentorium cerebellum. During uncal herniation, the medial temporal lobe compresses the ipsilateral third nerve as it exits the midbrain, causing an ipsilateral oculomotor palsy. Also, the herniating temporal lobe can compress the contralateral cerebral peduncle against its adjacent tentorium, forming a so-called Kernohan's notch in that peduncle. The damaged cerebral peduncle results in motor weakness on the opposite side of the body—the side of the herniating temporal lobe and oculomotor palsy.

Finally, internal to the perirhinal and entorhinal cortices, label the parahippocampal white matter; and then label the white matter along the lateral border of the cornu ammonis as the alveus; and show that along the superomedial border of the cornu ammonis, the alveus becomes the fimbria.[3,6–9,12]

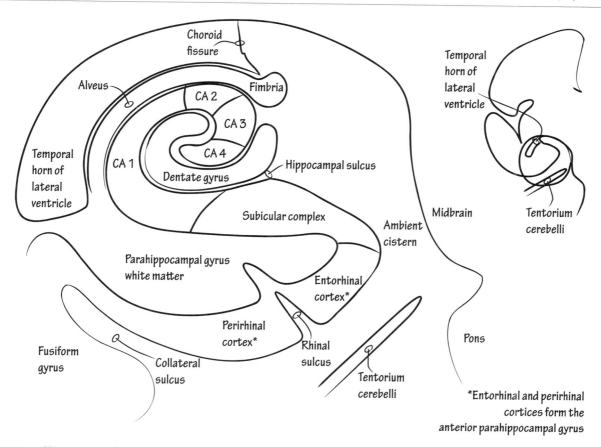

Choroid
fissure

Alveus

Fimbria

CA 2

CA 3

CA 4

CA 1

Dentate gyrus

Temporal
horn of
lateral
ventricle

Hippocampal sulcus

Subicular complex

Parahippocampal gyrus
white matter

Entorhinal
cortex*

Ambient
cistern

Midbrain

Fusiform
gyrus

Collateral
sulcus

Perirhinal
cortex*

Rhinal
sulcus

Tentorium
cerebelli

Pons

Temporal
horn of
lateral
ventricle

Tentorium
cerebelli

*Entorhinal and perirhinal
cortices form the
anterior parahippocampal gyrus

DRAWING 21-3 **Hippocampus: Anatomy**

Hippocampus: Circuitry

Here, we will draw the fundamental extra- and intra-hippocampal circuitry. We begin with the extra-hippocampal circuitry, namely the Papez circuit. First, in sagittal view draw the following structures: the corpus callosum, cingulate gyrus, basal forebrain, thalamus, and parahippocampal gryus with its anterior gyral fold—the uncus. Next, let's show the steps in the Papez circuit. First, indicate that the entorhinal cortex (in the anterior parahippocampal gyrus) projects to the hippocampus, which projects via the fornix to the mammillary nuclei. Divide the fornix as follows: the crus of the fornix is its vertical ascent; the body of the fornix is its anterior projection underneath the corpus callosum; and the column of the fornix is its descent. Note that the fornix descends both anterior and posterior to the anterior commissure. The anterior projection is called the precommissural fornix and the posterior projection through the hypothalamus (shown here) is called the postcommissural fornix. Next, indicate that the mammillary nuclei project to the anterior thalamic nuclei via the mammillothalamic fasciculus (aka the Vicq d'Azyr bundle), and then show that the anterior thalamic nuclei project to the cingulate gyrus. Finally, show that the cingulate gyrus projects back to the entorhinal cortex via the cingulum to close the Papez circuit loop. When James Papez introduced this circuit in 1937, he believed it played a fundamental role in emotional processing; however, now the Papez circuit is understood to be the cornerstone of memory consolidation, instead.

Neuronal input reaches the hippocampus through widespread neocortical, limbic, diencephalic, and brainstem neurobehavioral areas. Here, we will show two examples of how these areas reach the hippocampus. First, simply show that the cingulate gyrus has reciprocal connections with the neocortex that project via the cingulum to the entorhinal cortex, which then projects to the hippocampus. Second, indicate that widespread neocortical areas project to the posterior parahippocampal gyrus, which then projects to the perirhinal cortex, and subsequently to the entorhinal cortex and on to the hippocampus. Note that although not shown as such, here, many areas skip synapsing in the posterior parahippocampal gyrus and directly synapse in the perirhinal or entorhinal cortices or even directly in the hippocampus, itself.

Now, let's draw the intrahippocampal circuitry, namely the perforant pathway. First, in coronal view, redraw the medial temporal lobe. Include the dentate gyrus, cornu ammonis, subiculum, entorhinal cortex, alveus, and fimbria. Then, add the posterior length of the hippocampus. Show that the fimbria becomes the crus of the fornix, which makes its vertical ascent at the splenium of the corpus callosum. The intrahippocampal circuitry is distinct in that it follows a very specific unidirectional progression—unlike most cortical projections, which are generally bidirectional. Show that the entorhinal cortex projects through the subiculum (it perforates it) to synapse in the dentate gyrus. Then, indicate that the dentate gyrus projects to CA3, which projects to CA1 via Schaffer collaterals. CA1 then projects to the subiculum, which projects along the alveus to the fimbria, which passes posteriorly and becomes the crus of the fornix. The fornix ultimately projects, most notably, to the mammillary nuclei (as shown in the Papez circuit portion of the diagram). Finally, show that the subiculum also projects back to the entorhinal cortex. Note that CA3 and CA1 also send direct projections to the fimbria that skip the intervening steps in this pathway, and also note that many other intrahippocampal projections also exist, including subiculum projections to the other components of the subicular complex (ie, the pre-subiculum and parasubiculum).[13] Lastly, consider that because of the anatomic relationship between the entorhinal cortex, dentate gyrus, cornu ammonis, and subiculum, these structures are often collectively referred to as the hippocampal formation.[3,6–9,12]

EXTRA-HIPPOCAMPAL CIRCUITRY
& THE PAPEZ CIRCUIT

INTRA-HIPPOCAMPAL CIRCUITRY
& THE PERFORANT PATHWAY

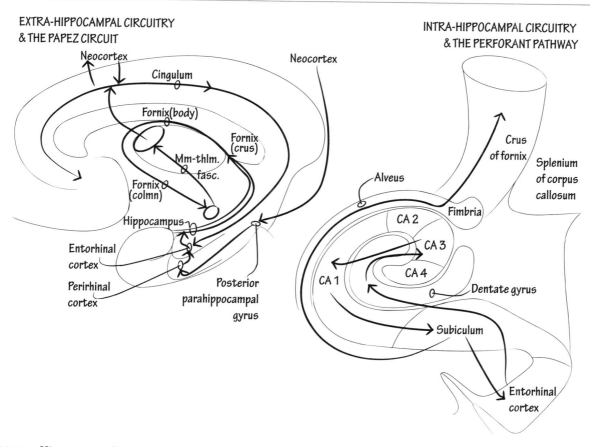

DRAWING 21-4 **Hippocampus: Circuitry**

Olfactory System, Part 1

Here, we will draw the olfactory system; we will focus on the olfactory nerve, bulb, tract, and striae, here, and learn the olfactory cortex in Drawings 21-7 and 21-8. Begin with a sagittal view of the midline nasal cavity; include the following anatomic landmarks: the cribriform plate, which separates the cranial vault from the nasal cavity; the medial anterior frontal lobe and temporal lobe; and the anterior corpus callosum. Note that fracture to the cribriform plate (or more commonly to the ethmoid air cells posterolateral to the cribriform plate) is a common cause of rhinorrhea—a cerebrospinal fluid leak from the nasal cavity. Now, along the upper nasal cavity, draw the olfactory epithelium. Next, just above the cribriform plate, draw an olfactory bulb, and underneath the frontal lobe, draw the olfactory tract. Then, within the olfactory epithelium, draw a bipolar primary olfactory neuron and show that its centrally mediated axon, the olfactory nerve, extends through the cribriform plate to innervate the olfactory bulb. Note that this is the extent of cranial nerve 1, the olfactory nerve. The olfactory bulb and tract are telencephalic extensions of the cerebrum, itself. Next, within the olfactory bulb, draw a bipolar secondary olfactory cell, and show that it connects with the olfactory nerve in the inferior olfactory bulb and also sends an axon down the olfactory tract. Then, at the posterior end of the olfactory tract, at the olfactory trigone, show that the olfactory tract divides into a medial olfactory stria, which innervates the medial olfactory area in the subcallosal (aka septal) region, and a lateral olfactory stria, which innervates the primary olfactory cortex in the basal frontal and anteromedial temporal lobes. Note that (as we will draw later) olfactory impulses also extend across the anterior commissure to the opposite side of the cerebrum.[14–17]

Next, let's draw an expanded view of the olfactory nerve and bulb. Draw the olfactory epithelium, cribriform plate, olfactory bulb, and the anterior segment of the connected olfactory tract. Next, draw a representative primary olfactory neuron (aka olfactory receptor cell), which is bipolar. Show that at one end, it projects an apical dendrite to the epithelial surface. Indicate that cilia from the apical dendrite interact with the mucus layer of the olfactory epithelial surface. Next, indicate that an unmyelinated nerve bundle, which is the olfactory nerve, itself, projects from the other end of the primary olfactory neuron through the cribriform plate to the olfactory bulb. As we will soon show, it interacts with dendrites from the secondary olfactory neuron at the glomerular layer of the olfactory bulb. Other constituents of the olfactory epithelium include the sustentacular cells, which are olfactory supporting cells; the basal cells, which renew the primary olfactory neurons and sustentacular cells; and the Bowman's glands, which secrete a serous, watery fluid that serves as an odor dissolvent.[18]

Now, within the olfactory bulb, draw a representative bipolar secondary olfactory neuron. Two principal forms of secondary olfactory neuron exist: tufted cells and mitral cells; less notable interneurons (eg, periglomerular and granule cells) also exist within the olfactory bulb. Indicate that dendrites from the secondary olfactory neurons communicate with the primary olfactory axons within the inferior olfactory bulb. These nerve processes intermingle within spherical glomeruli—thus, this layer is called the glomerular layer. Lastly, show that the secondary olfactory neurons project axons that travel either directly down the olfactory tract to synapse in the olfactory cortex or first to the anterior olfactory nucleus, which then projects down the olfactory tract to the olfactory cortex.[10,14,17,18]

OLFACTORY SYSTEM
SAGITTAL VIEW

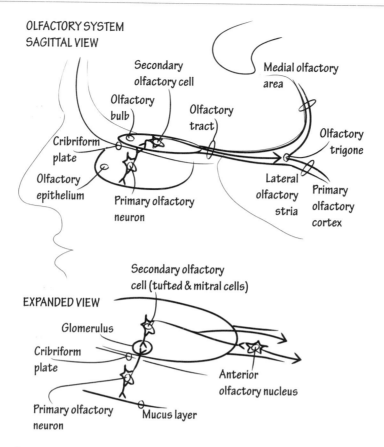

DRAWING 21-5 **Olfactory System, Part 1**

Olfactory System, Part 2 (*Advanced*)

Next, let's show the flow of olfactory information from the olfactory bulb to the olfactory cortex. Note that this flow of information is actually bidirectional, although we show it one direction, only, here. Also, note that the olfactory system bypasses the thalamus in its projection to the cerebral cortex, which is unique. Consider that auditory, visual, somatosensory, and gustatory sensory pathways all relay within the thalamus prior to synapsing in the cerebral cortex. Draw an inferior view of the frontal and anterior-temporal lobes and, for anatomic reference, include the optic chiasm, pituitary stalk, and mammillary bodies. Also, in front of the optic chiasm, draw the diagonal band of Broca, which is a prominent cholinergic gray and white matter structure (see Drawing 21-7). Next, in the frontal lobes, draw the bilateral olfactory bulbs and tracts, which lie within the olfactory sulci. Note that the olfactory bulb is often distinguished as the main olfactory bulb because the majority of vertebrates also have an accessory olfactory system.[19,20] However, the role and existence of the accessory olfactory system (aka vomeronasal system) in humans is disputed.

Now, show that at the olfactory trigone the olfactory tract splits into lateral and medial striae. The bilateral medial striae communicate at the anterior commissure. In between the olfactory trigone and the diagonal band of Broca, label the anterior perforated substance; the perforated appearance of this gross anatomic area gives it its name. Next, indicate that behind the olfactory trigone, overlying the anterior perforated substance, is a gray matter structure called the olfactory tubercle, which is

innervated by a third, not yet introduced, olfactory stria: the intermediate olfactory stria. The existence and significance of the intermediate stria in humans is controversial. Next, return to the olfactory tract and show that the anterior olfactory nucleus lies along its anteroposterior length. The anterior olfactory nucleus has cortical cytoarchitecture and, thus, is often referred to as the anterior olfactory cortex, and it is commonly considered to be part of the primary olfactory cortex (see Drawing 21-8).[8,21,22]

Finally, we're ready to show the flow of information from the olfactory bulb to the primary olfactory cortex. First, show an impulse pass from the olfactory bulb down the olfactory tract into the lateral olfactory stria to the primary olfactory cortex. Note that we define the structures of the primary olfactory cortex in Drawing 21-8. From the primary olfactory cortex, information projects to secondary olfactory regions, which include the orbitofrontal cortex, lateral hypothalamus, insula, anterior hippocampus, and indusium griseum. Next, show an impulse pass from the anterior olfactory nucleus down the ipsilateral olfactory tract to the ipsilateral medial stria. Show that it decussates in the anterior commissure to the contralateral medial stria and that it then passes anteriorly along the contralateral olfactory tract to the olfactory bulb. Again, note that olfactory sensory impulses are bidirectional, which means that the olfactory cortex also communicates with the olfactory bulb in a reciprocal manner to what we have drawn, here.[16,17]

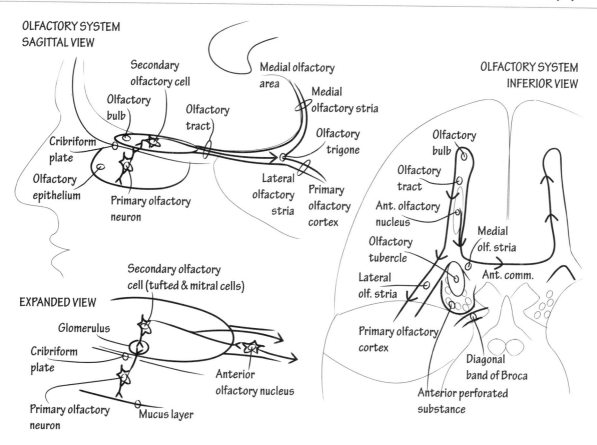

OLFACTORY SYSTEM
SAGITTAL VIEW

Secondary
olfactory cell
Olfactory
bulb
Olfactory
tract
Medial olfactory
area
Medial
olfactory stria
Olfactory
trigone
Cribriform
plate
Olfactory
epithelium
Primary olfactory
neuron
Lateral
olfactory
stria
Primary
olfactory
cortex

OLFACTORY SYSTEM
INFERIOR VIEW

Olfactory
bulb
Olfactory
tract
Ant. olfactory
nucleus
Olfactory
tubercle
Lateral
olf. stria
Primary olfactory
cortex
Medial
olf. stria
Ant. comm.
Diagonal
band of Broca
Anterior perforated
substance

EXPANDED VIEW

Secondary olfactory
cell (tufted & mitral cells)
Glomerulus
Cribriform
plate
Primary olfactory
neuron
Mucus layer
Anterior
olfactory nucleus

DRAWING 21-6 **Olfactory System, Part 2**

Olfactory Cortex & Basal Forebrain, Part 1

Here, we will draw two coronal sections through the basal frontal and medial temporal lobes to learn the anatomy of the olfactory cortex and basal forebrain. First, let's establish the anteroposterior positions of our two coronal sections: indicate that one section lies along the plane of the optic chiasm, which is the more anterior diagram, and the other lies along the plane of the optic tract, just posterior to the plane of the optic chiasm. In the optic chiasm diagram, draw the putamen, caudate, and their ventral connection: the nucleus accumbens. Then, label the intervening internal capsule. Also, for reference, include the frontal horn of the lateral ventricle and the corpus callosum. In the optic tract diagram, again draw the caudate and putamen, but here show that they are completely separated by the internal capsule (the nucleus accumbens lies anterior to this plane). Next, medial to the putamen, draw the globus pallidus. Now, again include the frontal horn of the lateral ventricle and the corpus callosum. Next, in each diagram, draw the border of the basal frontal and medial temporal lobes and draw the inferior border of the insula.

Now, let's complete the diagram through the optic chiasm. First, for further reference, show that the medial hypothalamus connects the optic chiasm to the basal frontal lobe. Next, along the basal perimeter, from medial to lateral, label the subcallosal gyrus, olfactory tubercle, and piriform cortex. Then, draw the periamygdaloid cortex in between the piriform cortex, laterally, and the entorhinal cortex, medially. Now, in the center of the medial temporal lobe, draw the amygdala; separate it into corticomedial and basolateral divisions. Finally, in between the subcallosal gyrus and the nucleus accumbens, label the diagonal band of Broca.

Next, let's complete the more posterior diagram: the one through the optic tract. In the middle of the diagram, inferiorly, label the hypothalamus. Superiorly, in midline, label the septal nuclei and the bed nucleus of the stria terminalis below them. Next, in the basal frontal lobe, lateral to the hypothalamus and beneath the basal ganglia, label the substantia innominata. Above the substantia innominata and below the basal ganglia, label the anterior commissure. Within the substantia innominata, label the basal nucleus of Meynert. Note that the basal nucleus of Meynert is variably considered to be either synonymous with the substantia innominata or to reside within this "unnamed substance" as it is drawn, here. Then, just below the anterior commissure, label the ventral pallidum. Now, in the medial temporal lobe, draw the amygdala, but show that in this more posterior section, the amygdala extends to the surface of the temporal lobe. Again, divide the amygdala into corticomedial and basolateral divisions. Finally, along the medial rim of the temporal lobe, medial to the amygdala, label the entorhinal cortex.

Certain basal forebrain structures share important cholinergic properties that are understood to play a substantive role in memory. Of the listed structures, those with the most notable cholinergic properties are the medial septal nuclei, the diagonal band of Broca, and the basal nucleus of Meynert. As a clinical corollary, acetylcholinesterase inhibitors, which prevent the breakdown of acetylcholine, were developed to promote cholinergic health in the basal forebrain with the hope of slowing the progression of Alzheimer's disease.[23] Unfortunately, although these medications are widely used, they have limited clinical efficacy.[6,9,10,24]

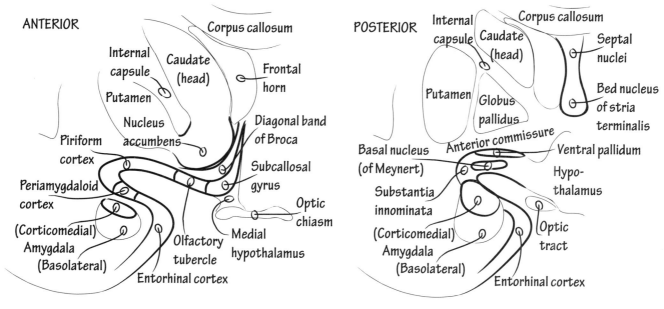

DRAWING 21-7   **Olfactory Cortex & Basal Forebrain, Part 1**

Olfactory Cortex & Basal Forebrain, Part 2 (*Advanced*)

Now, let's group the anatomic structures we have drawn into olfactory and basal forebrain listings. Begin with the olfactory cortex. Divide it into medial, intermediate, and primary (or lateral) cortices, which are innervated by the medial, intermediate, and lateral striae, respectively. Indicate that the medial olfactory cortex comprises, most notably, the subcallosal and paraterminal gyri, which are collectively referred to (in this context) as the medial olfactory area. Next, show that the intermediate stria terminates in the olfactory tubercle within the anterior perforated substance, which makes the olfactory tubercle part of the intermediate olfactory cortex. However, note that the olfactory tubercle is variably considered part of the primary olfactory cortex, as well. Now, show that the primary olfactory cortex comprises the piriform cortex, periamygdaloid cortex, corticomedial amygdala, and a small portion of the entorhinal cortex, anteriorly. Note that as we discussed previously, the anterior olfactory nucleus is also variably listed as part of the primary olfactory cortex. Also, note that the distinction between the primary and secondary olfactory cortices is highly variable; as an example, certain texts include the entorhinal cortex as secondary olfactory cortex rather than as primary cortex—many other discrepancies can also be found.[8,14,25]

Finally, let's address the basal forebrain. The list of structures that constitute the basal forebrain is inconsistently defined throughout the literature; therefore, here we will focus only on those structures that are nearly universally grouped within the basal forebrain and will disregard the less commonly affiliated structures. Indicate that the following structures are commonly considered part of the basal forebrain: the septal nuclei, diagonal band of Broca, ventral pallidum, basal nucleus of Meynert, substantia innominata, the corticomedial amygdala, and the extended amygdala, which refers to those areas of the basal forebrain with prominent connections to the corticomedial amygdala: most notably, the bed nucleus of the stria terminalis and the nucleus accumbens. Note that the ventral pallidum and nucleus accumbens are alternatively (or additionally) categorized as part of the basal ganglia. Also note that the corticomedial amygdala is commonly organized along with both the olfactory cortex and basal forebrain. And as a final note, consider that the piriform cortex in rats, the animal model for olfaction, is extensive and functionally important, but its size and significance in humans remains to be determined.[6,9,10,24,26,27]

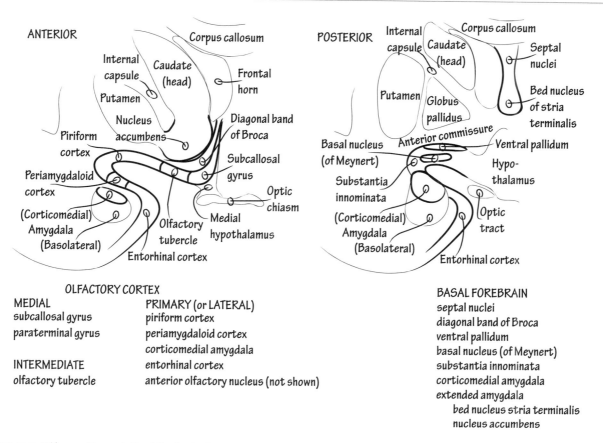

ANTERIOR

Corpus callosum
Internal capsule
Caudate (head)
Putamen
Nucleus accumbens
Piriform cortex
Periamygdaloid cortex
(Corticomedial)
Amygdala (Basolateral)
Frontal horn
Diagonal band of Broca
Subcallosal gyrus
Optic chiasm
Olfactory tubercle
Medial hypothalamus
Entorhinal cortex

POSTERIOR

Internal capsule
Caudate (head)
Putamen
Globus pallidus
Basal nucleus (of Meynert)
Anterior commissure
Substantia innominata
(Corticomedial)
Amygdala (Basolateral)
Corpus callosum
Septal nuclei
Bed nucleus of stria terminalis
Ventral pallidum
Hypo-thalamus
Optic tract
Entorhinal cortex

OLFACTORY CORTEX

MEDIAL
subcallosal gyrus
paraterminal gyrus

INTERMEDIATE
olfactory tubercle

PRIMARY (or LATERAL)
piriform cortex
periamygdaloid cortex
corticomedial amygdala
entorhinal cortex
anterior olfactory nucleus (not shown)

BASAL FOREBRAIN
septal nuclei
diagonal band of Broca
ventral pallidum
basal nucleus (of Meynert)
substantia innominata
corticomedial amygdala
extended amygdala
    bed nucleus stria terminalis
    nucleus accumbens

DRAWING 21-8 **Olfactory Cortex & Basal Forebrain, Part 2**

References

1. Psarros, T. G. & Moore, S. P. *Intensive neurosurgery board review: neurological surgery Q & A,* p. 37 (Lippincott Williams & Wilkins, 2006).

2. Ramamurti, R. *Textbooks of operative neurosurgery,* Vol. 1, p. 635 (BI Publications Pvt. Ltd., 2005).

3. Brodal, P. *The central nervous system: structure and function,* 4th ed., Chapter 31 (Oxford University Press, 2010).

4. Tonkonogii, I. M. & Puente, A. E. *Localization of clinical syndromes in neuropsychology and neuroscience,* p. 592 (Springer Pub., 2009).

5. Tsokos, M. *Forensic pathology reviews,* Vol. 5 (Humana Press, 2008).

6. Mai, J. K., Voss, T. & Paxinos, G. *Atlas of the human brain,* 3rd ed. (Elsevier/Academic Press, 2008).

7. Duvernoy, H. M. & Cattin, F. *The human hippocampus: functional anatomy, vascularization and serial sections with MRI,* 3rd ed. (Springer, 2005).

8. Afifi, A. K. & Bergman, R. A. *Functional neuroanatomy: text and atlas,* 2nd ed., Chapter 21 (Lange Medical Books/McGraw-Hill, 2005).

9. Naidich, T. P. & Duvernoy, H. M. *Duvernoy's atlas of the human brain stem and cerebellum: high-field MRI: surface anatomy, internal structure, vascularization and 3D sectional anatomy* (Springer, 2009).

10. Nieuwenhuys, R., Voogd, J. & Huijzen, C. V. *The human central nervous system,* 4th ed. (Springer, 2008).

11. Saleem, K. S. *A combined MRI and histology atlas of the rhesus monkey brain in stereotaxic coordinates,* pp. 13–16 (Elsevier Ltd., 2007).

12. Andersen, P. *The hippocampus book,* Chapter 2 (Oxford University Press, 2007).

13 . Burwell, R. D. & Agster, K. L. Anatomy of the hippocampus and the declarative memory system. Chapter 10 in *Concise learning and memory: the editor's selection* (ed John H. Byrne) (Elsevier Ltd., 2009).

14. Binder, D. K., Sonne, D. C. & Fischbein, N. J. *Cranial nerves: anatomy, pathology, imaging,* Chapter 1 (Thieme, 2010).

15. Brazis, P. W., Masdeu, J. C. & Biller, J. *Localization in clinical neurology,* 6th ed., p. 163 (Wolters Kluwer Health/Lippincott Williams & Wilkins, 2011).

16. Miller, J. H. *Eighty Years Behind the Masts,* p. 106 (AuthorHouse, 2011).

17. Wilson-Pauwels, L. *Cranial nerves: function and dysfunction,* 3rd ed., Chapter 1 (People's Medical Pub. House, 2010).

18. Young, B. & Wheater, P. R. *Wheater's functional histology: a text and colour atlas,* 5th ed., p. 401 (Churchill Livingstone Elsevier, 2006).

19. Davis, S. F. & Buskist, W. *21st century psychology: a reference handbook,* p. 222 (SAGE Publications, 2008).

20. Ågmo, A. *Functional and dysfunctional sexual behavior: a synthesis of neuroscience and comparative psychology.* 1st ed., pp. 105–108 (Elsevier/Academic Press, 2007).

21. Shepherd, G. M. *The synaptic organization of the brain,* 5th ed., p. 416 (Oxford University Press, 2004).

22. Gazzaniga, M. S. *The cognitive neurosciences,* 3rd ed., p. 263 (MIT Press, 2004).

23. Papanicolaou, A. C. & Billingsley-Marshall, R. *The amnesias: a clinical textbook of memory disorders,* pp. 45–47 (Oxford University Press, 2006).

24. Federative Committee on Anatomical Terminology. *Terminologia anatomica: international anatomical terminology* (Thieme, 1998).

25. Andrew John Taylor, D. D. R. *Flavor perception,* pp. 212–214 (Blackwell Publishing Ltd., 2004).

26. Heilman, K. M. & Valenstein, E. *Clinical neuropsychology,* 4th ed., p. 533 (Oxford University Press, 2003).

27. Bruni, J. E. & Montemurro, D. G. *Human neuroanatomy: a text, brain atlas, and laboratory dissection guide* (Oxford University Press, 2009).

22

Vision

Know-It Points

The Eye

- The outer layer comprises the cornea and the sclera.
- The middle layer comprises the iris, choroid, and ciliary body.
- The inner layer is the retina and, from inner to outer, lies the nerve fiber layer, the synaptic and cell body layers, and the photoreceptor cell segment layer (the rods and cones).
- The lens is transparent and focuses a target on the retina.
- During near accommodation, the ciliary bodies contract (ie, shorten), which relaxes the zonule and rounds the lens (ie, thickens it), and the near object is brought into focus.
- Ciliary epithelia actively secrete aqueous humor, which is reabsorbed at the iridocorneal filtration angle into the canal of Schlemm.

- The vitreous chamber contains vitreous humor, which helps maintain the eye's shape.
- The retina transitions into optic nerve where it exits the eye, posteriorly, at the lamina cribrosa.
- In the center of the optic nerve head sits the optic cup: a white-appearing hole through which the central retinal vessels (artery and vein) emanate.
- The optic disc is the pink-colored ring of nerve tissue that surrounds the optic cup.
- Impaired axoplasmic transport at the lamina cribrosa results in optic disc swelling (disc edema).
- The fovea lies in the center of the retina and is the area of highest visual acuity.
- The optic nerve head corresponds to the blind spot.

Visual Pathways: Axial View

- The right visual field projects to the temporal left hemiretina and the nasal right hemiretina.
- The left temporal hemiretina projects ipsilaterally to the left lateral geniculate nucleus.
- The right nasal hemiretina sends crossing fibers through the optic chiasm to the contralateral lateral geniculate nucleus (the left lateral geniculate nucleus).

- The left lateral geniculate nucleus sends optic radiations to the left occipital cortex.
- The optic projections between the retina and the optic chiasm are the optic nerve.
- The projections between the optic chiasm and the lateral geniculate nucleus are the optic tract.

Visual Pathways: Sagittal View

- The superior visual world projects to the inferior portion of the retina.
- The inferior visual world projects to the superior portion of the retina.
- Central vision comprises the majority of the lateral geniculate body and lies posterior.
- Peripheral vision comprises the minority of the lateral geniculate body and lies anterior.
- The superior optic radiation bundle projects to the superior primary visual cortex.

- The inferior optic radiation bundle projects to the inferior primary visual cortex.
- Injury to an optic radiation disrupts visual perception of a single visual quadrant, called quadrantanopia.
- Cortical representation of central (or macular) vision lies in the posterior calcarine sulcus and occupies a large cortical area relative to its small retinal expanse.
- Cortical representation of peripheral vision lies in the anterior calcarine sulcus and encompasses a small cortical area relative to its broad retinal expanse.

Cortical Visual Processing

- The ventral stream comprises the "what," object recognition pathway (or P pathway).
- The dorsal stream comprises the "where," spatial localization (or M pathway).
- The cone photoreceptors are responsible for color detection and excite parvocellular ganglion cells of the "what" pathway.
- The rod photoreceptors are responsible for motion detection and excite magnocellular ganglion cells of the "where" pathway.
- The primary visual cortex in each hemisphere encodes the visual field from the opposite half of the world.
- The secondary visual cortex processes illusory boundaries: contours that cannot actually be visualized but that are implied by the context of a larger scene.
- Area V4 is the color processing area; it demonstrates color constancy.
- The lateral occipital complex responds disproportionately strongly for object recognition and displays perceptual constancy.
- The fusiform face area is the most well-studied area for facial processing.
- Non-face body parts are processed separate from faces: most notably, in the extrastriate body area in the lateral occipitotemporal cortex.
- The parahippocampal place area processes places: environmental scenes and buildings.
- The motion-processing center lies at the occipital-temporal-parietal junction.
- The parietal lobes contain numerous visual cortical areas dedicated to the processing of spatial awareness, collectively called the "parietal dorsal stream area," which comprises the "where" pathway.
- High-level processing of vision allows for the preservation of depth perception in the setting of monocular (one-eye) vision.

The Eye

Here, we will draw the eye. First, we will draw the outer and middle layers of the eye and then we will draw the inner layer of the eye—the retina. Begin with the cornea, which is the anterior portion of the eye's outer layer. The cornea is avascular and transparent to optimize the passage of light. Its contour, smoothness, transparency, and refractive index all play an important role in focusing light on the retina, and they all demand a healthy endothelium and epithelium.

Next, show that where the cornea ends, the outer layer becomes the sclera. In contrast to the cornea, the sclera is opaque and blocks the transmission of light. We refer to the portion of the sclera we can see as the "white of the eye"; conjunctiva covers it. Posterior to the conjunctiva, the six extraocular muscles insert into the sclera. Note that both the cornea and sclera comprise a fibrous histology that gives the outer eye a semi-elasticity and high tensile strength to allow it to endure the extraocular muscle forces placed upon it and to protect the eye from physical harm.

Now, draw the biconvex lens. Like the cornea, the lens is transparent and serves to focus a target on the retina. The cornea and lens bend the target's light rays so that they strike the retinal area of maximal visual acuity: the fovea. This light ray manipulation is called optic refraction. Unfortunately, opacities, called cataracts, commonly develop in the lens and produce hazy vision, reduced color intensity, increased glare, and worsened visual acuity.

In front of the lens, draw the iris, and show it in coronal view, as well. Indicate that the open region within the center of the iris is the pupil. The pigmented epithelium of the iris blocks light transmission and funnels light through the pupil. The iris forms an adjustable diaphragm that opens and closes based on the illumination demands of the eye. In bright light, show that parasympathetically innervated, circumferentially arranged, iris sphincter muscles contract and constrict pupil size; whereas, in darkness, sympathetically innervated, radially arranged, pupillary dilator muscles activate and widen pupil size (also, see Drawing 23-6).

Lateral to the iris, draw the ciliary body, and posterior to it, draw the choroid. Indicate that these three structures form the middle layer of the eye, called the uvea. The choroid is a thin, brown, highly vascular layer sandwiched between the sclera and retina; it nourishes the retina and removes heat produced during phototransduction, which is the process wherein the photoreceptors transform light into neural signal.

The functions of the ciliary body are twofold. First, show that it anchors suspensory ligaments, collectively called zonule, which stretch the lens and alter its refractive power. As mentioned, the refraction of light adjusts where a visual object falls on the retina, and the adjustment for near or far objects is called accommodation. Accommodation for near objects occurs from relaxation of the zonule. During far vision, the ciliary bodies are relaxed, the zonule are stretched, and the lens is flattened. During near accommodation, the ciliary bodies contract (ie, shorten), which relaxes the zonule and rounds the lens (ie, thickens it), and the near object is brought into focus.

To demonstrate this principle for yourself, do the following. Extend your right index finger to represent a relaxed ciliary body. Then make a V with your left hand's thumb and index finger and touch their tips to the ends of the relaxed ciliary body. The V represents the taut zonular fibers. Imagine that your left hand is the lens; feel the pull of the zonule on your left hand and imagine the lens being flattened. Then, contract the ciliary body (ie, collapse your stretched right index finger); the zonule fold in on themselves, which causes your left hand to relax, and you can imagine the lens rounding.

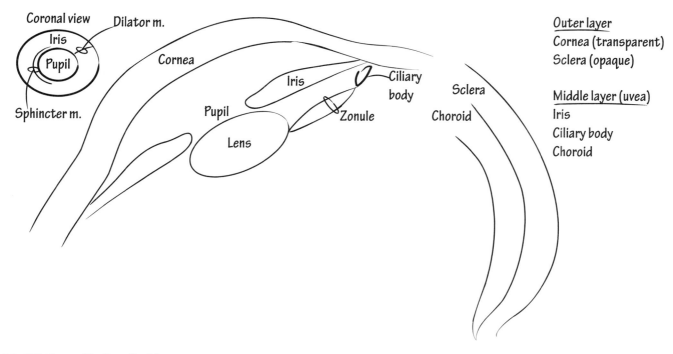

Coronal view

Iris

Pupil

Dilator m.

Sphincter m.

Cornea

Pupil

Lens

Iris

Zonule

Ciliary body

Sclera

Choroid

<u>Outer layer</u>
Cornea (transparent)
Sclera (opaque)

<u>Middle layer (uvea)</u>
Iris
Ciliary body
Choroid

DRAWING 22-1 **The Eye—Partial**

The Eye (Cont.)

In addition to being an anchor for the zonule, the ciliary bodies also produce aqueous humor, which is a low-protein, aqueous (ie, watery) fluid. Show that the ciliary epithelia actively secrete aqueous humor into the posterior chamber (the space between the lens and iris) and show that the aqueous humor then flows through the pupil into the anterior chamber (the space between the iris and cornea), and finally show that the aqueous humor is then reabsorbed at the iridocorneal filtration angle through the trabecular meshwork into the canal of Schlemm. The trabecular meshwork and canal of Schlemm (along with the scleral spur) lie within the internal scleral sulcus, which sits at the inner surface of the sclera–corneal junction, called the limbus. The trabecular meshwork gates the reabsorption of aqueous humor through the canal of Schlemm, which drains directly into the venous system. Note that an alternative reabsorption pathway also exists in which aqueous humor is directly reabsorbed through the ciliary body into the uveal vessels.

Pathology in the aqueous system produces increased intraocular pressure, called glaucoma. Although there are many causes of glaucoma, glaucoma is commonly divided into two forms: open-angle (i.e., wide-angle) and angle-closure (i.e., narrow-angle) glaucoma. In open-angle glaucoma, the more common form, there is failure of adequate aqueous reabsorption through the canal of Schlemm, most commonly due to aberrancy in the trabecular meshwork, itself. In angle-closure glaucoma, the rarer form, there is apposition of key anterior structures, which trap the flow of aqueous humor. For instance, there is abutment of the iris and cornea or lens and iris. Common pharmacologic therapies for glaucoma either reduce aqueous humor production or promote aqueous humor reabsorption.

Next, draw the vitreous chamber, which contains vitreous humor. Like aqueous humor, vitreous humor is primarily water, but the presence of glycosaminoglycans and collagen within this substance gives it its gel-like composition, which helps maintain the eye's shape.[1-3]

Now, draw the retina internal to the choroid. We will parse the retina into its specific layers later, but first let's draw the optic nerve. Indicate that the retina transitions into optic nerve where it exits the eye, posteriorly, at the lamina cribrosa, which is an opening in the sclera. Next, indicate that in the center of the optic nerve lie the central retinal artery and vein. Now, label the optic nerve head and draw a coronal view of it. Indicate that in the center of the optic nerve head sits the optic cup, a white-appearing hole through which the central retinal vessels emanate. Next, label the optic disc, the pink-colored ring of nerve tissue that surrounds the optic cup. Then, back in our main diagram show that the subarachnoid space and dura mater, which is an extension of the sclera, extend along the optic nerve. The presence of the subarachnoid space, here, allows increased intracranial pressure to translate along the optic nerve and impair its axoplasmic transport. Impaired axoplasmic transport at the lamina cribrosa results in optic disc swelling, which is called disc edema or, rather, papilledema when it occurs in the setting of increased intracranial pressure. Papilledema causes disc margin blurring (i.e., blurring of the nerve layer around the disc), venous congestion, and optic disc hyperemia from capillary dilatation secondary to reduced venous return.

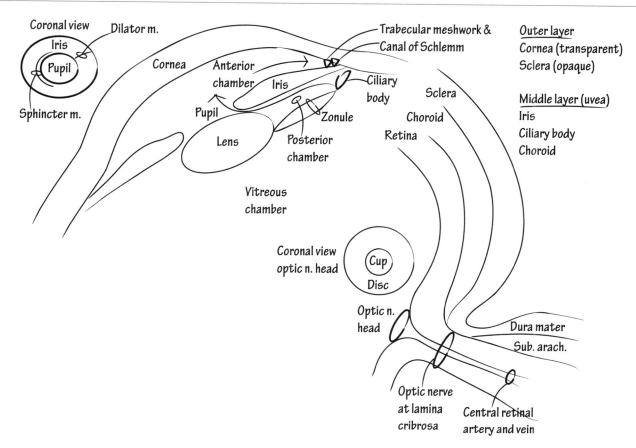

Coronal view
Iris
Pupil
Dilator m.
Sphincter m.

Cornea
Anterior chamber
Iris
Pupil
Lens
Zonule
Posterior chamber
Vitreous chamber

Trabecular meshwork &
Canal of Schlemm
Ciliary body
Sclera
Choroid
Retina

Outer layer
Cornea (transparent)
Sclera (opaque)

Middle layer (uvea)
Iris
Ciliary body
Choroid

Coronal view
optic n. head
Cup
Disc

Optic n. head

Dura mater
Sub. arach.

Optic nerve
at lamina
cribrosa
Central retinal
artery and vein

DRAWING 22-2 **The Eye—Partial**

The Eye (Cont.)

Now, we will address the specific layers of the retina, discuss the passage of light through the retina, and discuss the transformation of light into neural signal, called phototransduction. By convention, the retina contains ten distinct layers, which are reviewed in detail in Drawing 22-4; here, we will simply group the retinal layers into four different functional layers and skip the retinal membranes. First, let's orient ourselves: indicate that internal to the retina lies the vitreous chamber, and external to it lies the choroid. Next, label the innermost retinal layer as the nerve fiber layer; then, label the surrounding layers as the synaptic and cell body layers; then, label the surrounding layer as the photoreceptor cell segment layer (the rods and cones); and finally, label the outermost layer as the retinal pigmented epithelium. Indicate that light passes through the retina and is captured by the photoreceptor cell segments. Show that the phototransduction cascade occurs, here, which transforms light into neural signal, and indicate that the signal is passed back through the retina and passed out of the eye through the optic nerve. The nerve fiber layer is unmyelinated to avoid blocking the passage of light: the nerve fibers become myelinated only after they exit the eye as the optic nerve. Note that the pigmented epithelium captures light not picked up by the photoreceptors and that the photoreceptor cell segments are metabolically dependent upon the pigmented epithelium for photoreceptor regeneration and waste disposal.

Finally, show that the fovea lies in the center of the retina. Draw the center of the fovea as a pin-sized depression; in this central pit, the ganglion and bipolar cells are pushed aside so as not to impede the path of light rays to the photoreceptor layer. This unimpeded path, in combination with the pure cone composition of the central foveal photoreceptor layer, makes the center of the fovea the area of highest visual acuity. Note that in contrast, the optic nerve head is devoid of photoreceptors and we do not perceive the visual region that corresponds to the optic nerve: it forms the blind spot. As a corollary, when disc edema occurs (ie, when the optic nerve head swells), the blind spot enlarges. Enlarged blind spots are commonly observed in the clinical syndrome of idiopathic intracranial hypertension (aka pseudotumor cerebri).

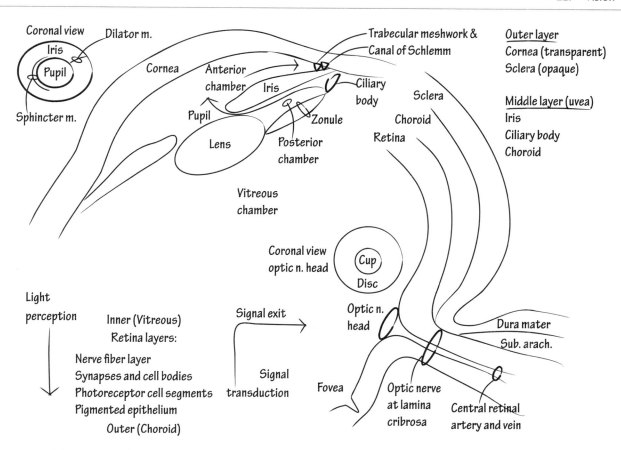

Coronal view
Iris
Pupil
Dilator m.
Sphincter m.

Cornea
Anterior chamber
Pupil
Lens
Iris
Posterior chamber
Zonule
Ciliary body

Trabecular meshwork & Canal of Schlemm

Sclera
Choroid
Retina

Outer layer
Cornea (transparent)
Sclera (opaque)

Middle layer (uvea)
Iris
Ciliary body
Choroid

Vitreous chamber

Coronal view optic n. head
Cup
Disc

Light perception

Inner (Vitreous)
Retina layers:

Nerve fiber layer
Synapses and cell bodies
Photoreceptor cell segments
Pigmented epithelium
Outer (Choroid)

Signal exit

Signal transduction

Fovea

Optic n. head

Optic nerve at lamina cribrosa

Dura mater
Sub. arach.

Central retinal artery and vein

DRAWING 22-3 **The Eye—Complete**

The Retina (*Advanced*)

Here, let's address the organization of the ten distinct layers of the retina in further detail. Label the top of the page as internal to the retina (the vitreous chamber) and the bottom of the page as external to it (the choroid). From inner to outer, the retinal layers are the inner limiting membrane; nerve fiber layer; ganglion cell layer; inner plexiform layer; inner nuclear layer; outer plexiform layer; outer nuclear layer; outer limiting membrane; photoreceptor cell segment layer; and retinal pigmented epithelium.

Once again, indicate that light passes through the retina and is captured by the photoreceptor cell segments. Show that the phototransduction cascade occurs here, which transforms light into neural signal, and indicate that the signal is passed back through the retina and passed out of the eye through the optic nerve. Note that the photoreceptor cell segments are metabolically dependent upon the pigmented epithelium.

Indicate that the inner limiting membrane is a thin, basal lamina that separates the nerve fiber layer from the vitreous chamber and that the outer limiting membrane is a row of intercellular junctions that separates the photoreceptor cell segments from the outer nuclear layer. Müller glial cells extend across the retina: their proximal endings oppose the inner limiting membrane and their distal processes help form the outer limiting membrane.

Next, show that the ganglion cell layer contains ganglion cell bodies, the axons of which form the nerve fiber layer. Then, indicate that the plexiform layers are synaptic zones: the inner plexiform layer is relatively thick whereas the outer plexiform layer is much thinner. Now, show that the nuclear layers contain cell bodies: the inner nuclear layer comprises retinal interneuronal cell bodies and the outer nuclear layer comprises photoreceptor cell bodies.

Lastly, let's further define the five neuronal cell types that exist within the retina. The outermost cells are the rods and cones, which are the photoreceptor cells, and the innermost cells are the ganglion cells, whose unmyelinated axons form the nerve fiber layer. Sandwiched in between the photoreceptor cells and ganglion cells are the bipolar cells, which pass forward visual information from the photoreceptor cells to the ganglion cells, and also the horizontal and amacrine cells, which enhance visual contrast. It is well recognized that the visual system relies more on visual contrast than the overall level of illumination for visual perception: The visual system attends to the borders between light and dark areas or color differences more so than light intensity. As long as we can read the page of a book comfortably, we perceive the words on it just the same in varying levels of illumination; it is the contrast of the ink from the page that makes the largest impression in our mind.

Inner (Vitreous)

Light
perception

Retinal layers:

Structure/function:

Signal exit
through the
optic nerve

Inner limiting membrane — Thin, basal lamina

Nerve fiber layer — Axons of ganglion cells

Ganglion cell layer — Ganglion cell bodies

Inner plexiform layer — Thick synaptic zone

Inner nuclear layer — Retinal interneuronal cell bodies

Outer plexiform layer — Thin synaptic zone

Outer nuclear layer — Photoreceptor cell bodies

Outer limiting membrane — Row of intercellular junctions

Photoreceptor cell segment layer — Light capture & phototransduction

Retinal pigmented epithelium — Photoreceptor metabolism

Outer (Choroid)

DRAWING 22-4 **The Retina**

Visual Pathways: Axial View

Here, we will draw an axial view of the visual pathways from the retinae to the occipital cortices. We will show only the right visual field projection to the left visual cortex for simplicity—the left visual field projects to the right visual cortex in mirror-image fashion. First, let's address the visual fields: the visual fields represent the person's view of the world. Draw axial sections through the left and right eyes and draw projections from central vision to the fovea of each eye. Using the fovea as the midpoint of the retina, subdivide the retinae into nasal and temporal hemiretinae. Now, we are ready to march through the optic projections from the right visual field to the left visual cortex.

First, show that the right visual field projects to the temporal left hemiretina and the nasal right hemiretina. Next, let's establish the key structures along the path of the optic projections. Draw the optic chiasm, the lateral geniculate nuclei, and the visual cortices. Indicate that the left visual cortex receives the right visual field and that the right visual cortex receives the left visual field. Now, show that the left temporal hemiretina projects ipsilaterally to the left lateral geniculate nucleus, and then, show that the right nasal hemiretina sends crossing fibers through the optic chiasm to the contralateral lateral geniculate nucleus (the left lateral geniculate nucleus). Finally, show that the left lateral geniculate nucleus sends optic radiations to the left occipital cortex. We have now completed the path from the right visual field to the left visual cortex.

Next, let's define the optic nerve and optic tract. Encircle the optic projection between the retina and the chiasm and label it as the optic nerve, and encircle the projection between the optic chiasm and the lateral geniculate nucleus and label it as the optic tract. Optic nerve injuries are prechiasmatic and optic tract injuries are postchiasmatic.

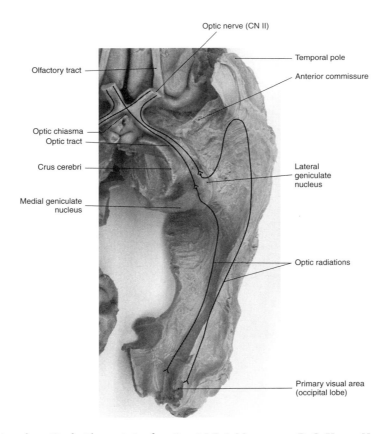

FIGURE 22-1 **Axial view of optic pathway.** Used with permission from Bruni, J. E. & Montemurro, D. G. *Human Neuroanatomy: A Text, Brain Atlas, and Laboratory Dissection Guide.* New York: Oxford University Press, 2009.

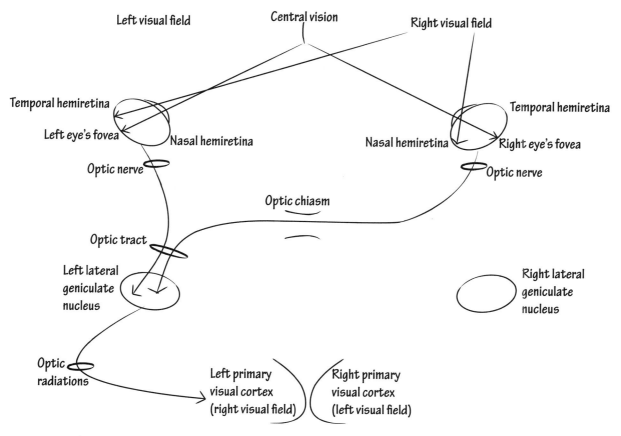

Left visual field

Central vision

Right visual field

Temporal hemiretina

Temporal hemiretina

Left eye's fovea

Nasal hemiretina

Nasal hemiretina

Right eye's fovea

Optic nerve

Optic nerve

Optic chiasm

Optic tract

Left lateral geniculate nucleus

Right lateral geniculate nucleus

Optic radiations

Left primary visual cortex (right visual field)

Right primary visual cortex (left visual field)

DRAWING 22-5 **Visual Pathways: Axial View**

Visual Pathways: Sagittal View

Here, we will draw the visual pathways in sagittal view. First, draw a sagittal view of a cerebral hemisphere and include an eye. Indicate that the superior visual world projects to the inferior portion of the retina and that the inferior visual world projects to the superior portion of the retina. Next, show that the retina projects to the lateral geniculate nucleus. Then, indicate that the stretch of the pathway anterior to the optic chiasm is optic nerve, and the stretch posterior to the optic chiasm is optic tract.

Now, draw an enlarged retinotopic map of the lateral geniculate body. Indicate that central vision comprises the majority of the lateral geniculate body and lies posterior, whereas peripheral vision localizes within the most anterior portion of the lateral geniculate body. Next, let's draw the optic radiations. First, define the occipital horn of the lateral ventricle and show that the superior optic radiation bundle, which carries superior retinal input (from the inferior visual world), projects along the occipital horn through the superior temporal and inferior parietal lobes and terminates in the superior primary visual cortex. Then, define the temporal horn of the lateral ventricle and show that the inferior optic radiation bundle, which carries inferior retinal input (from the superior visual world), fans out in Meyer's loop over the temporal horn and projects back through the inferior temporal lobe to the inferior primary visual cortex. Injury to the inferior bundle is more common than to the superior bundle, so superior visual field defects are more common than inferior field defects. Injury to one optic radiation or the other is called quadrantanopia because it results in injury to a single visual quadrant with preservation of the other three quadrants. For instance, a lesion to the left inferior radiation will affect vision from the right, superior visual quadrant, only. The anterior extent of the inferior optic radiation is important because surgeons must be mindful of the optic radiations during anterior temporal lobe resection.[4]

Lastly, draw an enlarged retinotopic map of the primary visual cortex. Indicate that the cortical representation of central (or macular) vision lies in the posterior calcarine sulcus and occupies a large cortical area relative to its small retinal expanse, whereas representation of peripheral vision lies in the anterior calcarine sulcus and encompasses a small cortical area relative to its broad retinal expanse. Visual cortex is also called "calcarine cortex" because it lies within the dorsal and ventral banks of the calcarine sulcus, which separates the cuneus from the lingual gyrus. The upper bank of the calcarine sulcus encodes the lower half of the visual fields whereas the lower bank encodes the upper half of the visual fields.

Now, let's address the neuroscience of the lateral geniculate body. The lateral geniculate body has both parvocellular and magnocellular components and also koniocellular components; we will address only the parvocellular and magnocellular components, here, because the koniocellular components are less well understood. Layers 3 through 6, the most posterior layers, are parvocellular, whereas layers 1 and 2, the most anterior layers, are magnocellular. The parvocellular layers receive input from the cone layers of the retina and the magnocellular layers receive input from the rod layers. Cones lie within the central retina (the macula) and communicate with X retinal ganglion cells called midget cells, which have small fields and are responsible for visual acuity and color vision. Rods lie in the periphery of the retina and communicate with Y retinal ganglion cells called parasol cells, which have large fields and are sensitive to motion. Thus, because the X and Y division of the retinal ganglion output cells is preserved within the lateral geniculate nucleus as parvocellular and magnocellular regions, respectively, the X and Y ganglion cells are synonymously referred to as P (for parvocellular) and M (for magnocellular) cells, respectively. Note, however, that the X-Y and P-M comparison is imperfect—the differences are beyond our scope, here.[4-11]

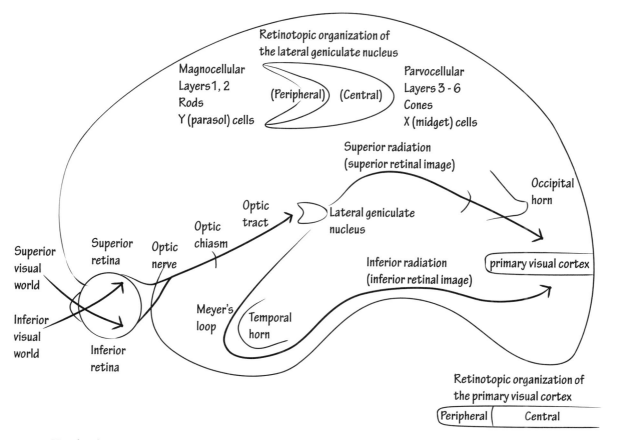

DRAWING 22-6 **Visual Pathways: Sagittal View**

Visual Field Deficits

Here, we will learn the different visual field deficits. First, let's set up our axial diagram of the visual pathways. Label the left and right visual fields, then draw the eyes, the optic chiasm, the lateral geniculate nuclei, and the primary visual cortices. Next add the pathways. On the right-hand side of the page, for each case, we will draw a pair of eyes with their left and right visual fields.

Case I

Patient presents with loss of vision in the left eye. Exam reveals absent vision in the left eye, only. The right eye is normal.

Our diagnosis is a left optic nerve lesion. The unilaterality of the injury localizes the deficit to a prechiasmatic lesion, either in the optic nerve or in the retina, itself. We learn how to distinguish retinal and optic nerve lesions later. Note that a relative afferent pupillary defect would almost certainly accompany this optic nerve injury (see Drawing 23-6).

Case II

Patient presents with right eye loss of vision. Exam reveals left visual field loss in the right eye, only. The left eye is normal.

Our diagnosis is a right lateral optic chiasm lesion. Again, the deficit is limited to one eye; therefore, the injury is anterior to the optic tract. The deficit is in the visual field contralateral to the affected eye, which means that the temporal retinal fibers are selectively affected. Note that this pattern of injury could also occur along the optic nerve, but it is in the optic chiasm that the nasal and temporal retinal fibers split apart: this case highlights the separation of the nasal and temporal retinal fibers within the optic chiasm.

Case III

Patient presents with bilateral loss of vision. Exam reveals bitemporal hemianopia.

Our diagnosis is an optic chiasm lesion. The optic chiasm contains crossing fibers from the bilateral nasal hemiretinae. The nasal hemiretinae receive the temporal visual fields, which means that the left nasal retina perceives the left visual field and the right nasal retina perceives the right visual field. Bitemporal hemianopia is an important exam finding because it often suggests the presence of a sellar mass, such as a pituitary adenoma or craniopharyngioma. Often it is stated that this lesion produces a constriction of vision and a sensation of "wearing horse blinders"; however, more accurately, bitemporal hemianopia produces a loss of binocular fusion, which results in "hemifield slide."[12]

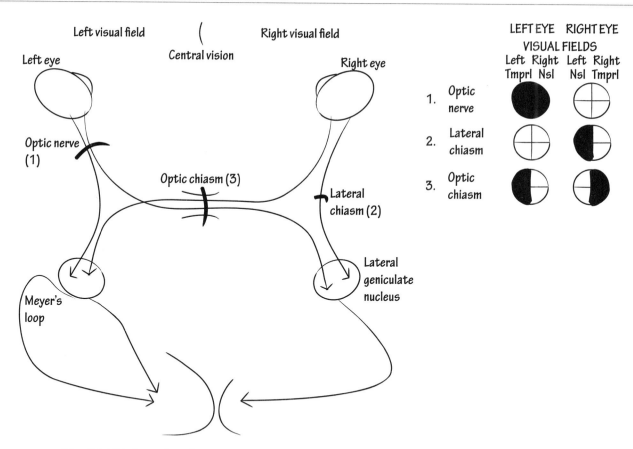

DRAWING 22-7 **Visual Field Deficits—Partial**

Visual Field Deficits (Cont.)

Case IV

Patient presents with difficulty seeing the right half of the world, which is bilateral (both eyes affected). Exam reveals a right homonymous hemianopia: right visual field blindness in both eyes.

Our diagnosis is a lesion of the left postchiasmatic pathway. Disruption of fibers from both the nasal right hemiretina and temporal left hemiretina produces a right homonymous hemianopia. These retinal fibers first bundle posterior to the optic chiasm within the optic tract; however, a lesion anywhere along the postchiasmatic pathway—in the left optic tract, left lateral geniculate nucleus, left optic radiations, or left visual cortex—will produce the described right homonymous hemianopia.

Case V

Patient presents with difficulty seeing the right half of the world, which is bilateral (both eyes affected). Exam reveals a right homonymous inferior quadrantanopia.

Our diagnosis is a left superior optic radiation lesion. The lateral geniculate nucleus projects through superior and inferior optic radiations to the visual cortex. These radiations maintain the same superior–inferior retinotopic organization found in the retina; therefore, a superior optic radiation lesion produces an inferior field defect. The hemianopia lateralizes to the right side, which means that the lesion is postchiasmatic on the left.

Case VI

Patient presents with difficulty seeing the right half of the world, which is bilateral (both eyes affected). Exam reveals a right homonymous superior quadrantanopia.

Our diagnosis is a left inferior optic radiation lesion. As described in the previous case, projections from the lateral geniculate nucleus to the visual cortex maintain the same superior–inferior retinotopic organization as found in the retina; therefore, an inferior radiation lesion produces a superior field defect. Also, as described previously, the hemianopia lateralizes to the right side, so the lesion is postchiasmatic on the left.

Case VII (*Advanced*)

Patient presents with difficulty seeing the right half of the world, which is bilateral (both eyes affected). Exam reveals a right homonymous hemianopia with preserved central vision, called macular sparing.

Our diagnosis is a left occipital lobe lesion. Our current patient has a right homonymous hemianopia with preserved central vision through sparing of left macular cortical representation. According to the vascular model for macular sparing, the posterior cerebral artery supplies the occipital cortex except for the occipital pole, which the middle cerebral artery supplies. Therefore, in the setting of posterior cerebral artery infarction, the middle cerebral artery maintains perfusion of the occipital pole, which spares macular cortical representation.

Additionally, or alternatively, macular sparing is argued to occur from redundant macular representation in both occipital cortices in much the same way that auditory information is redundantly localized to both transverse temporal gyri (of Heschl).[13]

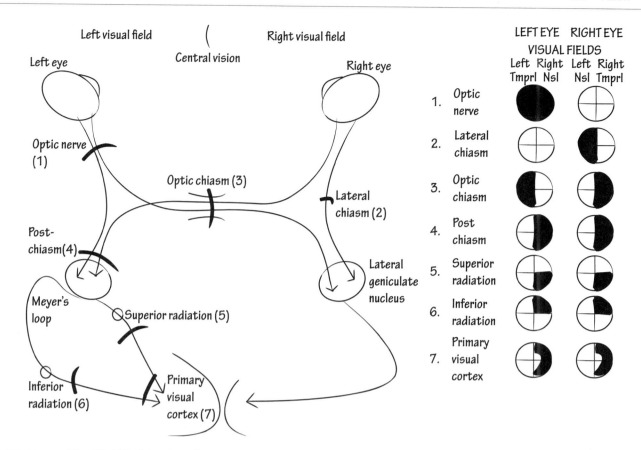

DRAWING 22-8 **Visual Field Deficits—Partial**

Visual Field Deficits (Cont.)

Case VIII (*Advanced*)

Patient presents with blurry vision in the right eye. Exam reveals a central scotoma in the right eye, only.

Our diagnosis is a right-side retinal lesion, specifically a lesion within the macula. The restriction of the deficit to one eye makes this a prechiasmatic lesion, localizing to either the retina or optic nerve. However, the limited pattern of visual field defect allows us to further localize this as a retinal lesion (with the caveat noted at the end). Retinal lesions typically parse into the following categories: central or cecocentral scotomas from injury to the papillomacular bundle; arcuate field defects, which obey the horizontal meridian; and temporal wedge defects from nasal retinal wedge fiber injury. We must appreciate, however, that a partial optic nerve injury can potentially assume the same deficit pattern as any retinal layer injury, and we must go beyond visual field testing to distinguish the localization of a prechiasmatic lesion.[14]

Case IX (*Advanced*)

Patient presents with bilateral visual loss. Exam reveals a central scotoma on the right and a left superior quadrantanopia.

Our diagnosis is a junctional scotoma. To understand the pathogenesis of junctional scotoma, show a fiber project from the left nasal hemiretina through the optic chiasm, and then bend anteriorly into the contralateral optic nerve (the nerve on the right) before projecting posteriorly into the right optic tract. Indicate that this bend is called Wilbrand's knee, and show that it carries inferonasal fibers. Wilbrand's knee has actually been proven to be an artifact of pathologic processing and not a true anatomic entity; however, it is still commonly discussed and still teaches us about the separation of the inferior and superior nasal projections. Although the bend into the optic nerve does not exist, the inferonasal fibers do collect in the anterior optic chiasm and the superonasal fibers do collect in the posterior optic chiasm.[15,16]

Junctional scotoma is a lesion at the junction between the optic nerve and optic chiasm. Two forms of anterior junctional defect are commonly recognized: junctional scotoma (aka anterior junction syndrome) and junctional scotoma of Traquair. Both forms of anterior junctional defect involve the ipsilateral optic nerve. Junctional scotoma results in an ipsilateral central scotoma (from subtotal involvement of the ipsilateral optic nerve) and contralateral superior temporal quadrantanopia from injury to the crossed inferonasal fibers from the opposite eye. Whereas, junctional scotoma of Traquair is an anterior junction injury with isolated ipsilateral optic nerve deficit and results in an ipsilateral temporal hemifield defect, only.[15,17,18]

Let's not let the differences of the junctional scotoma and junctional scotoma of Traquair distract us from a key similarity between the two. Both syndromes are perichiasmatic, and yet they both can easily be mistaken for optic nerve lesions. Distinguishing perichiasmatic from optic nerve lesions is important because perichiasmatic lesions are almost universally secondary to parasellar tumors or aneurysms, whereas optic nerve lesions occur from both compressive and also noncompressive causes.[15,17,18]

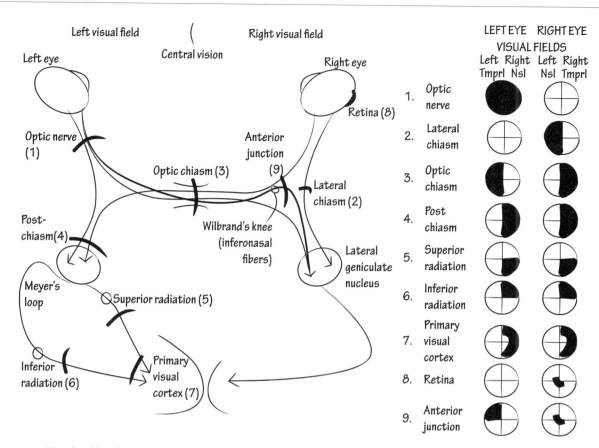

DRAWING 22-9 **Visual Field Deficits—Complete**

Cortical Visual Processing (*Advanced*)

Here, we will create a diagram for the organization of the visual cortex. To create an overview of cortical visual processing, draw a lateral cerebral hemisphere. First, label the posterior, occipital region as the occipital area. In this region, initial cortical visual processing occurs. For our purposes, here, consider this region to encompass the primary visual cortex (aka striate cortex) and the secondary and tertiary visual cortices. Next, label the inferior temporal lobe as the ventral stream and the parietal lobe as the dorsal stream. The ventral stream comprises the "what," object recognition pathway (or P pathway), and the dorsal stream comprises the "where," spatial localization (or M pathway). Note that the division between these pathways begins within the photoreceptors of the retinae: the cone photoreceptors are responsible for color detection and excite parvocellular ganglion cells of the "what" pathway, and the rod photoreceptors are responsible for motion detection and excite magnocellular ganglion cells of the "where" pathway. As visual information is fed forward within the cortex, the "what" and "where" properties of vision separate topographically into ventral and dorsal visual streams. Within the ventral stream, components of objects are integrated to allow for cohesive object identification, and within the dorsal stream, numerous different visuospatial processing centers exist. To complete this overview diagram, draw the frontal eye fields, which are responsible for the cortical initiation of many different classes of eye movements.

Next, let's label the most well-studied cortical visual areas. Draw the posterior aspect of the medial and lateral hemispheres. Then, draw the following anatomic landmarks. Within the medial hemisphere, draw the calcarine sulcus and then the collateral sulcus (which separates the parahippocampal gyrus, medially, from the fusiform gyrus, laterally); then, within the lateral hemisphere, label the Sylvian fissure and the temporo-parietal-occipital junction. Now, show that V1 (the primary visual cortex) lies along the calcarine sulcus of the medial face of the occipital lobe, and also show that it lies at the very tip of the lateral occipital pole. The primary visual cortex is known as V1 because visual cortical stimuli first collect in this area. V1 is often referred to by its Brodmann designation—Brodmann area 17. Also, it is commonly referred to as the striate cortex because of the heavy myelination of its fourth cytoarchitectural layer, which produces a white stripe called the stria of Gennari. Within layer 4, sublayer 4Ca is the primary recipient of magnocellular input and sublayer 4Cb is the primary recipient of parvocellular input. The primary visual cortex processes the most basic visual properties: for example, line orientation, motion direction, luminance orientation, and color. The primary visual cortex in each hemisphere encodes the visual field from the opposite half of the world: right V1 encodes the left visual field and left V1 encodes the right visual field. The cortical representation of central, or macular, vision lies in the posterior calcarine sulcus and occupies a large cortical area relative to its small retinal expanse, whereas representation of the peripheral retina lies in the anterior calcarine sulcus and encompasses a small cortical area relative to its broad retinal expanse. The upper bank of the calcarine sulcus encodes the lower half of the visual field and the lower bank encodes the upper half of the visual field. Interestingly, patients with injury to area V1 often report having blindsight—an unconscious utilization of visual information from the visual field in which they are blind.[19–24]

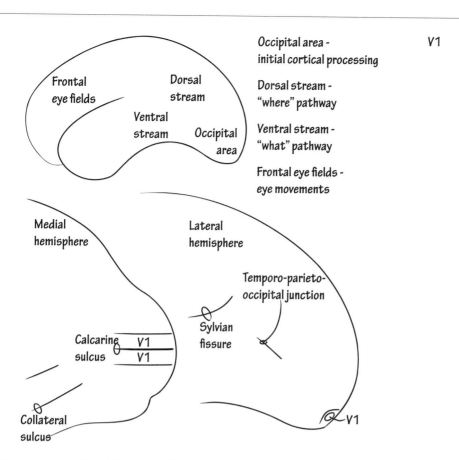

Occipital area -
initial cortical processing

Dorsal stream -
"where" pathway

Ventral stream -
"what" pathway

Frontal eye fields -
eye movements

V1   Primary visual cortex
(Primary processing)

DRAWING 22-10 Cortical Visual Processing—Partial

Cortical Visual Processing (*Advanced*) (Cont.)

Next, let's draw the secondary and tertiary visual cortices. Secondary visual cortex is called V2 and corresponds to Brodmann area 18; tertiary visual cortex is called V3 and corresponds to Brodmann area 19. Indicate that on the medial face of the cerebral hemisphere, V2 lies above and below V1, and V3 lies above and below V2. Note that the ventral part of V3 is commonly referred to as VP instead of V3 because controversy exists as to whether the ventral part of V3 is a unique visual cortical area or whether the dorsal and ventral parts of V3 are both part of a common visual cortical area. Also note that the dorsal and ventral parts of the visual cortices are often denoted by the abbreviations "d" for dorsal and "v" for ventral; for instance, the ventral part of V2 is often denoted as "V2v." Next, on the lateral surface of the hemisphere, indicate that V2 comprises a small strip of the posterior occipital lobe, just anterior to V1; and then show that V3 lies in front of V2—leave a small space inferior to V3 for V4 (drawn next). The secondary and tertiary visual cortices process simple visual properties akin to those processed in V1; notably, however, V2 processes illusory boundaries, contours that cannot actually be visualized but that are implied by the context of a larger scene. Stand in the doorway with one half of your body in the room and the other half outside of view; no one will misperceive that only half of you exists. Through grouping principles of proximity, continuity, and similarity, we naturally incorporate the hidden half of your body into our Gestalt—our general makeup of the world. We generate an illusory boundary of your body based on the characteristics of you that we are able to visualize.[19-24]

Now, let's label the color-processing area V4, which, for practical purposes, can be considered a transitional zone in the visual pathway wherein the ventral stream (the "what" pathway) begins to topographically separate from the dorsal stream; note that we take liberty in designating V4 as part of the ventral stream—the ventral stream is commonly considered to begin anterior to V4. On the medial and lateral surfaces of the cerebral hemisphere, in the ventral-occipital lobe, label the region inferior to V3 as V4. Note that debate exists regarding the anatomy of V4, and also note that an additional visual area separate from V4, called V8, has also been introduced into the literature; for this reason, the ventro-occipital region is often referred to as the V4/V8 region. Also, note that a similar term for V8 has been introduced called VO, which stands for the "ventral occipital" cluster.[19-24]

One important aspect of color processing found within area V4 is that of color constancy, which is the property of color vision wherein regardless of the illumination cast on an object, the object maintains its perceived color. It has been shown that a red patch will maintain its perceived red color and a white patch will maintain its perceived white color even when the level illumination cast on the two different colors is adjusted so that they should be perceived as the same color. To demonstrate this for yourself, consider the color of your pants. Now, look closely at them and see that your pants are not a single color or even a discrete combination of colors but, instead, they comprise a vast array of colors from the different levels of illumination cast onto them—yet we are able to retain a uniform impression of our clothing color due to the high-level color vision processing that occurs within area V4. As a clinical corollary for color processing, before functional MRI studies could identify the ventral occipital cortical response to color patterns, clinical-pathologic case studies demonstrated that ventral occipito-temporal injury caused abnormalities in color processing, called achromatopsia, which results in the visual world appearing gray or drained of color; note, however, that injury to area V4, alone, may or may not be sufficient to cause achromatopsia.[25]

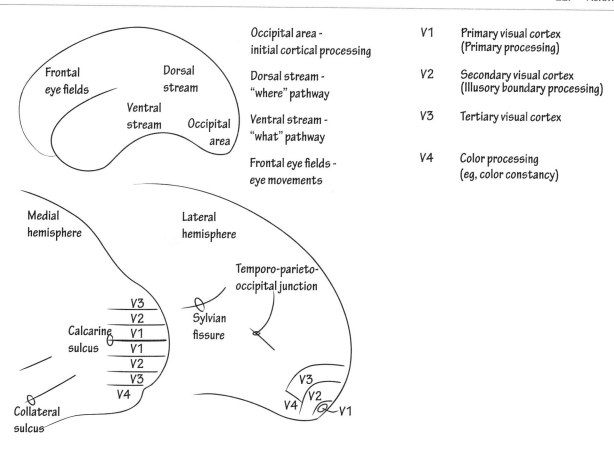

Occipital area -
initial cortical processing

Dorsal stream -
"where" pathway

Ventral stream -
"what" pathway

Frontal eye fields -
eye movements

V1   Primary visual cortex
(Primary processing)

V2   Secondary visual cortex
(Illusory boundary processing)

V3   Tertiary visual cortex

V4   Color processing
(eg, color constancy)

DRAWING 22-11 **Cortical Visual Processing—Partial**

Cortical Visual Processing (*Advanced*) (Cont.)

Now, in the lateral hemisphere diagram, in the lateral occipital cortex, anterior to V4, label the lateral occipital complex. This area responds disproportionately strongly for object recognition. It displays perceptual constancy, meaning an object can be recognized equally well regardless of such properties as object viewpoint, size, or illumination; it also displays form-cue invariance, meaning, for example, that an object is equally identifiable whether it is viewed in the form of a drawing or a photograph.[26]

Next, label the fusiform face area within the right, lateral posterior fusiform gyrus; the fusiform face area is the most well-studied area for facial processing, but additional facial processing centers for different attributes of facial recognition do exist—they include the occipital face area as well as a region of the superior temporal sulcus. Also, note that a longstanding debate is whether the fusiform face area is specific for the recognition of human faces or whether it responds to any over-trained visual stimulus (eg, cars in car salesmen or birds in bird-watchers). As a clinical corollary, injury to the fusiform face area can result in prosopagnosia: a deficit for the recognition of familiar faces (ie, friends and family).[27]

Now, show that non-face body parts are processed separate from faces, most notably, in the extrastriate body area in the lateral occipitotemporal cortex. When we view a human figure, the person's face and body are projected onto the retina contiguously, as they are perceived in the visual world, and they maintain this contiguous relationship when they are projected to the primary visual cortex and, presumably, as they step through the secondary and tertiary visual cortices. But for higher-level visual processing, at least in part, the body is separated from the face and is processed near the V5 motion-sensitive area (discussed next), presumably because of the relationship between body parts and movement. Note, however, that just as multiple centers for facial processing exist, so, too, multiple body part analysis centers also exist, such as the fusiform body area.[22,28]

Next, show that the processing of places lies within the parahippocampal place area, which lies within the posterior parahippocampal and anterior lingual cortices. The parahippocampal place area responds to environmental scenes and buildings. Injury to the parahippocampal place area can potentially cause landmark agnosia, which is the inability to recognize fundamental navigation landmarks: for example, one's own house. Landmark agnosia is often categorized under the more broad clinical phenomenon of topographic disorientation, which is the inability to find one's way through an environment, because patients with landmark agnosia naturally have substantial navigational disorientation. Note, also, that the parahippocampal place area is separate from the parietal dorsal stream area, which is responsible for encoding orientation of the body in space.[26,29–32]

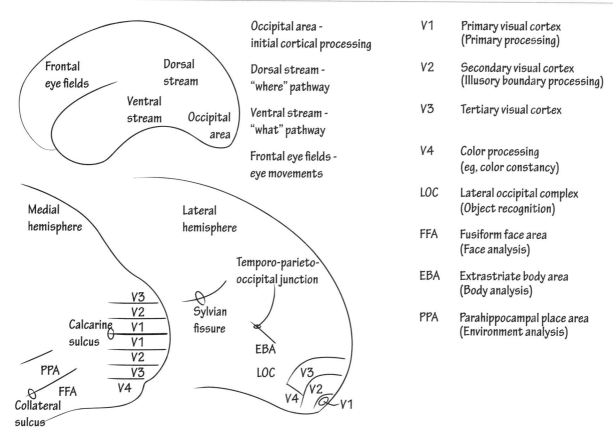

Occipital area -
initial cortical processing

Dorsal stream -
"where" pathway

Ventral stream -
"what" pathway

Frontal eye fields -
eye movements

V1	Primary visual cortex (Primary processing)
V2	Secondary visual cortex (Illusory boundary processing)
V3	Tertiary visual cortex
V4	Color processing (eg, color constancy)
LOC	Lateral occipital complex (Object recognition)
FFA	Fusiform face area (Face analysis)
EBA	Extrastriate body area (Body analysis)
PPA	Parahippocampal place area (Environment analysis)

DRAWING 22-12 **Cortical Visual Processing—Partial**

Cortical Visual Processing (*Advanced*) (Cont.)

Now, at the occipital-temporal-parietal junction, label area V5, which is the motion-processing center and which is often referred to as hMT because it represents the human correlate to the macaque middle temporal visual area. Visual perception of motion is processed in this region; this visual area is part of our model for the circuitry of smooth pursuit eye movements (see Drawing 23-5)—it plays a fundamental role in the tracking of a moving target. Note that motion processing also involves other brain regions, including area V5a, the human corollary for the macaque medial superior temporal visual area, which lies adjacent (just superior) to V5. Note, as well, that for practical purposes, just as we consider V4 to be the first step in the topographic separation of the ventral stream from the dorsal stream, so, too, here, we take the practical liberty of considering V5 to be the first step in the separation of the dorsal stream from the ventral stream—even though the dorsal stream, itself, is commonly limited to the parietal visual areas (discussed next). Finally, as a clinical corollary, patients with injury to V5 demonstrate akinetopsia, which is an inability to visualize moving objects despite a preserved ability to accurately visualize stationary objects.

Next, label the lateral parietal lobe as P-DSA, which stands for "parietal dorsal stream area." The parietal lobes contain numerous visual cortical areas dedicated to the processing of spatial awareness, and they comprise the "where" pathway. Some of the specific visual areas that are identified within the parietal dorsal stream area are the parietal reach region in the intraparietal sulcus, which activates during reach and pointing movements; the anterior parietal area in the anterior parietal sulcus, which activates during fine motor movements; the ventral parietal area in the depths of the intraparietal sulcus, which activates during multimodal motion detection of moving stimuli; the lateral intraparietal area in the posterior intraparietal sulcus, which activates during visually guided saccadic eye movements; and the superior and inferior parietal lobules, which function in attention control and spatial awareness. We can think of the parietal dorsal stream area as the "show me the way" area; it instructs the motor cortex where to move.[22]

As a final point, consider that an important aspect of visual processing is depth perception, which, as it turns out, is more than simply a product of stereoscopic vision (the reconciliation of binocular disparity); it also involves high-level processing of numerous visual cues. This visual processing allows for the preservation of depth perception in the setting of monocular (one-eye) vision. As a prominent example of the capability of monocular vision to provide depth perception, consider that Wiley Post was a highly regarded pilot who won the 1930 Los Angeles to Chicago Air Derby with the use of only one eye.[33–35]

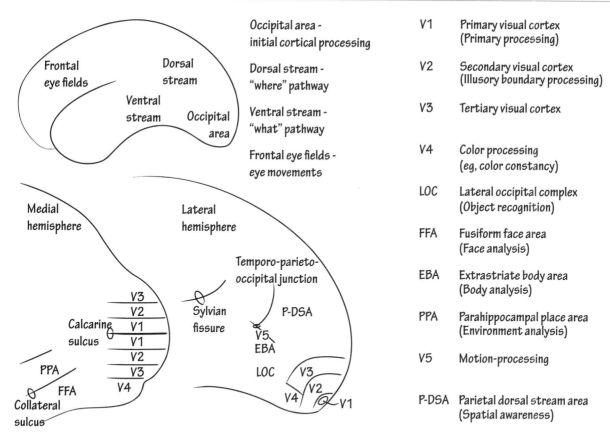

Occipital area - initial cortical processing

Dorsal stream - "where" pathway

Ventral stream - "what" pathway

Frontal eye fields - eye movements

V1	Primary visual cortex (Primary processing)
V2	Secondary visual cortex (Illusory boundary processing)
V3	Tertiary visual cortex
V4	Color processing (eg, color constancy)
LOC	Lateral occipital complex (Object recognition)
FFA	Fusiform face area (Face analysis)
EBA	Extrastriate body area (Body analysis)
PPA	Parahippocampal place area (Environment analysis)
V5	Motion-processing
P-DSA	Parietal dorsal stream area (Spatial awareness)

DRAWING 22-13 **Cortical Visual Processing—Complete**

References

1. Atchison, D. A. & Smith, G. *Optics of the human eye*, pp. 11–12 (Butterworth-Heinemann, 2000).

2. Krachmer, J. H., Mannis, M. J. & Holland, E. J. *Cornea*, 2nd ed., pp. 3–27 (Elsevier Mosby, 2005).

3. Jenkins, A. J. *Drug testing in alternate biological specimens*, p. 118 (Humana Press, 2008).

4. Sherbondy, A. J., Dougherty, R. F., Napel, S. & Wandell, B. A. Identifying the human optic radiation using diffusion imaging and fiber tractography. *J Vis* 8, 12.1–11 (2008).

5. Alonso, J. M., Yeh, C. I., Weng, C. & Stoelzel, C. Retinogeniculate connections: A balancing act between connection specificity and receptive field diversity. *Prog Brain Res* 154, 3–13 (2006).

6. Fitzpatrick, D., Itoh, K. & Diamond, I. T. The laminar organization of the lateral geniculate body and the striate cortex in the squirrel monkey (*Saimiri sciureus*). *J Neurosci* 3, 673–702 (1983).

7. Glees, P. & le Gros Clark, W. E. The termination of optic fibres in the lateral geniculate body of the monkey. *J Anat* 75, 295–308 (1941).

8. Guido, W. Refinement of the retinogeniculate pathway. *J Physiol* 586, 4357–4362 (2008).

9. Kaplan, E. & Shapley, R. M. X and Y cells in the lateral geniculate nucleus of macaque monkeys. *J Physiol* 330, 125–143 (1982).

10. Murray, K. D., Rubin, C. M., Jones, E. G. & Chalupa, L. M. Molecular correlates of laminar differences in the macaque dorsal lateral geniculate nucleus. *J Neurosci* 28, 12010–12022 (2008).

11. Schiller, P. H. & Malpeli, J. G. Functional specificity of lateral geniculate nucleus laminae of the rhesus monkey. *J Neurophysiol* 41, 788–797 (1978).

12. Schiefer, U., Wilhelm, H. & Hart, W. M. *Clinical neuro-ophthalmology: a practical guide*, p. 8 (Springer, 2007).

13. Leff, A. A historical review of the representation of the visual field in primary visual cortex with special reference to the neural mechanisms underlying macular sparing. *Brain Lang* 88, 268–278 (2004).

14. Walsh, F. B., Hoyt, W. F. & Miller, N. R. *Walsh and Hoyt's clinical neuro-ophthalmology: the essentials*, 2nd ed., Chapter 2 (Lippincott Williams & Wilkins, 2008).

15. Horton, J. C. Wilbrand's knee of the primate optic chiasm is an artefact of monocular enucleation. *Trans Am Ophthalmol Soc* 95, 579–609 (1997).

16. Lee, J. H., Tobias, S., Kwon, J. T., Sade, B. & Kosmorsky, G. Wilbrand's knee: does it exist? *Surg Neurol* 66, 11–17 (2006).

17. Schiefer, U., et al. Distribution of scotoma pattern related to chiasmal lesions with special reference to anterior junction syndrome. *Graefes Arch Clin Exp Ophthalmol* 242, 468–477 (2004).

18. Karanjia, N. & Jacobson, D. M. Compression of the prechiasmatic optic nerve produces a junctional scotoma. *Am J Ophthalmol* 128, 256–258 (1999).

19. Brown, J. M. Visual streams and shifting attention. *Prog Brain Res* 176, 47–63 (2009).

20. Grill-Spector, K. & Malach, R. The human visual cortex. *Annu Rev Neurosci* 27, 649–677 (2004).

21. Wandell, B. A., Dumoulin, S. O. & Brewer, A. A. Visual field maps in human cortex. *Neuron* 56, 366–383 (2007).

22. Rajimehr, R. & Tootell, R. Organization of human visual cortex. In *The senses: a comprehensive reference* (ed A. I. Basbaum) (Elsevier Inc., 2008).

23. Fukushima, T., Kasahara, H., Kamigaki, T. & Miyashita, Y. High-level visual processing. In *The senses: a comprehensive reference*. (ed A.I. Basbaum) (Elsevier Inc., 2008).

24. Downing, P. E., Chan, A. W., Peelen, M. V., Dodds, C. M. & Kanwisher, N. Domain specificity in visual cortex. *Cereb Cortex* 16, 1453–1461 (2006).

25. Walsh, V. & Kulikowski, J. J. *Perceptual constancy: why things look as they do*, pp. 359–362 (Cambridge University Press, 1998).

26. Banich, M. T. *Cognitive neuroscience*, 10th ed., pp. 190–191, 225 (Wadsworth/Cengage Learning, 2010).

27. Calder, A. *Oxford handbook of face perception*, new book ed., pp. 115–117 (Oxford University Press, 2011).

28. Astafiev, S. V., Stanley, C. M., Shulman, G. L. & Corbetta, M. Extrastriate body area in human occipital cortex responds to the performance of motor actions. *Nat Neurosci* 7, 542–548 (2004).

29. Dudchenko, P. A. *Why people get lost: the psychology and neuroscience of spatial cognition*, pp. 221–249 (Oxford University Press, 2010).

30. D'Esposito, M. *Neurological foundations of cognitive neuroscience*, pp. 89–90 (The MIT Press, 2002).

31. Devinsky, O. & D'Esposito, M. *Neurology of cognitive and behavioral disorders*, pp. 248–249 (Oxford University Press, 2004).

32. Aguirre, G. K. & D'Esposito, M. Topographical disorientation: a synthesis and taxonomy. *Brain* 122 (Pt 9), 1613–1628 (1999).

33. Davis, J. R. *Fundamentals of aerospace medicine*, 4th ed., p. 16 (Lippincott Williams & Wilkins, 2008).

34. Gibb, R., Gray, R. & Scharff, L. *Aviation visual perception: research, misperception and mishaps*, pp. 80–81 (Ashgate, 2010).

35. Vickers, J. N. *Perception, cognition, and decision training: the quiet eye in action*, pp. 22–23 (Human Kinetics, 2007).

23

Eye Movements

Final Common Pathway

Horizontal Saccade Circuitry

Horizontal Saccade Details (Advanced)

Vertical Saccades (Advanced)

Smooth Pursuit

Pupillary Light Reflex

Know-It Points

Final Common Pathway

- The abducens nucleus of cranial nerve 6 comprises pools of motoneurons and interneurons.
- The motoneurons innervate the ipsilateral lateral rectus muscle, which drives the attached eye laterally.
- The interneurons project fibers across midline that ascend the medial longitudinal fasciculus and synapse in the oculomotor nucleus.
- The oculomotor nucleus innervates the ipsilateral medial rectus muscle, which drives the attached eye medially.

- Through the final common pathway, the abducens nucleus and the contralateral oculomotor nucleus act in tandem.
- In a complete abducens nuclear injury, there is loss of gaze to the side of the lesion.
- In an internuclear ophthalmoplegia (or MLF syndrome), the ipsilateral eye is unable to adduct and the opposite eye has horizontal nystagmus when it abducts.

Horizontal Saccade Circuitry

- The superior colliculus is commonly divided into a dorsal, "visuosensory" division and a ventral, "motor" division.
- The frontal eye fields directly excite contralateral excitatory burst neurons.
- The frontal eye fields also send an indirect excitatory pathway through the superior colliculus, which also excites the contralateral excitatory burst neurons.
- The excitatory burst neurons (of the paramedian pontine reticular formation) excite the ipsilateral abducens nucleus.

- The excitatory burst neurons also excite the ipsilateral inhibitory burst neurons (of the medullary reticular formation), which inhibit the contralateral abducens nucleus.
- The omnipause cells tonically inhibit the excitatory burst neurons and also the inhibitory burst neurons.
- The excitatory burst neurons inhibit the omnipause neurons and inactivate their tonic suppression of the burst neurons.
- The neural integrator receives fibers from and projects fibers to a wide array of nuclei, including the excitatory and inhibitory burst neurons, to sustain gaze.

Vertical Saccades (*Advanced*)

- The rostral interstitial nuclei of the medial longitudinal fasciculus (riMLF) comprise the excitatory burst neurons for vertical and torsional saccades.
- The interstitial nuclei of Cajal (INC) are the neural integrator for vertical and torsional saccades.

- The riMLF produces bilateral projections for upward gaze but only ipsilateral projections for downward gaze.
- From the subject's point of view, the right riMLF produces clockwise torsional rotation of the eyes, and the left riMLF produces counterclockwise torsional rotation of the eyes.

Smooth Pursuit

- Each hemisphere is responsible for ipsilateral smooth pursuit eye movements; for instance, the right hemisphere detects and tracks images as they move to the right.
- M retinal ganglion cells receive rod photoreceptor detection of the target's movement.
- The primary visual cortex projects to visual area V5 (the human homologue to the macaque middle temporal [MT] area).
- Area V5 projects to visual area V5a (the human homologue to the macaque medial superior temporal [MST] area).
- Area V5a projects to the posterior parietal cortex, which projects to the frontal eye fields.

- The frontal eye fields (and other cortical visual areas, as well) project to the ipsilateral pontine nuclei.
- The pontine nuclei project across midline to the opposite side of the cerebellum, most notably to the vestibulocerebellum.
- The cerebellum projects to the ipsilateral medial vestibular nucleus in the medulla.
- The medial vestibular nucleus projects to the contralateral abducens nucleus (on the side of the brain that detected the movement), which excites the final common pathway for horizontal eye movements.

Pupillary Light Reflex

- Optic fibers of the pupillary light reflex synapse in the pretectal olivary nucleus of the pretectal area rather than the lateral geniculate nucleus.
- The prectectal olivary nucleus projects directly to the ipsilateral Edinger–Westphal nucleus and to the contralateral Edinger–Westphal nucleus via the posterior commissure.

- Each Edinger–Westphal nucleus projects to its ipsilateral ciliary ganglion.
- The ciliary ganglion sends short ciliary nerves to innervate the sphincter pupillae muscles to produce pupillary constriction.

Final Common Pathway

Here, we will draw the anatomy of the final common pathway for conjugate horizontal eye movements. Note that our diagram is a simplified schematic: the topographic anatomy of the oculomotor and abducens nuclei is more accurately depicted in Chapters 11 & 12. First, draw a coronal view of the brainstem and label the midbrain, pons, and medulla. Then, draw axial sections through the eyes. Now, label the left side of the page as left and the right side as right, and also denote the midline of the diagram. Next, attach a lateral rectus muscle to the left eye and a medial rectus muscle to the right eye.

Now, let's draw the cranial nerve nuclei involved in the final common pathway for horizontal eye movements. In the pons, on the left side, draw the abducens nucleus of cranial nerve 6. Show that it comprises pools of motoneurons and interneurons. Indicate that the motoneurons innervate the left eye's lateral rectus muscle, which drives the left eye to the left (laterally). Next, draw the right oculomotor nucleus of cranial nerve 3 in the midbrain. Now, let's show the internuclear connection between these two nuclei: the right medial longitudinal fasciculus. Then, show that the left abducens interneurons project fibers across midline that ascend the right medial longitudinal fasciculus and synapse in the right oculomotor nucleus. Finally, show that the right oculomotor nucleus innervates the right eye's medial rectus muscle and drives the right eye to the left (medially).

Next, to enhance our understanding of this pathway, let's address the common lesions that disrupt it. First, redraw our diagram. Then, show that injury to the abducens motoneurons causes loss of ipsilateral eye abduction. Next, show that injury to the abducens interneurons causes loss of contralateral eye adduction. Finally, encircle the entire abducens nucleus to indicate that in a complete abducens nuclear injury, there is loss

of gaze to the side of the lesion: for example, in a left abducens nuclear injury, the eyes are unable to deviate to the left.

Now, again, redraw our diagram. Show that when the medial longitudinal fasciculus is injured, the ipsilateral eye is unable to adduct. This is called an internuclear ophthalmoplegia (or MLF syndrome)—the ipsilateral eye is unable to adduct and the opposite eye has horizontal nystagmus when it abducts.

Next, redraw our diagram, again, but here include the bilateral eye movement circuitry: draw the bilateral medial and lateral recti muscles and draw eye movements for both horizontal directions of gaze. Then, show that when both medial longitudinal fasciculus tracts are injured, neither eye can adduct: the right eye can't turn horizontally to the left and the left eye can't turn horizontally to the right. This is called bilateral internuclear ophthalmoplegia. Pathologic processes that cross midline, such as demyelinating plaques, hemorrhages, or tumors, can cause this form of injury because the medial longitudinal fasciculus tracts run close together in the midline of the brainstem.

For the last diagram, redraw the bilateral final common pathway arrangement. Show that when the left abducens nucleus is injured, there is loss of gaze toward the side of the lesion (left gaze palsy), and then show that when the adjacent medial longitudinal fasciculus is injured, the ipsilateral eye (the left eye) can't adduct. Thus, when both the abducens nucleus and the adjacent medial longitudinal fasciculus are injured, the only intact movement is right eye abduction (and it has nystagmus from the left medial longitudinal fasciculus injury); thus, one-and-a-half of the two complete eye movements are impaired, so the injury pattern is called one-and-a-half syndrome.[1,2]

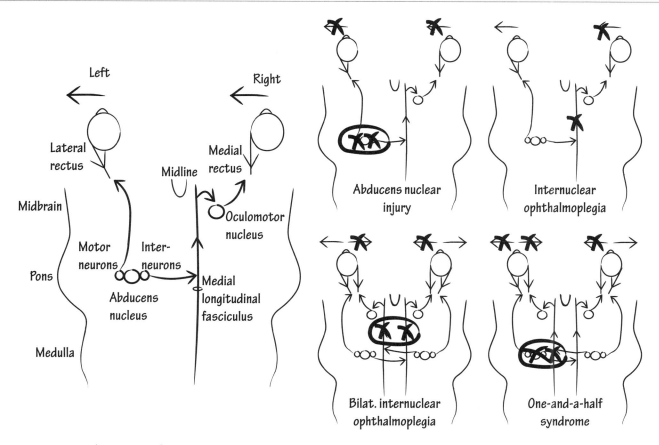

DRAWING 23-1 **Final Common Pathway**

Horizontal Saccade Circuitry

Here, we will draw the supra-ocular circuitry for horizontal saccadic eye movements (aka horizontal saccades). First, draw a brainstem in coronal view and divide it into its midbrain, pons, and medulla, and then label its anatomic left and right sides. Next, above the brainstem, draw a right cerebral hemisphere and label the frontal eye fields. Now, in the upper midbrain, draw the right superior colliculus. For a long time, the importance of the superior colliculus went unrecognized because isolated lesions of the superior colliculus are rare, but experimental inactivation of the superior colliculus has proven its significance. The superior colliculus is commonly divided into a dorsal, "visuosensory" division and a ventral, "motor" division. The dorsal division receives an organized retinotopic map of the contralateral visual hemifield from retinal ganglion cells and also receives afferent input from visual cortical regions, as well, including the striate, extrastriate, and frontal cortices. The ventral division projects to the contralateral abducens nucleus (as drawn next).

Now, draw the bilateral abducens nuclei, which span from the mid-pons to the low pons. For the remainder of the diagram, we will draw the left brainstem ocular nuclei, only. Next, in the mid-pons, draw the excitatory burst neurons of the paramedian pontine reticular formation; they lie anterior to the superior aspect of the abducens nucleus. Then, draw the inhibitory burst neurons of the medullary reticular formation; they lie within the rostral medulla anterior to the plane of the abducens nucleus. Now, show that the neural integrator lies along the dorsal tegmentum of the upper medulla; it lies just anterior to the fourth ventricle. Finally, draw the omnipause neurons in midline, which lie in between the rootlets of the abducens nerves in the pontine tegmentum.

Next, let's add the functional circuitry for horizontal saccades. First, show that the frontal eye fields directly excite contralateral excitatory burst neurons, and then show that the frontal eye fields also send an indirect excitatory pathway that synapses within the superior colliculus, which, in turn, excites the contralateral excitatory burst neurons. Note that the indirect pathway is actually more robust than the direct pathway. Now, draw excitatory projection fibers from the excitatory burst neurons to the ipsilateral abducens nucleus. This excitation stimulates the final common pathway for horizontal saccades (see Drawing 23-1).

Next, let's interrupt our diagram to demonstrate with our fists that the right hemisphere drives the eyes to the left and that the left hemisphere drives the eyes to the right. Hold your fists in front of you; they represent the frontal eye fields. Point your index fingers inward in a V shape to show that each cerebral hemisphere drives the eyes in the opposite direction. Next, drop your right fist to show that a destructive lesion, such as a stroke, causes a loss of innervation from the right frontal eye fields, and as a result, the left frontal eye fields drive the eyes to the right. Then, shake your right hand to show that an excitatory event, such as a seizure, causes overstimulation of the right frontal eye fields, and so the right frontal eye fields overpower the left and drive the eyes to the left.

Now, let's continue with our diagram. Show that in addition to exciting the abducens nucleus, the excitatory burst neurons also excite the ipsilateral inhibitory burst neurons, which inhibit the contralateral abducens nucleus. Thus, when the left abducens nucleus is stimulated, the right abducens nucleus is inactivated, which prevents both nuclei from firing at the same time.

Next, show that the omnipause cells tonically inhibit the excitatory burst neurons and also the inhibitory burst neurons. Then, indicate that the excitatory burst neurons inhibit the omnipause neurons and inactivate their tonic suppression of the burst neurons. Finally, indicate that the neural integrator receives fibers from and projects fibers to a wide array of nuclei, including the excitatory and inhibitory burst neurons, to sustain gaze, as detailed further in Drawing 23-3.[1–3]

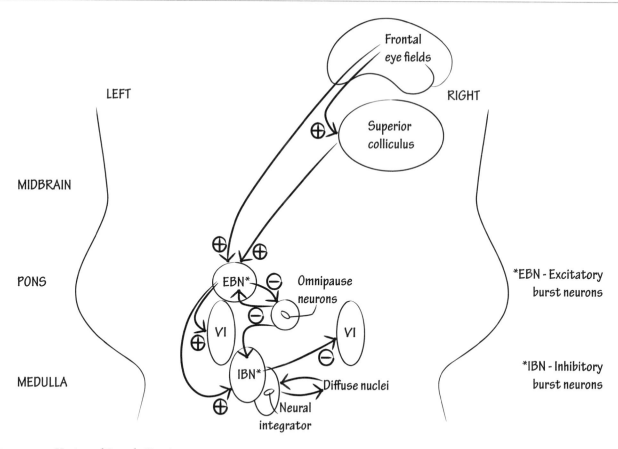

DRAWING 23-2 **Horizontal Saccade Circuitry**

Horizontal Saccade Details (*Advanced*)

Here, we will review and elaborate on our discussion of the anatomy and control of horizontal saccades. Across the top of the diagram, write the following headings: center, anatomy, action, and deficit. First, list the supra-ocular command centers for horizontal saccades. Begin with the frontal eye fields, which comprise the frontal eye *field*, a discrete region in the anterior precentral sulcus near the superior frontal sulcus that is homologous to the location of the frontal eye field of the macaque monkey; and then show that the frontal eye fields also comprise, most notably, the supplementary eye field and dorsolateral prefrontal cortex. Other important supra-ocular command centers include the superior colliculus and cerebellum, and also the anterior cingulate cortex and basal ganglia. Now, in regards to their action, indicate that the frontal eye fields and superior colliculus drive the eyes to the contralateral side, and then show that injury to these structures produces contralateral *volitional* horizontal gaze palsy.[4,5] Note that horizontal saccades via the vestibulo-ocular reflex are spared in the setting of frontal eye field or superior colliculus injury.

Next, let's address the excitatory burst neurons; indicate that they lie within the nucleus reticularis pontis caudalis of the paramedian pontine reticular formation (PPRF)—the nucleus reticularis pontis caudalis lies within the mid-pons, anterior to the superior aspect of the abducens nucleus. Indicate that the excitatory burst neurons activate the ipsilateral abducens nucleus, and also show that they activate the ipsilateral inhibitory burst neurons, which inhibit the contralateral abducens nucleus. Then, show that the excitatory burst neurons also inhibit the omnipause neurons and innervate the neural integrator, as well. Next, show that injury to the PPRF produces ipsilateral horizontal gaze palsy. When the PPRF is selectively injured, the final common pathway will be spared; however, due to its proximity to the abducens nucleus, PPRF injury is most often associated with abducens nucleus injury, which disrupts the final common pathway.

Now, let's address the inhibitory burst neurons; show that they lie within the nucleus paragigantocellularis dorsalis of the medullary reticular formation—the nucleus paragigantocellularis dorsalis lies within the rostral medulla anterior to the plane of the abducens nucleus. Indicate that the inhibitory burst neurons, most notably, suppress the contralateral abducens nucleus from firing, which prevents antagonist forces on the intended horizontal saccade movement. Injury to the inhibitory burst neurons is hypothesized to produce ocular flutter, high-frequency conjugate horizontal saccades without an intersaccadic interval.[1]

Next, let's address the neural integrator; show that it lies within the medial vestibular nucleus and the nucleus prepositus hypoglossi of the perihypoglossal complex, which lie along the dorsal tegmentum of the upper medulla just anterior to the fourth ventricle. Indicate that the neural integrator produces gaze holding. Show that injury to the neural integrator causes a leaky integrator, which means that the eyes do not remain in the intended direction of gaze but instead drift back to center, prompting a corrective saccade.

Finally, let's address the omnipause neurons; show that they lie within the nucleus raphe interpositus, which sits in midline in between the rootlets of the abducens nerves in the pontine tegmentum. Indicate that omnipause cells tonically suppress the excitatory and inhibitory burst neurons except immediately before and during saccadic eye movements. The predicted deficit in omnipause cell injury is opsoclonus: multidirectional saccadic oscillations without an intersaccadic interval, but what is actually observed, instead, is a slowing of saccades. Opsoclonus is often ascribed to cerebellar injury; the cerebellum receives projections from the frontal eye fields and superior colliculus, which first relay, most notably, within the nucleus reticularis tegmenti pontis, which lies within the mid- to upper antero-central pontine tegmentum.[1-3]

CENTER	ANATOMY	ACTION	DEFICIT
Supraocular command centers	Frontal eye fields: frontal eye field, supplementary eye field, dorsolateral prefrontal cortex. Superior colliculus, cerebellum, anterior cingulate cortex, & basal ganglia.	Frontal eye fields & superior colliculus produce contra-lateral horizontal saccades	Contralateral volitional horizontal gaze palsy
Excitatory burst neurons (EBN)	Nucleus reticularis pontis caudalis (of the paramedian pontine reticular formation)	Activate ipsilateral abducens nucleus & ipsilateral inhibitory burst neurons, inhibit omnipause neurons, & innervate neural integrator	Ipsilateral horizontal gaze palsy
Inhibitory burst neurons (IBN)	Nucleus paragigantocellularis dorsalis (of the medullary reticular formation)	Inhibit the contralateral abducens nucleus	Ocular flutter
Neural integrator	Medial vestibular nucleus & nucleus prepositus hypoglossi (of the perihypoglossal complex)	Gaze holding	Leaky integrator
Omnipause neurons	Nucleus raphe interpositus	Tonic inhibition of excitatory & inhibitory burst neurons	Saccade slowing

DRAWING 23-3 **Horizontal Saccade Details**

Vertical Saccades (*Advanced*)

Here, we will draw the anatomic substrate for vertical and torsional saccades. First, draw a coronal section through the midbrain and pons. Label the left and right sides of the brainstem. At the top of the diagram, at the midbrain–diencephalic junction, in the plane of the mammillary bodies, near the midline of the diagram, draw the bilateral rostral interstitial nuclei of the medial longitudinal fasciculus (riMLF). Next, just beneath the bilateral riMLF, still in the midbrain–diencephalic junction, near midline in the dorsal tegmentum, draw the bilateral interstitial nuclei of Cajal (INC). Now, beneath the bilateral INCs, show that the oculomotor complex straddles the midline of the mid- to upper midbrain; it lies within the dorsal tegmentum just anterior to the periaqueductal gray area. Note that although we often represent the oculomotor nuclei as comprising two discrete nuclei, it actually forms a single oculomotor complex consisting of many subnuclei (see Drawing 12-5). Next, beneath the oculomotor complex, in the lower midbrain (in the plane of the inferior colliculi), draw the bilateral trochlear nuclei, which also lie within the dorsal tegmentum, near midline. Lastly, draw the nucleus raphe interpositus in midline in the pontine tegmentum; it lies in between the rootlets of the abducens nerves.

Now that we have completed an anatomic view of the relevant ocular nuclei for vertical and torsional saccades, let's describe their supranuclear control. Write out the headings: nucleus and function. Then, indicate that the riMLF comprises the excitatory burst neurons for vertical and torsional saccades; it acts in similar fashion to the nucleus reticularis pontis caudalis of the PPRF for horizontal saccades. Now, show that the INC is the neural integrator for vertical and torsional saccades, similar to the medial vestibular nucleus and nucleus prepositus hypoglossi for horizontal saccades. Next, show that the nucleus raphe interpositus contains the omnipause neurons for vertical and torsional saccades just as it does for horizontal saccades. Lastly, note that certain texts describe the INC as containing the inhibitory burst neurons for vertical and torsional saccades whereas others describe the riMLF as containing them; as a reminder, for comparison, the nucleus paragigantocellularis dorsalis of the medullary reticular formation contains the inhibitory burst neurons for horizontal saccades.

Next, we will list the high points of vertical and torsional saccade circuitry. First, indicate that the riMLF produces bilateral projections for upward gaze but only ipsilateral projections for downward gaze. Thus, a unilateral riMLF lesion will cause isolated downward gaze palsy (observed as slowing of downward gaze), but redundant innervation for upward gaze preserves the function and speed of upward gaze. Next, indicate the laterality of riMLF innervation for torsional saccades. Show that from the subject's point of view, the right riMLF produces clockwise torsional rotation of the eyes, whereas the left riMLF produces counterclockwise torsional rotation of the eyes. Stated differently, from the subject's perspective, the top poles of the eyes rotate toward the riMLF that is activated. To demonstrate this, hold your fists in front of you and point your index fingers straight up. Now, activate the right riMLF and rotate your fingers to the right; then, activate the left riMLF and rotate your fingers to the left. Note that the torsional deficits observed in unilateral riMLF lesions are more substantial than the vertical deficits.

Finally, consider that whereas the frontal eye fields and superior colliculus project to the contralateral PPRF excitatory burst neurons for horizontal saccades, they project to the ipsilateral riMLF for vertical and torsional saccades.[1–3,6]

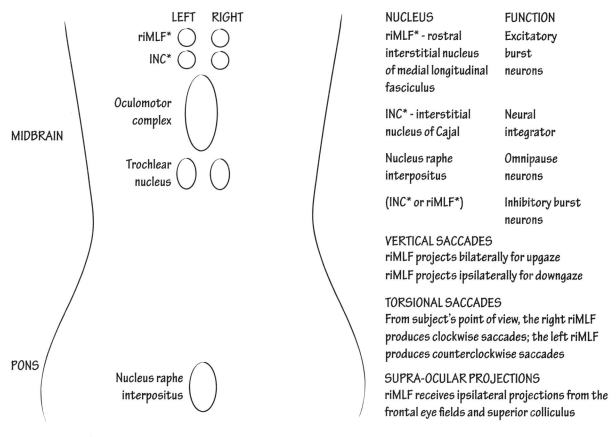

LEFT   RIGHT

riMLF*

INC*

Oculomotor
complex

MIDBRAIN

Trochlear
nucleus

PONS

Nucleus raphe
interpositus

NUCLEUS	FUNCTION
riMLF* - rostral interstitial nucleus of medial longitudinal fasciculus	Excitatory burst neurons
INC* - interstitial nucleus of Cajal	Neural integrator
Nucleus raphe interpositus	Omnipause neurons
(INC* or riMLF*)	Inhibitory burst neurons

VERTICAL SACCADES
riMLF projects bilaterally for upgaze
riMLF projects ipsilaterally for downgaze

TORSIONAL SACCADES
From subject's point of view, the right riMLF produces clockwise saccades; the left riMLF produces counterclockwise saccades

SUPRA-OCULAR PROJECTIONS
riMLF receives ipsilateral projections from the frontal eye fields and superior colliculus

DRAWING 23-4 **Vertical Saccades**

Smooth Pursuit

Here, we will draw a model for smooth pursuit eye movements. Smooth pursuit eye movements allow us to keep a moving target in our fovea and clearly visualize it. To begin our diagram, show a target object move from left to right. Each hemisphere is responsible for ipsilateral smooth pursuit eye movements, meaning the right hemisphere detects and tracks images as they move to the right and the left hemisphere detects and tracks images as they move to the left.[6–8] Within the circuitry for smooth pursuit, the contralateral cerebellum and medulla and the ipsilateral pons are incorporated via a double decussating pathway.

Now, divide the remainder of the page into left and right sides, making the right side larger than the left. Next, indicate that M retinal ganglion cells receive rod photoreceptor detection of the target's movement. Note that the visual system is generally divided into the pathway for detection of movement (the magnocellular [or M] pathway, which receives rod photoreceptor stimulation) and the pathway for detection of color (the parvocellar [or P] pathway, which receives cone photoreceptor stimulation). Show that visual detection of the target's movement from left to right is projected from the retinae to the right lateral geniculate nucleus and then to the right primary visual cortex (V1). Next, let's show the notable cortical visual processing steps for motion detection. Show that the primary visual cortex projects to visual area V5 (the human homologue to the macaque middle temporal [MT] area), which then projects to visual area V5a (the human homologue to the macaque medial superior temporal [MST] area)—in humans, both V5 and V5a lie at the temporo-occipito-parietal junction. Then, indicate that visual area V5a projects to the posterior parietal cortex, which projects to the frontal eye fields. Note that although we have shown this projection pathway as being sequential and unidirectional, many non-sequential, bidirectional connections exist. For instance, visual area V5 also projects directly to

the frontal eye fields without projecting through any of the intervening connections; also, reciprocal connections between visual areas exist—for instance, the posterior parietal cortex both receives projections from and sends projections to visual area V5a.

Now, show that the frontal eye fields (and other cortical visual areas, as well) project to the ipsilateral dorsolateral pontine nuclei (DLPN) in the high pons and the ipsilateral nucleus reticularis tegmenti pontis (NRTP) in the upper pons. Next, show that the right DLPN and right NRTP project across midline to the left side of the cerebellum, specifically to the flocculus and paraflocculus of the vestibulocerebellum and also to the dorsal vermis. Then, show that the vestibulocerebellum and dorsal vermis project to the ipsilateral medial vestibular nucleus in the medulla. Finally, show that the left medial vestibular nucleus projects to the contralateral abducens nucleus in the right mid- to low pons, which completes the double decussation. The right abducens nucleus then initiates horizontal pursuit eye movements to the right. Note that y-group vestibular nuclear connections to the oculomotor and trochlear nuclei also exist, which are involved in vertical pursuit movements.[9]

Lastly, let's use axial pontine sections to draw the topographic anatomy of the DLPN, NRTP, and abducens nucleus. First, draw the posterior–anterior and right–left planes of orientation for an anatomic, axial view of the pons. Then, draw an outline of the pons and remind ourselves of the territories of the pontine basis and tegmentum. In each section of the following pontine diagrams, we will include the anatomy of the fourth ventricle for reference. Now, show that the abducens nucleus of cranial nerve 6 lies near midline within the posterior tegmentum of the mid- to low pons. Next, show that the NRTP lies in the anterior, midline tegmentum of the upper pons. Lastly, show that the DLPN lies within the posterior lateral aspect of the high pontine basis.[3]

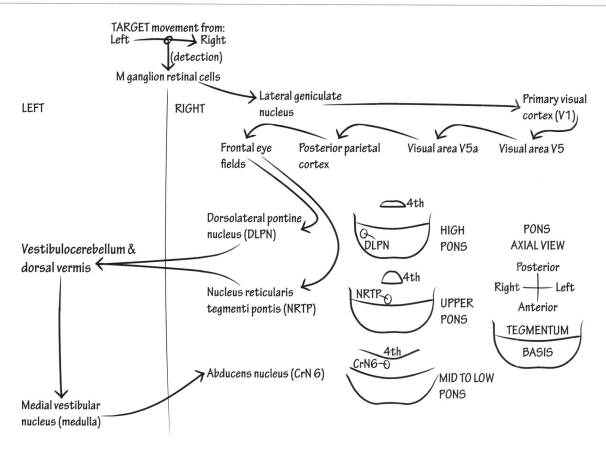

DRAWING 23-5 **Smooth Pursuit**

Pupillary Light Reflex

Here, we will draw a diagram of the pupillary light reflex. First, in axial view, draw the eyes and the midbrain, and, then, lateral to the posterior midbrain tegmentum, draw the lateral geniculate nucleus. Then, within the eyes, draw the lenses, and within the midbrain, draw the red nuclei and label the superior colliculi, for reference. Next, draw a sagittal view of the midbrain and diencephalon and indicate that our axial section lies at the level of the midbrain–diencephalic junction. Now, draw the following pupillary light reflex landmarks: the pretectal olivary nucleus of the pretectal area, which lies anterolateral to the superior pole of the superior colliculus; the posterior commissure, which forms the roof of the cerebral aqueduct (of Sylvius); the paired Edinger–Westphal nuclei of the oculomotor complex; the bilateral ciliary ganglia in the posterior orbit, each of which lies in between the related optic nerve and lateral rectus muscle; and the sphincter pupillae of the iris, which are small circumferential rings of smooth muscle in the pupillary margin of each eye. Next, to better illustrate the anatomy of the sphincter pupillae muscle, draw a coronal view of the iris and pupil. Show that the parasympathetic-innervated sphincter pupillae muscle fibers are circumferentially arranged to constrict pupil size, whereas the sympathetic-innervated pupillary dilator muscle fibers are radially arranged to widen pupil size.

Now, let's draw the pupillary light reflex pathway. First, show that light activates the retinae. Then, show that the optic nerve fibers combine to form the optic tracts, which pass toward the lateral geniculate nucleus—we show the left optic tract, only, here, for simplicity. Next, show that whereas the majority of optic fibers synapse within the lateral geniculate nucleus, fibers of the pupillary light reflex, instead, synapse in the pretectal olivary nucleus of the pretectal area. Then, indicate that the prectectal olivary nucleus projects directly to the ipsilateral Edinger–Westphal nucleus and to the contralateral Edinger–Westphal nucleus via the posterior commissure. Now, show that each Edinger–Westphal nucleus projects to the ipsilateral ciliary ganglion. Then, using the left side of the diagram, only, show that the ciliary ganglion sends short ciliary nerves to innervate the sphincter pupillae muscles to produce pupillary constriction. The short ciliary nerves pass initially within the sclera and then within the suprachoroidal space as they wrap around the globe to innervate the sphincter pupillae. Note that the majority of short ciliary nerves actually innervate the ciliary muscle of the ciliary body (see Drawing 22-3), which assists in the accommodation reflex, rather than the sphincter pupillae muscles for the pupillary light reflex (drawn here).[5,10,11]

As a clinical corollary, in an Adie's tonic pupil, pathology within the ciliary ganglion or the short ciliary nerves prevents the pupil from constricting in reaction to light. On evaluation, cholinergic supersensitivity is present: a dose of pilocarpine (a cholinergic agonist) that would not affect a normal eye is able to produce pupillary constriction because the denervated sphincter pupillae in the Adie's pupil is supersensitive to acetylcholine. Finally, consider that unlike saccadic eye movement circuitry, which involves brainstem projections that pass inferior to the midbrain to enter the lower pons and upper medulla, the circuitry for the pupillary light reflex does not descend below the upper midbrain. Thus, impaired pupillary constriction is extremely important to detect because it can be an early warning sign of brainstem herniation.

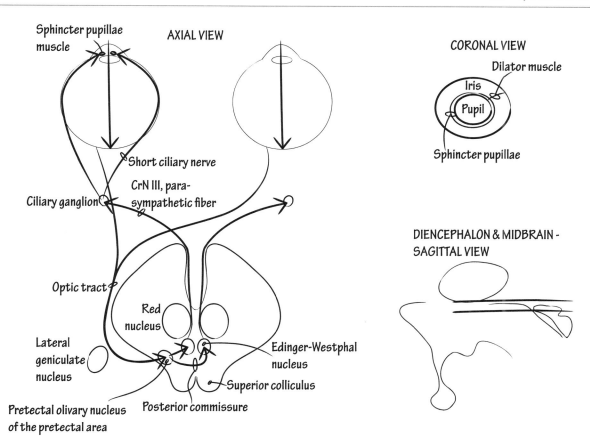

Sphincter pupillae muscle

AXIAL VIEW

CORONAL VIEW

Dilator muscle

Iris

Pupil

Sphincter pupillae

Short ciliary nerve

CrN III, para-sympathetic fiber

Ciliary ganglion

DIENCEPHALON & MIDBRAIN - SAGITTAL VIEW

Optic tract

Red nucleus

Lateral geniculate nucleus

Edinger-Westphal nucleus

Superior colliculus

Pretectal olivary nucleus of the pretectal area

Posterior commissure

DRAWING 23-6 **Pupillary Light Reflex**

References

1. Leigh, R. J. & Zee, D. S. *The neurology of eye movements* (Oxford University Press, 2006).

2. Wong, A. M. F. *Eye movement disorders* (Oxford University Press, 2008).

3. Naidich, T. P. & Duvernoy, H. M. *Duvernoy's atlas of the human brain stem and cerebellum: high-field MRI: surface anatomy, internal structure, vascularization and 3D sectional anatomy* (Springer, 2009).

4. Hall, W. C. & Moschovakis, A. *The superior colliculus: new approaches for studying sensorimotor integration*, pp. 36–37 (CRC Press, 2004).

5. Afifi, A. K. & Bergman, R. A. *Functional neuroanatomy: text and atlas*, 2nd ed., pp. 136–137, 143 (Lange Medical Books/McGraw-Hill, 2005).

6. Brazis, P. W., Masdeu, J. C. & Biller, J. *Localization in clinical neurology*, 6th ed., pp. 221–228 (Wolters Kluwer Health/Lippincott Williams & Wilkins, 2011).

7. Wright, K. W., Spiegel, P. H. & Thompson, L. S. *Handbook of pediatric strabismus and amblyopia*, pp. 29–30 (Springer, 2006).

8. Yanoff, M., Duker, J. S. & Augsburger, J. J. *Ophthalmology*, 3rd ed., p. 1004 (Mosby Elsevier, 2009).

9. Benarroch, E. E. *Basic neurosciences with clinical applications*, p. 503 (Butterworth Heinemann Elsevier, 2006).

10. Jankovic, D. & Harrop-Griffiths, W. *Regional nerve blocks and infiltration therapy: textbook and color atlas,* 3rd ed., p. 20 (Blackwell Pub., 2004).

11. Forrester, J. V. *The eye: basic sciences in practice,* 2nd ed., p. 28 (W.B. Saunders, 2002).

24

Cognition

Know-It Points

Language Disorders

- In 90% of individuals, the language centers lie within the left hemisphere.
- Broca's aphasia is a non-fluent aphasia with preserved comprehension and impaired repetition.
- Broca's aphasia localizes to Broca's area and also involves the precentral gyrus, basal ganglia, insula, and related white matter pathways.
- Wernicke's aphasia is a fluent aphasia with poor comprehension and impaired repetition.
- Wernicke's aphasia localizes to Wernicke's area and the neighboring supramarginal gyrus and angular gyrus and the surrounding temporal and parietal lobes and insula.
- Global aphasia, which is most easily thought of as a combined Broca's and Wernicke's aphasia, is due to extensive injury to the left middle cerebral artery territory.
- In transcortical aphasia, the perisylvian region is spared, which is presumably why repetition is unaffected.
- Conduction aphasia is a fluent aphasia with normal comprehension but impaired repetition; it classically localizes to the arcuate fasciculus.

Memory: Classes

- Sensory memory is the transitory retention of a primary sensory stimulus.
- Short-term memory lasts for roughly 3 to 30 seconds.
- Long-term memory refers to memories that are anywhere from older than 30 seconds to the most remote memories.
- Declarative (aka explicit) memories are those that are consciously recalled (eg, reciting a country's capitals).
- Nondeclarative (aka implicit) memories are those that are unconsciously retrieved (eg, riding a bicycle).
- Episodic memory refers to the recollection of episodes, typically autobiographical episodes, which have a strong contextual stamp.
- Semantic memory refers to our knowledge stores: our collection of facts or information, which have no contextual stamp.
- Procedural memory refers to skills learning, such as riding a bicycle.
- Priming refers to the improved ability to identify recently perceived stimuli in comparison to new stimuli.

Memory: Capacity & Consolidation

- Short-term memory is able to hold seven bits of information (plus or minus two) at any given time.
- Chunking is the process wherein we organize information into fewer chunks or bits.
- Encoding is the process in which information is transformed into a format that can be stored and retrieved.
- Storage is the stockpiling of memory into its stored state.
- Retrieval is the accessing of stored memories.
- According to multiple memory trace theory, every time an episodic memory is retrieved, the hippocampal–neocortical ensemble of that memory is strengthened.
- Anterograde amnesia is the inability to form new memories after the development of amnesia.
- Retrograde amnesia is the inability to retrieve memories that occurred prior to the development of the amnesia.

Apraxia & Neglect (*Advanced*)

- Overall, apraxias are more common with left brain injuries and neglect is more common with right brain injuries.
- Broadly, the frontally based executive apraxias affect movement and the posterior apraxias affect sensory skills and sensorimotor planning.
- Ideational apraxia is an inability to correctly conceptualize an action; for instance, patients might seal an envelope and then try to stuff a letter into it.
- Ideational apraxia localizes to the left hemispheric temporoparietal junction.
- Ideomotor apraxia is a failure to know how to perform a complex motor movement—for instance, patients might have trouble waving goodbye.
- Ideomotor apraxia localizes to the left inferior parietal lobule.
- Balint syndrome (optic ataxia, gaze apraxia, simultagnosia) is due to bilateral occipitoparietal lesions.
- Gerstmann syndrome is a four-part syndrome of left–right disorientation, finger agnosia, dyscalculia, and dysgraphia.
- Gerstmann syndrome localizes to the left hemispheric inferior parietal lobule with specific involvement of the angular gyrus.
- Hemispatial neglect involves a lack of regard for objects in the contralateral hemisphere.
- Right parietal lobe injuries can cause anosognosia, which is a lack of awareness of the presence of a deficit.

Language Disorders

Here, we will learn the major language disorders as a window into the neuroanatomy of language. First, draw an outline of a left lateral cerebral hemisphere and then list the following headings: aphasia, fluency, comprehension, and repetition. Note that in regards to the laterality of language, in 90% of individuals, the language centers lie within the left hemisphere, which is why we draw a left hemisphere, here.[1]

Begin with Broca's aphasia, which is a nonfluent aphasia with preserved comprehension and impaired repetition. Broca's aphasia is agrammatic, has a monotonous (or flat) melody, and is dysarthric, effortful, and hesitant. Show that Broca's aphasia localizes to the inferior frontal gyrus, which is the site of Broca's area, and also involves the precentral gyrus, basal ganglia, insula, and related white matter pathways.[2]

Now, list Wernicke's aphasia, which is a fluent aphasia with poor comprehension and impaired repetition. In Wernicke's aphasia, there is preserved melody and rhythm but the speech content is empty or meaningless, producing a word salad (a high-frequency, unintelligible jumble of words), and there are paragrammatic and paraphasic substitution errors, and even the production of new, meaningless words, called neologisms. Indicate that the site of injury in Wernicke's aphasia is the posterior superior temporal gyrus (Wernicke's area) and the neighboring supramarginal gyrus and angular gyrus and the surrounding temporal and parietal lobes and insula.[2]

Next, list global aphasia, which is most easily thought of as a combined Broca's and Wernicke's aphasia; it is a nonfluent aphasia with poor comprehension and impaired repetition. Indicate that global aphasia is due to extensive injury to the left middle cerebral artery territory.[3]

Now, list transcortical motor aphasia, which, like Broca's aphasia, is a nonfluent aphasia with preserved comprehension. However, in transcortical motor aphasia, unlike in Broca's aphasia, repetition is intact. In fact, make a notation that repetition is such a prominent aspect of the transcortical aphasias that they all can cause echolalia—the parrot-like tendency to repeat words and sentences.[4] Show that transcortical motor aphasia is commonly due to anterior and middle cerebral artery watershed injury with resultant injury to the dorsolateral prefrontal cortex and with sparing of the perisylvian region—the presumptive reason for the preserved repetition.[5-7]

Next, list transcortical sensory aphasia, which, like Wernicke's aphasia, is a fluent aphasia with poor single-word comprehension. However, in transcortical sensory aphasia, unlike in Wernicke's aphasia, repetition is intact. Indicate that transcortical sensory aphasia is due to middle and posterior cerebral artery watershed distribution injury with involvement of the temporo-parieto-occipital junction and with sparing of the perisylvian region.[5-7]

Now, list mixed transcortical aphasia, which, like global aphasia, is a nonfluent aphasia with poor comprehension. However, in mixed transcortical aphasia, unlike in global aphasia, repetition is intact. Indicate that mixed transcortical aphasia can occur with combined anterior and middle cerebral artery and middle and posterior cerebral artery watershed distribution strokes that spare the perisylvian region.[5-7]

Finally, list conduction aphasia, which is essentially the opposite of mixed transcortical aphasia; it is a fluent aphasia with normal comprehension but impaired repetition. In conduction aphasia, speech is hesitant and paraphasic, presumably from an inability to accurately transmit the intended word choice from the comprehension center to the speech production center. Indicate that conduction aphasia classically localizes to the arcuate fasciculus, most notably, and also to the associated supramarginal gyrus and insula.[2] Note, however, that although historically and still commonly we consider the arcuate fasciculus to be the tract that carries language from the comprehension center to the production center (as we have shown, here), this process may actually occur through the superior longitudinal fasciculus, middle longitudinal fasciculus, and the extreme capsule (see Drawing 17-2).[8]

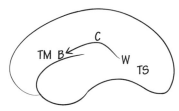

Broca's (B): Inferior frontal gyrus, precentral gyrus, basal ganglia, insula, & white matter

Wernicke's (W): Posterior superior temporal gyrus, & supramarginal & angular gyri, & neighboring parietal and temporal lobes, & insula

Global: Extensive left middle cerebral artery territory

Transcortical motor (TM): Dorsolateral prefrontal cortex with perisylvian sparing

Transcortical sensory (TS): Temporo-parietal-occipital junction with perisylvian sparing

Mixed transcortical: Ant./middle & middle/post. cerebral artery watersheds; perisylvian sparing

Conduction (C): Arcuate fasciculus (& supramarginal gyrus & insula)

DRAWING 24-1 **Language Disorders**

APHASIA	FLUENCY	COMPREHENSION	REPETITION
Broca's	Non-fluent	Preserved	Impaired
Wernicke's	Fluent	Poor	Impaired
Global	Non-fluent	Poor	Impaired
Transcortical motor	Non-fluent	Preserved	Intact
Transcortical sensory	Fluent	Poor single-word	Intact
Mixed transcortical	Non-fluent	Poor	Intact
Conduction	Fluent	Preserved	Impaired

*Echolalia can occur in all transcortical aphasias

*In 90% of individuals, language lateralizes to the left hemisphere

Memory: Classes

Here, we will create a diagram to categorize memory types based on their duration. Note that the terms used, here, demonstrate intertextual inconsistency because they are derived from multiple memory theories generated over many decades. To begin, let's divide memory into three different time spans: sensory, short-term, and long-term. Sensory memory is the transitory retention of a primary sensory stimulus; it is assumed that each sensation has its own time duration, but show that sensory memory as a class lasts from a fraction of a second to a few seconds. Visual sensory memory is retained for an exceedingly short period of time: a third of a second, meaning every fraction of a second, our snapshot of the world is refreshed. This explains why when we view a fan, the blades appear continuous—the rapidly moving stimuli (the blades) overlap in our visual memory and consequently blur. However, at slow enough fan speeds, if we blink, we can visualize the individual blades. Auditory sensory memory (aka echoic memory) retention is longer: a few seconds. Just as we ask people what they were saying we often "hear" them using our echoic memory.[9]

Now, show that short-term memory lasts for roughly 3 to 30 seconds. Note, however, that the decay of short-term memory begins within a few seconds; thus, we must rehearse what's available in our short-term memory in order to preserve it (eg, a newly learned telephone number). Therefore, indicate that we need to divide short-term memory into automatic processing, in which a memory is *not* consciously manipulated, and effortful processing (or as it is more commonly referred to, working memory), in which a memory is actively maintained through various processes, such as subvocal rehearsal. Indicate that working memory relies on at least two different storage mechanisms: the phonological loop, which stores acoustic information through subvocal rehearsal of words or sounds, and the visuospatial sketchpad, which stores visual and spatial information about object characteristics and localization. Note that we

leave out of our discussion, here, for simplicity, the concepts of the central executive and episodic buffer.[10]

Next, show that long-term memory refers to memories that are anywhere from older than 30 seconds to our most remote memories. Indicate that long-term memory is parsed based on the presentation type of the memory, basically its sensory form (ie, verbal, visual, olfactory, etc.), and whether or not there is awareness of the memory. Show that declarative (aka explicit) memories are those that are consciously recalled (eg, reciting a country's capitals) and that nondeclarative (aka implicit) memories are those that are unconsciously retrieved (eg, riding a bicycle).

Indicate that declarative memory is most commonly subdivided into episodic and semantic memory. Episodic memory refers to our recollection of episodes, typically autobiographical episodes, which have a strong contextual stamp, whereas semantic memory refers to our knowledge stores: our collection of facts or information, which have no contextual stamp. The memories of times spent with family are part of our episodic memory, whereas the dates of family members' birthdays and anniversaries are part of our semantic memory.

Nondeclarative memory encompasses several different unconscious forms of memory; indicate that three prominent forms of them are procedural memory, priming, and classical conditioning. Procedural memory refers to our skills learning, such as riding a bicycle. Priming refers to our improved ability to identify recently perceived stimuli in comparison to new stimuli; for instance, our processing speed for words recently read is faster than that of our processing speed for more unfamiliar words. Classical conditioning refers to the transformation of a neutral stimulus into a conditioned stimulus with a conditioned response; for instance, Pavlov observed that his laboratory dogs so strongly associated his laboratory workers with meat powder that the dogs would salivate at the site of them.[11]

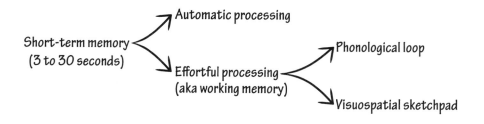

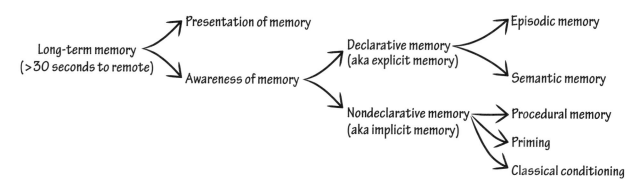

DRAWING 24-2 **Memory: Classes**

Memory: Capacity & Consolidation

Here, we will address the concept of memory capacity and we will create a workflow for the consolidation of memory. First, in regards to short-term memory capacity, indicate that short-term memory is able to hold seven bits of information (plus or minus two) at any given time. However, these bits of information are routinely manipulated to ease their memory burden. Show that the most commonly discussed example of information manipulation is the process of chunking, wherein we take a large amount of information and organize it into fewer chunks or bits. For instance, we can represent the string of digits in a telephone number as seven separate digits, which we may struggle to remember and have to frequently rehearse to avoid their decay, or we can use the principles of chunking to combine digits into larger chunks and reduce their memory burden. For example, even the 11-digit number 18005551212 can easily be memorized when we chunk it into just three bits of information: 1-800, 555, 1212.

Chunking can also occur through more abstract means, as well. As a remarkable example, albeit rare, through synesthesia, certain individuals unconsciously perceive information in sensorial rather than semantic fashion, which can have disastrous effects on comprehension but can allow for an astonishing ability to chunk extremely large quantities of information and dramatically boost memory capacity.[12,13] For the autistic savant Daniel Tammet, numbers appear to him as colors and sounds and carry personalities; he unconsciously creates landscape-like projections of numbers in his mind that allow him to remember staggering amounts of information.[14]

Now, let's shift our focus to the consolidation of memory. Show that memory consolidation relies upon encoding (the process in which information is transformed into a format in which it can be stored and retrieved), storage (the stockpiling of memory into its stored state), and retrieval (the accessing of stored memories).

In regards to the neuroanatomic circuitry for memory processing, draw a medial face of a cerebral hemisphere, and show that memories pass from the sensory association cortices to the limbic lobe where they are encoded (most notably, in the Papez and amygdaloid circuits), and then pass to the neocortex, where they are stored and from where they are retrieved. However, this model predicts noninvolvement of the limbic lobe (more specifically, the hippocampus) in the storage process, but multiple memory trace theory has shown that the hippocampal–neocortical bond for episodic memory does not decay but, instead, persists as part of a memory scaffold. Thus, indicate that every time an episodic memory is retrieved, an additional memory trace is formed, and the hippocampal–neocortical ensemble of that memory is strengthened.[15,16]

Lastly, let's learn about the clinical corollary of amnesia (ie, loss of memory), through the often-written-about patient Henry Gustav Molaison, universally referred to by the initials H.M., who in 1953 underwent bilateral medial temporal lobe resection for intractable epilepsy. The primary dysfunction in H.M. was the encoding of new memories; for example, people who came daily to visit H.M. were strangers anew every day. On the contrary, H.M.'s sensory memory was unaffected and his short-term memory was only partially affected. Indicate that anterograde amnesia is the inability to form new memories after the development of amnesia, whereas retrograde amnesia is the inability to retrieve memories that occurred prior to the development of the amnesia. H.M. had complete anterograde amnesia and also partial retrograde amnesia, which demonstrated a temporal gradient as follows: the degree of his retrograde amnesia was at its maximum for memories just prior to the operation and at its minimum for memories 11 years prior to the operation—note that the true duration of H.M.'s temporal gradient is debated.[17]

Short-term memory capacity: 7+/- 2 bits of information

Chunking: the process of reducing large amounts of information
into fewer chunks/bits

Encoding: the transformation of memory into a storagable state

Storage: the storing of memory

Retrieval: the accessing of stored memories

Multiple memory trace theory: episodic memory retrieval creates
memory traces that strenghthen the hippocampal–neocortical ensemble

Anterograde amnesia: the inability to form new memories post development of amnesia

Retrograde amnesia: the inability to retrieve memories from prior to development of amnesia

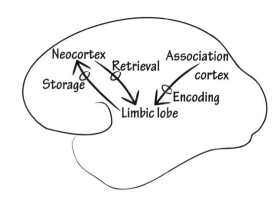

DRAWING 24-3 **Memory: Capacity & Consolidation**

Apraxia & Neglect (*Advanced*)

Here, we will learn about the anatomy of the apraxias and the phenomenon of neglect. Overall, apraxias are more common with left brain injuries and neglect is more common with right brain injuries; therefore, we will use a sagittal view of the left lateral hemisphere to draw the anatomy of the apraxias and a sagittal view of the right lateral hemisphere to draw the anatomy of neglect. However, we need to accept that apraxias can occur from right brain injury and neglect can occur from left brain injury, and we need to accept, as well, that although the laterality of the affected limb in the apraxias is often contralesional, it is variable. In simple terms, an apraxia is an inability to perform a purposeful action in the setting of preserved overall neurologic function. Broadly, the apraxias can be divided into the frontally based executive apraxias, which affect movement, and the posterior apraxias, which affect sensory skills and sensorimotor planning.[10]

First, in the left hemisphere, draw the following anatomic landmarks: the precentral sulcus, central sulcus, and intraparietal sulcus. Now, in regards to the executive apraxias, first, show that limb-kinetic apraxia occurs from injury to the premotor area. In limb-kinetic apraxia, there is impairment in finely graded finger movements and awkwardness of the arm and hand, manifesting with an inability to rhythmically open and close the affected hand. In speech apraxia, which is a slowing and incoordination of speech in the presence of otherwise normal language and sound vocalization, there is injury to what is referred to in this context as the left precentral gyrus of the insula (not shown).[10]

In regards to the posterior apraxias, first, show that injury to the left hemispheric temporoparietal junction produces ideational apraxia and then that left inferior parietal lobule injury produces ideomotor apraxia. Note that ideomotor apraxia also occurs through disconnection phenomena from injury to the premotor cortex and anterior corpus callosum. Variations in the definitions of ideational and ideomotor apraxia exist, but by at least one accepted definition, ideational apraxia is an inability to correctly conceptualize an action. For instance, patients with ideational apraxia might brush their teeth with a spoon or may be unable to sequence a complex action, meaning, for instance, rather than putting a letter into an envelope and sealing it, they might seal the envelope and then try to stuff the letter into it. Ideomotor apraxia is a failure to know how to perform a complex motor movement; gestures, such as waving goodbye, are more severely affected than concrete movements, such as using an actual tool.[18–21]

Now, let's show an example of a more restricted posterior apraxia. Indicate that injury to the superior parietal lobule has traditionally been considered the site of optic ataxia (aka visuomotor ataxia); note, however, that the actual lesion site for optic ataxia may lie more infero-posterior at the parieto-occipital junction. Optic ataxia manifests with an inability to accurately reach for objects due to visual guidance impairment. Optic ataxia is one of three important features of Balint syndrome, which is due to bilateral occipitoparietal lesions. The other two features of Balint syndrome are gaze apraxia (aka oculomotor apraxia or optic apraxia), which is an inability to direct the eyes toward the intended target (instead the eyes fixate on random objects or wander aimlessly), and simultagnosia, which is the visual fixation on a part of an object and an inability to see the object for its whole.[7,22,23]

Gerstmann syndrome occurs from injury to the left hemispheric inferior parietal lobule with specific involvement of the angular gyrus. It is a four-part syndrome of left–right disorientation; finger agnosia, which is a finger naming disorder; dyscalculia, which is a calculation disorder; and dysgraphia, which is a writing disorder.[24]

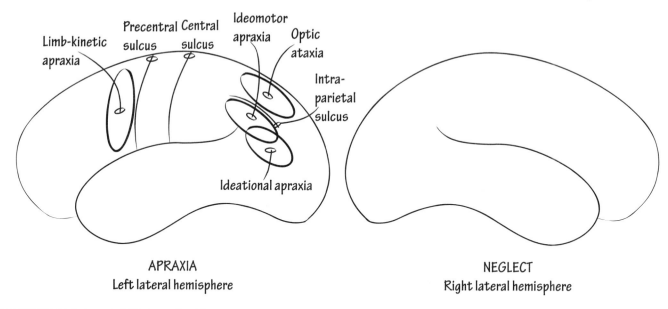

APRAXIA
Left lateral hemisphere

Limb-kinetic apraxia

Precentral sulcus

Central sulcus

Ideomotor apraxia

Optic ataxia

Intra-parietal sulcus

Ideational apraxia

NEGLECT
Right lateral hemisphere

DRAWING 24-4 **Apraxia & Neglect—Partial**

Apraxia & Neglect (*Advanced*) (Cont.)

Now, in regards to neglect, in the right cerebral hemisphere, draw the intraparietal sulcus and label the inferior parietal lobule as the site for hemispatial neglect. Hemispatial neglect involves a lack of regard for objects in the contralateral hemisphere. It may be as mild as to cause extinction to double simultaneous stimulation, meaning that patients will perceive a sensory stimulus on the left side when it is presented only to that side and neglect the stimulus when it is presented to both sides. Or it may be as severe as to cause failure to attend to the left half of the world, entirely.[21]

Finally, show that large right parietal lobe injuries can cause anosognosia, which is a lack of awareness of the presence of a deficit. When anosognosia accompanies occipital lobe injury, which results in a visual field deficit, patients may display a denial of their own blindness, called Anton syndrome. In a separate form of lack of awareness, patients may demonstrate autotopagnosia, which manifests with an unawareness of one's own body parts; for instance, in right hemispheric strokes with hemispatial neglect, patients with autotopagnosia may insist that their left hand is not their own but is instead the examiner's hand. Note that autotopagnosia can occur as a more restricted clinical phenomenon (separate from a broad neglect injury).[25,26]

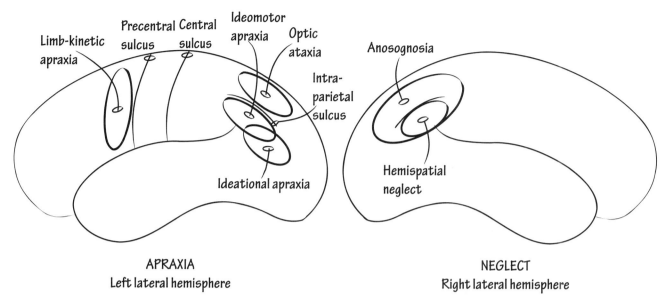

APRAXIA
Left lateral hemisphere

NEGLECT
Right lateral hemisphere

DRAWING 24-5 **Apraxia & Neglect—Complete**

References

1. Wilson, R. A. & Keil, F. C. *The MIT encyclopedia of the cognitive sciences*, p. 369 (MIT Press, 2001).

2. Murdoch, B. E. *Acquired speech and language disorders: a neuroanatomical and functional neurological approach*, 2nd ed., pp. 58–61 (Wiley-Blackwell, 2010).

3. Kent, R. D. & Massachusetts Institute of Technology. *The MIT encyclopedia of communication disorders*, pp. 243, 250 (MIT Press, 2004).

4. Berthier, M. L. *Transcortical aphasias*, pp. 154–155 (Psychology Press, 1999).

5. Festa, J. R. & Lazar, R. M. *Neurovascular neuropsychology*, pp. 27–29 (Springer, 2009).

6. Schaller, B. *State-of-the-art imaging in stroke*, Vol. 2, p. 144 (Nova Sciences Publishers, Inc., 2008).

7. Devinsky, O. & D'Esposito, M. *Neurology of cognitive and behavioral disorders*, pp. 147, 188–192 (Oxford University Press, 2004).

8. Schmahmann, J. D. & Pandya, D. N. *Fiber pathways of the brain* (Oxford University Press, 2006).

9. Hockenbury, D. H. & Hockenbury, S. E. *Psychology*, 4th ed., pp. 242–246 (Worth Publishers, 2006).

10. Cappa, S. F. *Cognitive neurology: a clinical textbook* (Oxford University Press, 2008).

11. Byrne, J. H. *Concise learning and memory: the editor's selection*, pp. 22–25 (Elsevier, 2008).

12. Cytowic, R. E. *Synesthesia: a union of the senses*, 2nd ed., pp. 103–104 (MIT Press, 2002).

13. Mills, C. B., Innis, J., Westendorf, T., Owsianiecki, L. & McDonald, A. Effect of a synesthete's photisms on name recall. *Cortex* 42, 155–163 (2006).

14. Tammet, D. *Born on a blue day: inside the extraordinary mind of an autistic savant*, p. 3 (Free Press: a Division of Simon & Schuster, Inc., 2006).

15. Nadel, L. & Moscovitch, M. Hippocampal contributions to cortical plasticity. *Neuropharmacology* 37, 431–439 (1998).

16. Nadel, L., Samsonovich, A., Ryan, L. & Moscovitch, M. Multiple trace theory of human memory: computational, neuroimaging, and neuropsychological results. *Hippocampus* 10, 352–368 (2000).

17. Spielberger, C. *Encyclopedia of applied psychology*, Vol. 3 (Elsevier, 2003).

18. Mohr, J. P. *Stroke: pathophysiology, diagnosis, and management*, 4th ed., pp. 152–154 (Churchill Livingstone, 2004).

19. Bock, G. & Goode, J. *Sensory guidance of movement*, p. 310 (John Wiley, 1998).

20. Banich, M. T. *Cognitive neuroscience*, 10th ed., p. 141 (Wadsworth/ Cengage Learning, 2010).

21. Campbell, W. W., DeJong, R. N. & Haerer, A. F. *DeJong's the neurologic examination: incorporating the fundamentals of neuroanatomy and neurophysiology*, 6th ed., pp. 93–95 (Lippincott Williams & Wilkins, 2005).

22. Clark, D. L., Boutros, N. N. & Mendez, M. F. *The brain and behavior: an introduction to behavioral neuroanatomy*, 3rd ed., p. 50 (Cambridge University Press, 2010).

23. Goldenberg, G. & Miller, B. L. *Neuropsychology and behavioral neurology*, p. 400 (Elsevier, 2008).

24. Mitchell, A. J. *Neuropsychiatry and behavioural neurology explained*, p. 84 (W.B. Saunders, 2004).

25. Brazis, P. W., Masdeu, J. C. & Biller, J. *Localization in clinical neurology*, 5th ed., p. 154 (Lippincott Williams & Wilkins, 2007).

26. Itti, L., Rees, G. & Tsotsos, J. K. *Neurobiology of attention*, p. 345 (Elsevier Academic Press, 2005).

Sleep and Wakefulness

Know-It Points

Sleep Neurocircuitry (*Advanced*)

- The area for non-REM sleep induction lies within the anterior hypothalamus, specifically in the ventrolateral preoptic area and the median preoptic nucleus.
- The thalamocortical networks generate sleep electroencephalographic (EEG) patterns: sleep spindles and slow-wave sleep.
- The reticular thalamic nuclei gate the flow of information between the thalamus and cortex.
- When the thalamocortical membrane hyperpolarizes more negatively than −65 mV, T-type calcium channels open, which generates a low-threshold spike.

- Through the phenomenon of sensory gating, sensory stimuli that might otherwise wake us from sleep fail to reach our cerebral cortex.
- The putative primary REM-promoting region lies within the pons in what is called the sublaterodorsal nucleus in the rat and the peri-locus coeruleus in the cat.
- The supra-olivary medulla is responsible for muscle atonia during REM sleep.

Suprachiasmatic Circuitry

- Our internal clock allows us to maintain a 24-hour cycle of behavioral activities even when we are placed in non-24-hour environments.
- The timing of our internal clock is affected by certain environmental cues, called zeitgebers, of which light is commonly considered the most potent.
- The retinohypothalamic pathway:
  - Dark phase:
    - Descending hypothalamospinal projections from the paraventricular nucleus excite the cervical spinal cord

    - The cervical spinal cord excites the superior cervical ganglion
    - The superior cervical ganglion activates the production of melatonin in the pineal body
  - Light phase:
    - The suprachiasmatic nucleus inhibits the paraventricular nucleus, thus inactivating the rest of the pathway
- Tumor necrosis factor-alpha and interleukin-1 are two well-studied substances with sleep-promoting properties.

Wakefulness Circuitry

- The laterodorsal tegmental and pedunculopontine nuclei lie within the lower midbrain and upper pons and are cholinergic.
- The locus coeruleus lies, most notably, within the posterior pons and is noradrenergic.
- The substantia nigra and ventral tegmental area lie within the anterior midbrain and are dopaminergic.
- The dorsal group of raphe nuclei lie within the central upper pons and midbrain and are serotinergic.

- The tuberomammillary nucleus lies within the hypothalamus and is the sole source of histamine in the brain.
- Cholinergic basal forebrain nuclei lie within the ventral surface of the frontal lobe.
- The intralaminar thalamic nuclei play an important role in the ascending arousal system.

Flip-Flop Switch (*Advanced*)

- The arousal center inhibits the sleep center.
- The orexigenic cells stabilize the arousal center.
- The sleep center inhibits the arousal center and also the orexigenic cells.

- Orexins are produced by a discrete neuronal population within the lateral hypothalamus.
- Loss of orexin results in the clinical condition of narcolepsy with cataplexy.

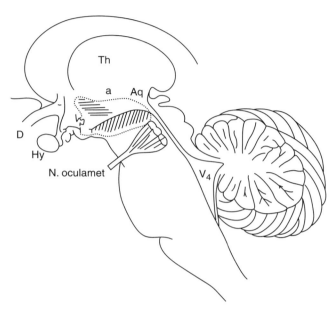

FIGURE 25-1 **Von Economo's clinical–pathologic correlation for the sleep and wakefulness centers. The center for sleep is designated by horizontal lines and the center for wakefulness is designated by vertical (diagonal) lines. Used with permission from Economo, Constantin von. "Sleep as a Problem of Localization."** *The Journal of Nervous and Mental Disease* **71, no. 3 (1930).**

Sleep Neurocircuitry (*Advanced*)

Here, we will learn the neurocircuitry of sleep: we will learn the anatomic location of the sleep center, the physiology of the thalamocortical circuits, and the pathway for the generation of REM sleep. Indicate that the area for non-REM sleep induction lies within the anterior hypothalamus, specifically in the ventrolateral preoptic area and the median preoptic nucleus. Baron Constantin von Economo first hypothesized that this area was the sleep induction center when in 1916–17 he studied the clinical–pathologic correlations of patients who had died from encephalitis lethargica (aka von Economo's encephalitis). The parkinsonian and oculomotor manifestations found in patients with that disorder led him to postulate that the sleep induction center lies within the anterior hypothalamus and the area for wakefulness lies, roughly, within the posterior hypothalamus/upper brainstem, and over the next several decades, he was proven, to a large extent, correct (see Figure 25-1).[1]

Now, let's shift our discussion to the physiology of sleep: specifically, we will show how the thalamocortical networks generate sleep electroencephalographic (EEG) patterns—sleep spindles and slow-wave sleep. First, let's draw the major cell populations responsible for this network; draw the thalamus and label the GABAergic reticular thalamic neurons, and then draw the T-type calcium channel thalamocortical neurons. Next, draw the cortical pyramidal cells. The reticular thalamic nuclei gate the flow of information between the thalamus and cortex, and the thalamocortical neurons drive cortical EEG patterns through, at least in part, the low-threshold spike.

To illustrate the physiology of the low-threshold spike, include in our diagram a graph of the membrane potential of the thalamocortical neurons. Label voltage on the Y-axis and time on the X-axis. Then, demarcate the −65 mV point. Now, show that excitation of the reticular thalamic nuclei causes GABAergic inhibition of thalamocortical cells. Then, indicate that eventually the thalamocortical membrane hyperpolarizes more

negatively than −65 mV, which causes the T-type calcium channels to open, which generates a low-threshold spike: a burst of action potentials. In our drawing, show that the thalamocortical burst acts both on the reticular thalamic cells to facilitate their rhythmic oscillation and also on the cortical pyramidal neurons, which generate the EEG patterns observed during sleep. Lastly, show that after the low-threshold spike, there is a refractory period for the thalamocortical neurons. Indicate that as a byproduct of the refractory period, there is cessation of the excitatory thalamocortical inputs to such relay neurons as the lateral geniculate nucleus, which results in the phenomenon of sensory gating: the process wherein sensory stimuli that might otherwise wake us from sleep fail to reach our cerebral cortex.[2–6]

Now, let's turn our attention to REM sleep. Note that no definitive model for REM sleep has been confirmed and our flow diagram, here, represents only a best hypothesis. First, indicate that the putative primary REM-promoting region lies within the pons, in what is called the sublaterodorsal nucleus in the rat and the peri-locus coeruleus in the cat. Indicate that this region excites the cortex to produce the characteristic EEG pattern of REM sleep, and also excites a constellation of nuclei called the supra-olivary medulla to produce muscle atonia during REM sleep. Now, indicate that during wakefulness and non-REM sleep, the ventrolateral periaqueductal gray area and the dorsal deep mesencephalic reticular nucleus tonically inhibit the sublaterodorsal nucleus/peri-locus coeruleus. Lastly, show that during REM sleep, the dorsal paragigantocellular nucleus (in the medulla) and the lateral hypothalamic melanin-concentrating hormone nuclei suppress the ventrolateral periaqueductal gray area and dorsal deep mesencephalic reticular nuclei, which disinhibits the sublaterodorsal nucleus/peri-locus coeruleus, freeing them to act on the supra-olivary medulla and cerebral cortex to produce REM sleep as previously described.[7–10]

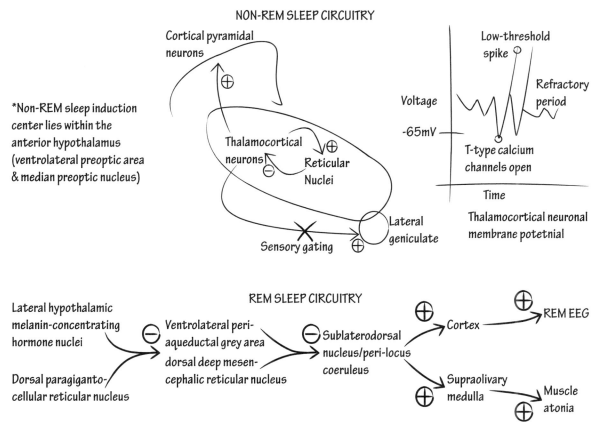

DRAWING 25-1 **Sleep Neurocircuitry**

Suprachiasmatic Circuitry

Here, we will draw the circuitry for the suprachiasmatic control of melatonin production and release. As a byproduct of 3.5 billion years of the Earth's daily rotation around its axis, all of us have a circadian rhythm of approximately 24 hours. Because of this internal clock, we maintain a 24-hour cycle of behavioral activities even when we are placed in non-24-hour environments. Importantly, the timing of our internal clock is affected by certain environmental cues, called zeitgebers, of which light is commonly considered the most potent. In this diagram, we will see how through the retinohypothalamic pathway, light acts on the suprachiasmatic nucleus (the master timekeeper) to adjust the production and release of melatonin and, in turn, the timing of our internal clock.

First, draw an outline of the hypothalamus—include the pituitary gland and mammillary bodies. Next, add the optic chiasm. Then, label the suprachiasmatic nucleus just above the optic chiasm in the anterior hypothalamus. Next, label the paraventricular nucleus. Now, add a cross-section through the cervical spinal cord. Then, show the superior cervical ganglion and the pineal gland.

Next, show that during the dark phase, descending hypothalamospinal projections from the paraventricular nucleus excite the cervical spinal cord, which, in turn, excites the superior cervical ganglion, which activates the production of melatonin from within the pineal body, causing its release into circulation, which helps promote sleep.

Now, show that during the light phase, light passes along the retinohypothalamic pathway to excite the suprachiasmatic nucleus. Then, indicate that the suprachiasmatic nucleus inhibits the paraventricular nucleus, which causes inhibition of the production and release of melatonin, thus promoting wakefulness.[11]

In addition to melatonin, several other substances have been shown to play an important role in sleep induction. At the beginning of the 20th century, Kuniomi Ishimori in Japan and Henri Piéron in France, independently but concurrently, performed experiments wherein they transferred brain matter (cerebrospinal fluid or brain tissue) from sleep-deprived dogs to well-rested dogs and observed that the well-rested dogs went to sleep. From this evidence, they both concluded that certain agents within the body must accumulate to promote sleep. Experiments over the past 30 years have identified several sleep-promoting substances. Tumor necrosis factor-alpha and interleukin-1 are two well-studied substances with sleep-promoting properties. They have been shown to cause sleepiness and fatigue as well as other somatic symptoms commonly associated with sleepiness: cognitive dysfunction, sensitivity to pain, impaired glucose tolerance, and chronic inflammation. Another sleep-promoting substance of particular interest is adenosine because caffeine, which is second only to oil in its importance as a global commodity, is believed to produce its wake-promoting effects through its actions on adenosine receptors.[12]

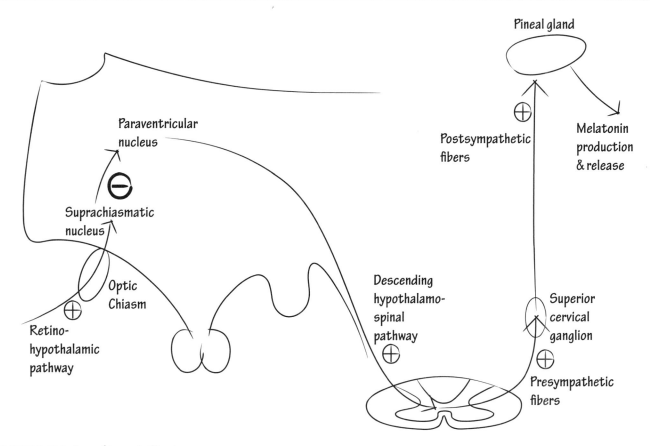

DRAWING 25-2 **Suprachiasmatic Circuitry**

Wakefulness Circuitry

Before the center for sleep was proven, the center for wakefulness was discovered. In the 1940s and 1950s neurophysiologists Giuseppe Moruzzi and H. W. Magoun performed a series of EEG studies to prove the existence of the wakefulness center. They described an active arousal generator in the brainstem reticular formation, coined the ascending reticular activating system, which was shown to directly and indirectly activate the cerebral cortex by way of diffuse projection fibers that projected directly to the cortex and also indirectly to the cortex through the thalamus. Over the past several decades, discovery of the specific brainstem, hypothalamic, thalamic, and basal forebrain cell populations responsible for the arousal system has elaborated and shaped our understanding of wakefulness anatomy. Numerous neurotransmitters and neuronal populations within the brainstem, hypothalamus, thalamus, and basal forebrain have been discovered, some of which we will specifically indicate here.

In the corner of the diagram, for reference, draw a mid-sagittal view of a brain. Next, in the center of the page, draw an expanded view of the basal forebrain, hypothalamus, and brainstem. To begin our process of labeling the wake-promoting cells, indicate the latero-dorsal tegmental and pedunculopontine nuclei in the lower midbrain and upper pons and show that they are cholinergic. Next, we will draw the upper brainstem monoaminergic nuclei. In the posterior pons, draw the locus coeruleus and label it as noradrenergic (the largest concentration of locus coeruleus neurons lies within the pons); in the anterior midbrain, group the substantia nigra and ventral tegmental area together and show that they are dopaminergic; and finally, in the central upper pons and midbrain, draw the dorsal group of raphe nuclei and indicate that they are serotinergic. Note that the locus coeruleus, substantia nigra, and raphe nuclei are drawn in greater detail in Chapter 9. Next, move to the hypothalamus. Draw the tuberomammillary nucleus in the hypothalamus; it is the sole source of histamine in the brain and it is important for wakefulness. Now, include the cholinergic basal forebrain nuclei in the ventral surface of the frontal lobe; they are important to wakefulness. Finally, consider that in Drawings 20-3 and 20-4, we showed that the intralaminar thalamic nuclei also play an important role in the arousal system.

As a pharmacologic corollary to the list of neurotransmitters involved in wakefulness, consider that amphetamines are adrenergic reuptake inhibitors and are stimulatory—they increase the amount of circulating monoamines; consider that *anti*histamines, such as diphenhydramine (Benadryl), cause drowsiness, as do *anti*cholinergic agents; and consider that tricyclic antidepressants can be especially sedating because they often have both *anti*cholinergic and *anti*histaminergic properties.[13]

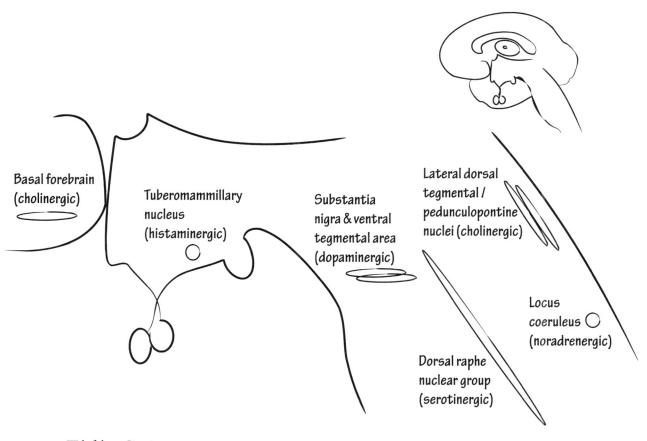

DRAWING 25-3 **Wakefulness Circuitry**

Flip-Flop Switch (*Advanced*)

Here, we will draw the flip-flop switch, which is the circuit for the transition between sleep and wakefulness. A flip-flop circuit is an electrical engineering term for a switch that avoids transitional states; the circuit is in either one of two states but not a blend of both. If you are tired when you lie down, you quickly fall asleep, and when you're ready to rise, you suddenly wake up. To begin, indicate the sleep and wake states and then draw the flip-flop switch, which transitions between them. In our first diagram, we will show the circuit in a state of wakefulness. Indicate the following important hypothalamic areas: the ventrolateral preoptic area and the median preoptic nucleus, which constitute the sleep center; the wake-promoting cells; and the perifornical-lateral hypothalamic orexigenic cells, which form the wakefulness stabilizer—discussed in detail at the end. Show that during wakefulness, the wake-promoting cells inhibit the sleep center and that the perifornical-lateral hypothalamic orexigenic cells excite the wake-promoting cells.

Next, let's show the flip-flop circuitry in the sleep state. Re-draw the sleep and wake states and the flip-flop switch, and then again include the previously listed structures. Now, show that in the sleep state, the sleep center inhibits the wake-promoting cells and also inhibits their stabilizer: the perifornical-lateral hypothalamic orexigenic cells.

In short, when we consider the sleep and wake states as a whole, the arousal center inhibits the sleep center; the orexigenic cells stabilize the arousal center; and the sleep center inhibits the arousal center and also the orexigenic cells.[14]

The story of the discovery of orexin is both interesting and illuminating. In 1998, two different research groups concurrently but independently identified a pair of hypothalamic neuropeptides, named orexins by Sakurai et al. and hypocretins by de Lecea et al. (we refer to them here as orexins). Orexins are produced by a discrete neuronal population within the lateral hypothalamus, and their functional role in the nervous system came as a surprise. A decade and a half prior to the identification of the orexins, in 1982, Baker et al. identified a candidate gene, designated canarc-1, for the clinical disorder of narcolepsy in a colony of Doberman Pinschers with canine narcolepsy. Despite extensive study of this gene, however, the protein responsible for narcolepsy was unable to be identified. In 1999, when researchers began studying the first orexin knockout mouse, they were not expecting to find any manifestations of narcolepsy; instead, they hypothesized that orexin would be shown to affect energy metabolism, given the already proven role of the lateral hypothalamus in energy homeostasis. However, study of homozygote orexin knockout mice, instead, demonstrated that the mice expressed a phenotype consistent with narcolepsy with cataplexy: they displayed cataplexy and abnormal wake-REM sleep transitions. Thus, orexin was discovered to play an unanticipated yet highly important role in the stabilization of wakefulness.[15]

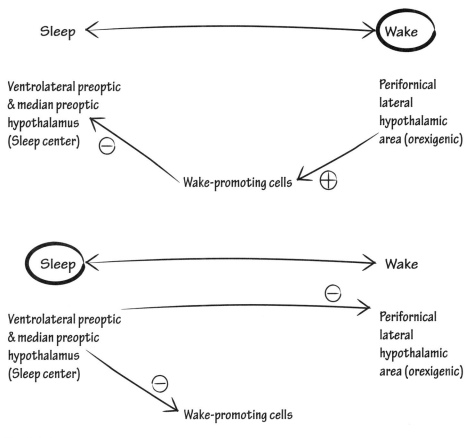

DRAWING 25-4 **Flip-Flop Switch**

References

1. Winkelman, J. W. & Plante, D. T. *Foundations of psychiatric sleep medicine*, Chapter 2 (Cambridge University Press, 2010).
2. Brazier, M. A. The history of the electrical activity of the brain as a method for localizing sensory function. *Med Hist* 7, 199–211 (1963).
3. Crunelli, V., Cope, D. W. & Hughes, S. W. Thalamic T-type Ca2 + channels and NREM sleep. *Cell Calcium* 40, 175–190 (2006).
4. Steriade, M., McCormick, D. A. & Sejnowski, T. J. Thalamocortical oscillations in the sleeping and aroused brain. *Science* 262, 679–685 (1993).
5. Livingstone, M. S. & Hubel, D. H. Effects of sleep and arousal on the processing of visual information in the cat. *Nature* 291, 554–561 (1981).
6. Anderson, M. P., et al. Thalamic Cav3.1 T-type Ca2 + channel plays a crucial role in stabilizing sleep. *Proc Natl Acad Sci USA* 102, 1743–1748 (2005).
7. Fort, P., Bassetti, C. L. & Luppi, P. H. Alternating vigilance states: new insights regarding neuronal networks and mechanisms. *Eur J Neurosci* 29, 1741–1753 (2009).
8. Hassani, O. K., Lee, M. G. & Jones, B. E. Melanin-concentrating hormone neurons discharge in a reciprocal manner to orexin neurons across the sleep-wake cycle. *Proc Natl Acad Sci USA* 106, 2418–2422 (2009).
9. Vetrivelan, R., Fuller, P. M., Tong, Q. & Lu, J. Medullary circuitry regulating rapid eye movement sleep and motor atonia. *J Neurosci* 29, 9361–9369 (2009).
10. Mallick, B. N. *Rapid eye movement sleep: regulation and function* (Cambridge University Press, 2011).
11. Benarroch, E. E. Suprachiasmatic nucleus and melatonin: reciprocal interactions and clinical correlations. *Neurology* 71, 594–598 (2008).
12. *Basics of sleep guide*, 2nd ed. (Sleep Research Society, 2009).
13. Moruzzi, G. & Magoun, H. W. Brain stem reticular formation and activation of the EEG. 1949. *J Neuropsychiatry Clin Neurosci* 7, 251–267 (1995).
14. Saper, C. B., Scammell, T. E. & Lu, J. Hypothalamic regulation of sleep and circadian rhythms. *Nature* 437, 1257–1263 (2005).
15. Chemelli, R. M., et al. Narcolepsy in orexin knockout mice: molecular genetics of sleep regulation. *Cell* 98, 437–451 (1999).

Index